VITAL SIGNS

Age	Weight (kg) approx	Surface area approx	RR/min	HR/min	Systolic BP mmHg	Mean BP mmHg
Premature	1-2		30-60	100-180	50-70	30-40
Newborn	3.5	0.23 m^2	30-60	100-180	50-70	40-60
6 mo	6	0.35 m^2	24-40	100-170	65-106	50-90
1 yr	10	0.47 m^2	20-40	90-160	72-110	50-100
3 yr	12	0.6 m^2	20-30	90-150	78-114	50-100
6 yr	18	0.8 m^2	18-25	80-140	80-116	60-90
8 yr	25	0.86 m^2	18-25	80-120	84-122	60-90
10 yr	30	1.05 m^2	16-20	80-120	90-130	60-90
12 yr	35	1.25 m^2	14-20	70-110	94-136	65-95
15 yr	50	1.37 m^2	12-20	60-100	100-142	65-95
18 yr	60	1.50 m^2	12-18	60-90	104-148	65-100

EQUIPMENT

Age	Endotracheal tube (uncuffed)	Distance mid-trachea to lip	Laryngoscope blade	Suction cath	NG tube	Foley catheter (fr)	Chest tube (fr)
Premature	2.5-3.0	6-7 cm	0 straight	5-6	5	5 feeding	8-10
Newborn	3-3.5	8-9 cm	1 straight	6	8	5 feeding	8-10
6 months	3.5-4.0	10 cm	1 straight	8	8	5 feeding	10-12
1 yr	4.0-4.5	11 cm	2 straight	8	10	8 foley	10-14
3 yr	4.5-5.0	13 cm	2 straight	8	10	10 foley	12-16
6 yr	5.0-5.5	15 cm	2 straight	10	12	10 foley	12-16
8 yr	5.5-6.0 (cuff)	16 cm	2 straight/curved	10	12	10 foley	14-20
10 yr	6.0-6.5 (cuff)	17 cm	3 straight/curved	12	14	12 foley	20-28
12 yr	6.0-6.5 (cuff)	18 cm	3 straight/curved	12	14	12 foley	20-28
15 yr	6.0-7.0 (cuff)	20 cm	3 straight/curved	12	16	14 foley	28-32
18 yr	6.5-7.0 (cuff)	20-22 cm	3 straight/curved	12	16	16 foley	32

Manual of Pediatric Emergencies and Critical Care

2nd Edition

Suchitra Ranjit MD
Senior Pediatric Intensivist and
Pediatric Intensive Care
and Emergency Services
Apollo Children's Hospital
Shafee Mohammed Road
Chennai

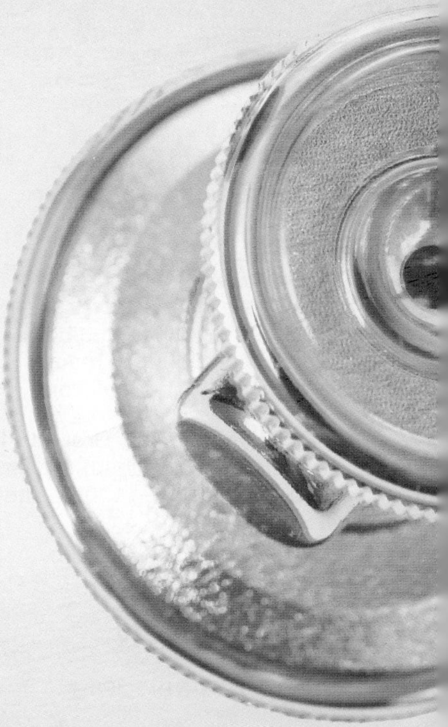

Paras Medical Publisher
Hyderabad ▪ New Delhi

Cover Design: Sonali Ranjit

Manual of Pediatric Emergencies & Critical Care

Published by
Divyesh Arvind Kothari
for Paras Medical Publisher
5-1-475, First Floor, Putlibowli
Hyderabad—500095, India.
parasmedpub@hotmail.com

Branch Office: 2/25, Ground Floor, Arun House, Daryaganj, Ansari Road, New Delhi—110002, India

First edition 2001
Second edition 2010

ISBN: 978-81-8191-308-1

PARAS

Enhancing Knowledge. Creating Possibilities

Note: As new information becomes available, changes become necessary. The editor/sub-editors/contributors and the publisher have, as far as it is possible, taken care to ensure that the information given in this book is accurate and up-to-date. In view of the possibility of human error or advances in medical science neither the editor nor the publisher nor any other party who has been involved in the preparation or publication of this work warrants that the information contained herein is in every respect accurate or complete. This book is being published with the understanding that the material provided by the author is original. This book is for sale in India only and cannot be exported without the permission of the publisher in writing. Any disputes and legal matters must be settled under Hyderabad jurisdiction only.

Printed in Hyderabad, India

FOREWORD

It gives me immense pleasure to write the 'Foreword' for the 2nd edition of the *Manual of Pediatric Emergencies and Critical Care*. The book reflects the maturation of the subspecialty, and increased knowledge about the organization and practice of pediatric emergency and critical care medicine.

I must contrast this scenario with the one in 1983, when Apollo Hospitals became operational in Chennai. I had insisted on a 24 hour Emergency Department with a large sign outside that proclaimed "EMERGENCY". However, because the term was unfamiliar at the time, a smaller board was placed below, which referred to a "Casualty" Department, a term that was more commonplace at the time. Over the next few decades, the concept of 24x7 Emergency Services became adopted by many other hospitals all over the country, and a quarter century later, the concept grew as a subspecialty with respect to children's health; Apollo Hospitals Group opened the first Apollo Children's Hospital in June 2009.

This book represents the vast clinical experience of Dr Suchitra Ranjit and her outstanding team in the Pediatric Intensive Care Unit and Emergency Department at the Apollo Children's Hospitals who believe that together they can create something greater than their individual efforts.

I understand that the first edition of this book was enormously successful as it was a comprehensive ready-reckoner, referenced for the care of the critically ill child. The 2nd edition continues to represent the "state of the art" on the care of the critically ill or injured child by presenting both evidence-based medicine as well as many years of clinical experience.

I congratulate the willingness of Dr Suchitra Ranjit and her team to share their collective experience and knowledge with the rest of the fraternity. I am certain that the 2nd edition of the *Manual of Pediatric Emergencies and Critical Care* will assist pediatric caregivers enormously when faced by critically sick children.

Padma Vibhushan Dr Prathap C Reddy
Founder Chairman, Apollo Hospitals Group

PREFACE

The 1st edition of the *Manual of Pediatric Emergencies and Critical Care* was originally developed because of the variety and complexity of patients in the PICU. Many non-intensivists including pediatricians, junior doctors and nurses are increasingly required to acquire skills in the recognition and stabilization of critically ill patients. Remembering the drugs of choice for arrhythmias, infections, electrolyte emergencies, sedation, poisonings, and a host of other problems has always been daunting. Oftentimes, definitive expertise may be unavailable. While many excellent textbooks in the subject exist, applying principles of Western literature to resource challenged areas is never easy, especially in the smaller hospitals and in the interior, where the bulk of desperately sick children are present. It was our aim to provide concise and easy to understand guidelines about relevant pathophysiology and essential "do's and don'ts" in order to optimize outcomes when confronted by critically unwell children.

As Critical Care Medicine is multidisciplinary specialty without borders, patients often present with many complex and difficult challenges that often interface with every branch of medical practice.

The doctor who practices in the ICU must have superb clinical skills plus a knowledge of some parts of many specialties. This is not to say that the Intensivist does not need the information and skills of others: an important function of the Intensivist is coordination of the skills and knowledge of other specialties.

Intensivists and Intensive Care may often be faced by an identity crisis—it might serve the Intensivist well to remember that their role as the primary caregiver in the ICU has to be earned and cannot be legislated. The ICU practitioner has the greatest chance of being accepted as the central caregiver of a critically ill child by other specialists if the Intensivist earns that right by demonstrating her/his commitment at the patient's bedside. Other essential ingredients that a successful Intensivist must have are superb clinical skills, knowledge, experience, enthusiasm and ability to work in a team.

The Second edition of *Manual of Pediatric Emergencies and Critical Care* is much larger than the First edition but continues to be a quick and concise reference for common emergencies and ICU issues and ideally should be used when rapid decisions need to be made. Our goal is to provide pediatricians dealing with acutely unwell children with simple, clinically useful and current evidence-based guidelines for the diagnosis and management of the most frequently encountered diseases in the ER and ICU.

This book will also be useful for Fellows in training in Intensive Care as many of the key clinical issues that are encountered both in the ICU and examination have been clearly delineated. However, it is not meant to be a substitute for standard well referenced textbooks on the subject. Also, it should not be used in the absence of clinical judgment: its recommendations are general and must be considered in light of a patient's specific circumstances

It is hoped that the Second edition of *Manual of Pediatric Emergencies and Critical Care* continues to be comprehensive, yet reader friendly, embracing both the new advances in science as well as the time-honored art of pediatric practice.

Suchitra Ranjit

CONTRIBUTORS

Celebrating the team—A salute to the Pediatric Critical Care Group, Chennai. Cheers and a huge *Thanks* to the Pediatric Critical Care Group, Chennai, each member of which has made substantial contributions to and elevated the standard of the second edition of the *Manual of Pediatric Emergencies and Critical Care.*

No task is insurmountable when you have a team that is willing to go the distance to move mountains and achieve nothing less than success. The Pediatric Critical Care Group, Chennai (PCCG), at the Apollo Children's Hospitals is an outstanding bunch of individuals whose simple philosophy is to achieve the highest level of excellence at work and in their personal spheres. Their spirit of teamwork constantly generates a high level of morale and unflagging enthusiasm resulting in excellent patient care outcomes plus a workplace that radiates positive energy and enjoyment.

In terms of this book, the team PCCG has effectively accomplished far more than it would have been possible for just me alone to do. All team members worked long hours to add new chapters and extensively revamp existing chapters underlining their commitment to bringing out the best ever Manual of Pediatric Emergencies and Critical Care.

Team PCCG has arrived, it has become empowered and is growing even further in confidence, skills and reputation and I'm so proud and privileged to be part of this outstanding group.

My gratitude to Indira Jayakumar, Senior Consultant in Pediatric Intensive Care, my capable partner in crime for more than a decade, a remarkable lady who radiates a zest for life, learning and teaching, epitomizes efficient multi-tasking and is the most charming and vital PR weapon on our team.

(Chapters contributed: Cardiogenic shock, Inotropes and vasoactive agents).

Kudos to Deepika Gandhi, Consultant in Pediatric Intensive Care, the most organized soul in the team with a formidable capacity for long term planning and execution-Deepika's documentation skills are almost an art form and she's been the key in successfully surmounting many major bureaucratic challenges.

(Chapters contributed: Major pediatric trauma, Head injury, Raised ICP)

A special thanks to Shrishu Kamath and Rajeshwari, Junior Consultants in Pediatric Intensive Care - both of whom have loyally supported the PICU right from their postgraduate days, and, as they imbibed key attitudes and skills during their overseas training stints, so they have strengthened our team with fresh ideas.

Shrishu is the ultimate team player; he carries everyone along with his infectious enthusiasm. He is blossoming into a professional, mature Intensivist who is constantly thinking of ways to improve the strengths and knowledge base of the Group.

(Chapters contributed: Hypertensive emergencies, ARDS, HFO, NIV, Drowning)

Rajeshwari is energetic, assertive, and has an immense capacity for absorbing newer ideas and concepts. She is a superior performer who relishes new challenges and has a talent for lateral thinking.

(Chapters contributed: Status epilepticus, RSI, Tracheostomy, Malaria, Pulse oximetry and capnography, Blood transfusion)

Also a Junior Consultant in Pediatric Intensive Care, Gayathri Subramanian's strengths are her highly developed communication skills, extreme professionalism and great leadership potential: she's efficient and fun loving and a role model for many of the newest entrants in the Unit.

(Chapters contributed: Acute liver failure, GI bleeds, Acute kidney injury, Burns)

Cool and composed characterizes VP Anitha, Consultant in Pediatric Intensive Care, who now jointly heads the PICU at the Mehta Children's Hospital, a place where many desperately sick kids arrive in the dead of the night; Anitha can be trusted to remain calm and efficiently commandeer available resources in order to optimize outcomes.

(Chapters contributed: Hospital acquired infections, Pancreatitis, Acute severe asthma, Care of the brain dead potential organ donor)

Sarfraz Navaz, Junior Consultant in Pediatric Intensive Care, has many strengths and is a great team player, his polished and articulate personality just about masks his punk rock band skills, he never refuses any task, be it minor or major.

(Chapters contributed: Oncologic emergencies, Fungal infections, DKA, co-contributed to PICU procedures)

Sunit Matha, who recently cleared the Pediatric Intensive Care Fellowship exam, is the vital PCCG Coordinator and amongst the strongest assets of our team. Sunit can move mountains; he is the person whom everyone wants when there is a major problem at hand; he gives his all to sick children, anytime of the day or night. His contribution to the *Manual of Pediatric Emergencies and Critical Care* has been the easily the largest and most important and he constantly scours the internet for anything that can add value to the book. Sunit has a wonderful attitude for PICU, great leadership potential and he is continually seeking ways to improve PICU quality, both at medical and nursing levels.

(Chapters contributed: Entire section compromising 10 chapters on Poisoning and envenomations, Entire Appendix compromising 21 sections, Sedatives, Procedural sedation, Muscles relaxants, Brain death, all 4 chapters on PICU procedures, enhanced various other chapters)

Amisha Rana is an efficient multi-tasker, has an eye and memory for important details and is capable and pleasant. Her task as PICU registrar was especially demanding as she had to juggle motherhood and family commitments along with her rota and exam pressures, but she's remained professional and carried out tasks assigned to her to the best of her abilities.

(Co-contributed chapter on metabolic disorders)

Anjul Dayal, Shivkumar Sarma, Samarth Burle and Dr Sukesh Mohta are no longer with the PCCG and have moved on as fully fledged PICU Consultants in other Units. Anjul, one of our first PICU registrars at Apollo, is an extremely capable organizer, quick witted, street smart, fun loving and a great achiever.

(Co-contributed chapters on Upper airway obstruction, Trauma)

Samarth has unique strengths in PICU, his highly developed planning and organizational abilities are matched by a cool controlled temperament. Samarth is able to make lightening fast assessments in emergencies and efficiently assign tasks to team members—these skills have enabled him to single-handedly pull off some amazing saves during emergencies and transports.

(Chapters contributed: Anaphylaxis, Hemodynamic monitoring, Upper airway obstruction, Co-contributed to Cardiogenic shock, Inotropes and vasoactive agents)

Shiv is quiet and soft spoken and has a strong core of professionalism, integrity and determination; he's a great team player, never shirks hard work.

(Chapters contributed: Approach to respiratory failure, Approach to shock)

Sukesh has a large appetite for ongoing learning, is willing to take risks and works hard. The worst crashes invariably landed up when he was on.

(Chapters contributed: CPR, Post-resuscitation care, Co-contributed to Arrhythmias)

Raghavendra Vanaki, ex PICU fellow, now an Assistant Professor in Karnataka, is a wonderfully dependable team player, popular and hard-working; we all still miss him.

(Chapters contributed: Bronchiolitis, Empyema)

Dr Natwar Lal Sharma, also ex PICU fellow, has now taken on the onerous challenge as academic co-ordinator of Pediatrics at Apollo Children's Hospital. Natwar can crack any exam that he sets his mind at passing, and now he takes his job or teaching and mentoring very seriously.

(Co-contributed to chapter on Fluids, Section on Poisoning)

I also thank our present PICU fellows at Apollo Children's Hospital, K Satish *(Chapter contributed: Diarrhea and dehydration)*, Praveen, Suresh Panda and Vijay. Also the PICU fellows at Mehta Children's Hospital, Dr Ayyammal, Dr Mumtaz and Dr Kavan Deshpande. You all have the enormous challenge of living up to the reputation of your seniors and raising the bar even further.

A special word of appreciation for Dr Sireesha in the Emergency Room at Apollo. Sireesha is universally admired and respected by the rest of the PCCG as she is so professional and efficient. Whether it's a difficult patient, parent or consultant, she can tackle them all with effortless poise and charm.

All of you in the PCCG are truly an amazing group of individuals, and I have felt honoured to know and work with you over the past few years. Thank you, the creation of this book would not have been possible without your passion and dedication.

ACKNOWLEDGEMENTS

I have always been inspired by the iconic vision and dynamicity of Dr Prathap C Reddy, Founder Chairman of the Apollo Hospitals Group. Dr Reddy, along with the Managing Director of Apollo Hospitals, Dr Preetha Reddy, believed in us pediatricians at Apollo and strongly endorsed and pushed for creating the superb Apollo Children's Hospitals (ACH) which became functional in mid 2009. Every nook and cranny at ACH bears testimony to Ms Preetha's graceful elegance matched by a passionate desire to make ACH amongst the best children's hospitals in the world. We are truly grateful for their unflinching encouragement and ongoing commitment to further elevate the standing and capacities of this exciting new hospital.

I also thank Dr Sathyabhama, Director of Medical Services, Apollo Hospitals, Chennai, for her zeal in overseeing every step in the creation of the Apollo Children's Hospitals and we value her continual support, valuable critiques and guidance at every juncture.

I am grateful to the Director of Medical Education and Head of Department Pediatrics, Dr Radha Rajagopalan for her encouragement, support and assistance in all our academic, research and teaching projects.

This book wouldn't have seen the light of day without the input of a group of talented individuals, all members of the Pediatric Critical Care group who find special mention in the Contributors section. To the awesome PCCG team—Hey! You guys save lives on a daily basis and yet manage to make each day such fun that I get withdrawal symptoms when I'm away.

It's always encouraging and heartening to have good friends who stand by one through good times and bad such as Dr Meena Thiagarajan and Dr Shyamala Jayamoorthy, Consultants at Apollo Children's Hospitals. Also, thanks to a compassionate human being and a wonderfully talented cardiac surgeon, Dr Neville Solomon; it's been a pleasure knowing him and having him during our morning rounds.

I have to thank the Consultants at the Apollo Children's Hospitals who provided valuable input and critiques for specific chapters in the book - Dr Revathy Raj, Consultant in Pediatric Hematology (Oncologic emergencies) and Dr CS Muthukumar, Consultant Pediatric Cardiologist (Arrhythmias in sick children). Dr Ramgopal Krishnan, Consultant, Infectious Disease (Empiric antimicrobials in sick children) and Dr Rema Menon,

Consultant in Transfusion Medicine (Blood product transfusion), also contributed their unique expertise. Dr BK Subramaniam, Pediatric Gastroenterologist provided wonderful input for a difficult chapter (Acute Liver Failure) during the short time that he was in Chennai.

I greatly value the long and close association of Dr Indumathy Santhanam, Assistant Professor in the Department of Pediatric Emergency Medicine, Institute of Child Health, Chennai, and also Dr Jayanthi Ramesh, Consultant in Telemedicine, KKCCTH, Chennai. I'm also grateful to Dr S Thangavelu, Consultant Pediatrician and Intensivist and Dr L Subramaniam, Senior Pulmonologist, both at the Mehta Children's Hospital. These two senior pediatricians have been a constant source of encouragement and advice to me for very many years.

It would be a crime if I fail to acknowledge the crucial role played by the dedicated nurses of PICU and Emergency Rooms at Apollo Children's Hospital and Mehta's Hospital. We salute your commitment without which even the best Intensivist's input would be futile. A special thanks to the senior Staff at ACH: The efficient and organized Sister Pushpa, Sister SriPriya and Sister Esther: all of you are the architects of nursing excellence at ACH.

I thank my husband and best friend, Dr MS Ranjit, who has supported me and hauled me out of trouble innumerable times and my daughters Sonali and Meghna who have enriched my life with their love and laughter. Kudos to Sonali for her unbelievable creative skills exemplified in the cover design of this book and "Wow!" to Meghna for her talent for all things electronic or computer related.

I owe my parents, G Manoharan and Mrs Kamala Manoharan a great deal for their bottomless love, strength and advice at every point in my life. Their unstinting support at many key junctures was instrumental in ensuring that I could do justice to a demanding and potentially stressful career. I also thank my wise twin sister, Sangeeta Jayadevan, who has given me many invaluable nuggets of management wisdom and advice.

Lastly, but importantly, I very much appreciate every single person who read the first edition of this book and applied its contents to save the lives of little children everywhere. I hope this edition won't let you down.

CONTENTS

Section 1 INTRODUCTION

Section 2 RESUSCITATION

Section 3 RESPIRATORY SYSTEM

Section 4 SPECIFIC RESPIRATORY PROBLEMS

Section 5 CARDIORESPIRATORY MONITORING

Section 6 MECHANICAL VENTILATION

Section 7 CARDIOVASCULAR SYSTEM

Section 8 CENTRAL NERVOUS SYSTEM

Section 9 GASTROINTESTINAL SYSTEM

Section 10 RENAL SYSTEM

Section 11 HEMATOLOGY IN PICU

Section 12 METABOLIC PROBLEMS IN PICU

Section 13 POISONING AND ENVENOMATION

Section 14 SYSTEMIC INFECTIONS IN PICU

Section 15 SEDATION AND ANALGESIA IN PICU

Section 16 TRAUMA AND BURNS

Section 17 PICU MONITORING AND PROCEDURES

Appendices

Index

1

ICU Daily Routine, Patient Assessment and Documentation

The care of patients in the ICU is increasingly complex with input being received from a number of different specialties. A major role for junior and senior staff in the ICU is the coordination of all aspects of patient care, and in particular the maintenance of good lines of communication between the different teams involved.

MOVING BETWEEN PATIENTS

- Wash hands thoroughly or use alcohol disinfectant scrub *before and after* patient contact.
- Do not share equipment such as stethoscopes.

ASSESSING A PATIENT

Each patient in ICU needs to be completely examined and assessed at least twice a day and more often if unstable. A large amount of information will be available from the charts, monitors and patient himself. Most conventional aspects of history taking and examination are either inappropriate or impractical.

It is important to have a uniform system for condensing the information easily so that patient assessment can be made, a plan formulated and communication between different teams and shifts facilitated.

1. **History**

   It is important to be aware of the detailed history of the patient, particularly when admitting a new patient. Important sources of information may be the family, patient notes, referring hospital or doctors.

   The patient's chart is an extension of the history and should be scanned for trends in the patient's condition since arrival to the ICU.

2. **Examining the patient**

   Before examining the patient, introduce yourself to the patient's family and explain any planned procedures, including risk.

   Examine the patient in the normal way, also ensuring that information from monitors and charts are assimilated.

   - *Cardiovascular: Obtain the following data.*
     - Trends and actual values of heart rate, *mean* blood pressure (check if age appropriate), CVP if available.
     - Adequacy of systemic perfusion: Capillary refill time (normal < 2 sec), peripheral pulse volume, cold/sweaty/warm peripheries.
     - Evidence of adequate organ perfusion: Consciousness level, urine output, metabolic acidosis.
     - Monitoring line sites: Clean or evidence of infection.
   - *Respiratory*
     - Check position and patency of endotracheal tubes (ETT), type and quantity of tracheal secretions. Check that the ETT is secured well.
     - Ensure that a peri-tubal leak is present at a PIP of 20-25 cm H_2O for both cuffed and

uncuffed tubes. For a cuffed ETT, check cuff inflation pressures thrice daily (should not exceed 25 mm Hg).
- Ventilatory settings, level of support, blood gas (assess in relation to FiO_2).
- Readiness for weaning: Patient's work of breathing, adequacy of spontaneous effort.
- A chest X-ray is considered an extension of the physical examination in most ICU patients, required daily in most *acute* patients, less frequently in chronic patients.

- *CNS*
  - Consciousness level, GCS, pupils.
  - For painful stimulus, press on nail bed or supra-orbital ridge.
  - Consider stopping/decreasing dose of all sedative/analgesic drugs to assess neurologic status.
  - Anticonvulsant: Are levels appropriate?
- *Abdomen*
  - Soft, tender or distended.
  - Gastric aspirates: type and volume.
  - Bowels sounds present/absent.
  - Bowels open, diarrhea.
- *Fluid/Electrolyte/Nutrition (FEN)*
  - Fluid intake/output and balance, urine output in ml/kg/hr, particularly in last 6 hours.
  - Renal indices, electrolytes.
  - Enteral/parenteral feeding: Calories and protein requirement met?
- *Infectious disease (ID) issues*
  - Hyper/hypothermia, possible septic focus.
  - White cell counts, culture results, day of antibiotics, review need for antibiotic.
- *Hematology*
  - Bleeds from skin, sites, tubes, gastro-intestinal.
  - Platelet count and coagulation status.
- *Limbs*
  - Perfusion, color, swelling, tenderness or compartment syndrome.
- *Invasive lines/catheters*
  - Days since inserted.
  - Inspect site for erythema, inflammation, exudates.
  - Decide if central lines/Foley catheter still required or will peripheral lines/weighing diapers suffice?
- *Wounds*
  - Surgical wounds/trauma sites: Expose and inspect for adequate healing.
  - Surgical drains: Volume and nature of drainage.

3. **Laboratory investigations**
   Review all hematology, biochemistry, microbiology investigations and all imaging studies.
4. **Prescription charts**
   Review drugs and dosages.
5. **Make an assessment** of the active problems/issues in relation to the diagnosis.
6. **Make a plan** which should systematically include all the above points.
7. **Communicate clearly** the plan to all members of the team including the nursing team and other consultants involved in the care of the patient.
8. **Educate and update the family** regarding the condition, expected course of illness and probable outcome.

2

The Pediatric MET (Medical Emergency Team)

- Cardiopulmonary arrests that occur outside the critical care units in pediatric hospitals have a poor survival rate. This high mortality rate makes prevention of in-hospital, out of ICU cardiopulmonary arrest particularly important.
- While some cardiac arrests are unpredictable, sometimes cardiac arrest is predictable, but:
  - Severity of illness is not recognized
  - Help is not requested until cardiac arrest
  - No assistance is available
  - Assistance is available but delayed
- **The MET (Medical Emergency Team) – known by some as the RRT (Rapid Response Team)** – is a team of clinicians who bring critical care expertise to the bedside of the patient (or wherever it is needed).
- *The main goal of the MET is to identify unstable patients and those patients likely to suffer cardiac or respiratory arrest. If identified in a timely fashion, their unnecessary deaths can often be prevented.*
- The MET team will respond immediately to call for assistance on wards/departments. They should have the skills to:
  - Manage medical/surgical emergencies.
  - Assess and treat the patient as required.
  - Discuss management of the patient with the members of the treating unit.
  - Admit the child to ICU or continue to help manage on ward as required.
- The members of the MET include physicians, nursing staff and other paramedicals such as respiratory therapists, etc.
- Prior to implementation of a MET, there is a need to educate and train the staff, particularly the nursing staff and the other members of the team. In addition to the skills of basic and advanced airway and circulation management, the training should include topics such as the benefits and myths of MET, criteria and procedure for calling the team, communication and team work, etc.
- In addition to education of the MET, training the hospital staff to recognize serious illness, understand calling criteria and providing feedback is important.
- The emphasis is on empowering nursing and medical staff. Ensure MET staff adopts a supportive attitude to ward staff initiating the MET call irrespective of perceived appropriateness.
- The MET is not intended to take the place of immediate consultation with the physician if needed.
- Each call to the MET should result in the completion of a documentation form or record, which should be kept in a central location and serve as a source of data.
- In addition, regular and timely assessment of the number of calls received by the MET should be done to monitor the progress of the team and to assess the change in the system and the outcome of patients, before and after the inception of the MET.

PEDIATRIC MET CRITERIA

1. Ward nurse or doctor WORRIED about clinical state
2. Airway threat: stridor/noisy breathing, snoring
3. Hypoxemia: $SpO_2 < 90\%$ in any amount of oxygen; $SpO_2 < 60\%$ in any amount of oxygen (cyanotic heart disease)
4. Severe respiratory distress, apnea or cyanosis
5. Tachypnea

Age	RR (breaths per min)
Term to 3 months	> 60
4-12 months	> 50
1-4 years	> 40
5-12 years	> 30
12+ years	> 30

6. Tachycardia or bradycardia

Age	HR too slow (beats per min)	HR too fast (bpm)
Term to 3 months	< 100	> 180
4-12 months	< 100	> 180
1-4 years	< 90	> 160
5-12 years	< 80	> 140
12+ years	< 60	> 130

7. Hypotension

Age	Systolic BP (mm Hg)
Term to 3 months	< 50
4-12 months	< 60
1-4 years	< 70
5-12 years	< 80
12+ years	< 90

8. Acute change in neurological status or convulsion
9. Cardiac or respiratory arrest

REFERENCE

1. Tibballs J, Kinney S, Duke T, Oakley E, Hennessy M. Reduction of paediatric in-patient cardiac arrest and death with a medical emergency team: preliminary results. Arch Dis Child. 2005;90:1148-1152.

3

Cardiopulmonary Resuscitation (CPR)

"Any attempt to resuscitate is better than none."

A cardiopulmonary arrest is the ultimate medical emergency and can occur because of two different scenarios:

1. **Hypoxia ± decompensated shock**: *This is the most common pathophysiological mechanism of cardiac arrest in infants and children through adolescence.* This is the terminal event of progressive respiratory failure or shock.
2. **Sudden cardiac arrest (SCA)**: This is uncommon in children. When it does occur, SCA is most often associated with ventricular fibrillation (VF), pulseless ventricular tachycardia (VT) or pulseless electrical activity (PEA).

The goal of therapeutic interventions in cardiac arrest is return of spontaneous circulation (ROSC), defined as restoration of a spontaneous and perfusing heart rhythm.

ROSC is detected by resumption of organized cardiac electric activity on cardiac monitor and corresponding clinical evidence of perfusion (e.g., palpable pulse, measurable blood pressure).

- **Basic Life Support (BLS)** is the term used to describe simple measures to maintain a patent airway and support breathing and circulation. While BLS has to be performed with the utmost urgency and expertise, it should be considered as a 'holding measure' to maintain brain and heart viability and buying time for specific measures to come into action.
- Priorities to be handled are:
  A : Airway
  B : Breathing
  C : Circulation

AIRWAY & BREATHING

- In an apneic unconscious patient, without evidence of head or neck trauma, use the *head tilt–chin lift* maneuvre to open the airway (Fig. 3.1 A-C).
- In the event of trauma, drowning or any patient with a suspected cervical spine injury, open the airway using *a jaw thrust without head tilt*. However, if jaw thrust does not open the airway sufficiently, use the head tilt– chin lift maneuvre as maintaining a patent airway and providing adequate ventilation takes the priority during CPR.
- While maintaining an open airway, *check whether the victim is breathing*, taking no more than 10 seconds:
  - *Look* for rhythmic chest and abdominal movement,
  - *Listen* for exhaled breath sounds at the nose and mouth, and
  - *Feel* for exhaled air on your cheek.
- Periodic gasping, also called *agonal gasps,* is not breathing.
- If the patient is not breathing, initiate rescue breathing with either bag-mask ventilation or direct mouth to mouth respiration. (Mouth to both mouth and nose respiration in neonates.)

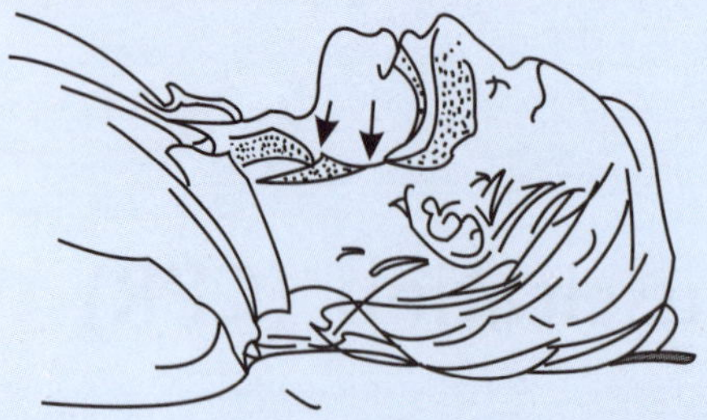

Fig. 3.1A Compromised airway in an unconscious patient due to neck flexion and tongue falling backwards

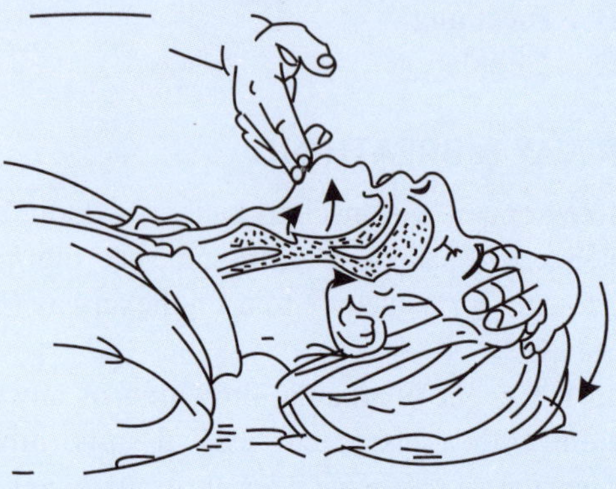

Fig. 3.1B Airway opening by head tilt and chin lift

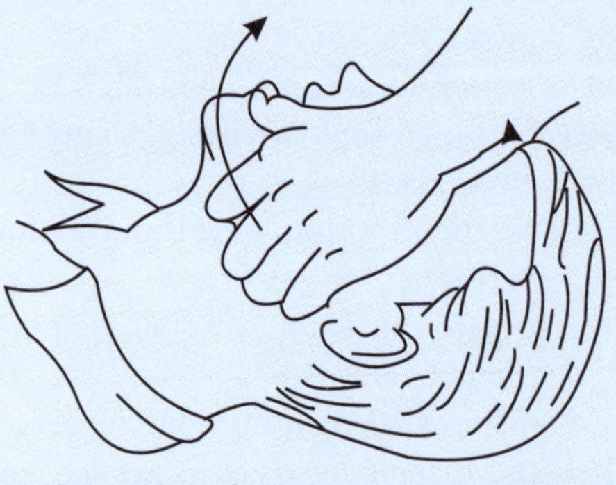

Grasp the angles of the lower jaw and lift with both hands, one on each side, moving the jaw forward. If victim's lips are closed, open the lower lip with your thumb

Fig. 3.1C Jaw thrust without head tilt

- Bag-mask ventilation can be as effective as endotracheal intubation and safer when providing ventilation for short periods.
- A self-inflating bag delivers only room air unless supplementary oxygen is attached, but even with an oxygen inflow of 10 L/min, the concentration of delivered oxygen varies from 30% to 50% and depends on the tidal volume and peak inspiratory flow rate.
- To deliver a high oxygen concentration (60% to 95%), attach an oxygen reservoir to the self-inflating bag and maintain an oxygen flow of 10 to 15 L/min.
- *Avoid hyperventilation:* Give each breath over 1 second.
- Excessive ventilation is detrimental because it:
  - Impedes venous return by increasing intrathoracic pressure. This in return leads to decreased cardiac output, cerebral blood flow, and coronary perfusion.
  - Can cause air trapping and barotrauma in patients with small airways obstruction.
  - Increases the risk of regurgitation and aspiration.
- *Minimize gastric inflation:*
  - Avoid excessive peak inspiratory pressures (e.g., by ventilating slowly and watching chest rise). Deliver only the volume needed to produce visible chest rise.
  - Apply cricoid pressure. It should be applied only in unresponsive victims. Avoid excessive pressure so as not to obstruct the trachea.
  - Pass a nasogastric (NG) or orogastric (OG) tube preferably *after* intubation because gastric tube stents open the gastro-esophageal sphincter, allowing possible regurgitation. Passing of NG or OG tube can initiate gag reflex and can cause aspiration.
- A rescuer should provide 12 to 20 rescue breaths per minute. One way to achieve this rate with a ventilating bag is to use the mnemonic "squeeze-release-release" at a normal speaking rate.

- *If the patient continues to remain apneic and/ or bradycardic, proceed to oral intubation.*
- While, traditionally, cuffed endotracheal tubes (ET) were recommended in children > 8 years, current recommendations of PALS/AHA 2005 state that *cuffed endotracheal tubes are as safe as uncuffed tube even in infants* (beyond the newborn period), provided that attention is paid to endotracheal tube size, position, and cuff inflation pressure. Keep cuff inflation pressure ≤ 20 cmH_2O.
- Cuffed tubes may be preferred in patients with poor lung compliance, high airway resistance or excessive airway secretions.

Table 3.1 The sizes of endotracheal tube (ETT) according to age

Age	Endotracheal tube size in mm	ETT : length at lips
1 month	3.0–3.5	9 cm
6 months	3.5–4.0	10 cm
1 year	4.0–4.5	11 cm
2 years	4.5	12 cm

Uncuffed endotracheal tube size (mm ID) > 2 years	: (Age in years/4) + 4
Cuffed endotracheal tube size (mm ID) > 2 years	: (Age in years/4) + 3
ETT fixation point at lip in cm	: (Age in years/2) + 12
ETT fixation point at lip in cm *in infancy*	: ET tube size x 3

- Keep additional tubes, with internal diameters that are 0.5 mm smaller and 0.5 mm larger than the size estimated ready at the bedside for use.
- Always keep suction apparatus ready.
- Immediately after intubation and again after securing the tube, confirm correct ET placement with the following techniques while positive pressure ventilation with a bag is being provided:
  - Look for bilateral chest movement and listen for equal breath sounds over both lung fields, especially over the axillae.
  - Listen for gastric insufflation sounds over the stomach (they should not be present if the tube is in the trachea).
  - Check for exhaled CO_2 (if available) only if there is a perfusing rhythm.
  - Check oxygen saturation with a pulse oximeter.
  - Obtain a chest X-ray to verify ET position.

☞ REMEMBER

- "Breath" sounds can be widely conducted over chest and abdomen in infants and young children.
- Effective pre-oxygenation may result in normal levels of oxyhaemoglobin saturation (SpO_2) that are sustained for as long as 3 minutes despite incorrect endotracheal tube position (e.g., tube misplacement or displacement).
- Conversely, in a patient with significant lung pathology (e.g., ARDS), SpO_2 may not rise satisfactorily despite ventilation via an appropriately placed ET.
- If still uncertain, perform direct laryngoscopy and visualize the ET passing between the cords (*the best confirmatory test).*

- Perform a chest X-ray (CXR) to verify that the tube is not in the right main bronchus (too low) or too high, i.e., at risk of easy displacement, although breath sounds may be equal. The ideal tube position is where the tip of ETT

ENDOTRACHEAL DRUG ADMINISTRATION

- If vascular access cannot be established rapidly, lipid soluble drugs such as lidocaine, epinephrine, atropine, and naloxone ("LEAN") can be given via the endotracheal tube.
- Flush with a minimum of 5 ml normal saline followed by 5 assisted manual ventilations.
- If CPR is in progress, chest compressions should briefly be discontinued during ET administration of medications.
- Administration of resuscitation drugs into the trachea results in lower blood concentrations than the same doses given intravenously. *For drugs administration during CPR, any vascular access (IO or intravenous) is preferred to ET.*

REFERENCES

1. Pediatric Basic Life Support. Circulation 2005;112:IV, 156-166
2. Pediatric Advanced Life Support. *Circulation* 2005; 112: IV, 167-187
3. Recognition and Management of Cardiac Arrest. Pediatric advanced life support provider's manual (Professional) 2006.

See also : Post Resuscitation Care (Chapter 4).

4

Post-Resuscitation Care

INTRODUCTION

- The goals of post-resuscitation management are:
  - Optimize and stabilize cardiopulmonary function. Restore and maintain vital organ perfusion (especially brain) and thereby prevent secondary organ injury.
  - Identify and treat the condition that has caused the sudden cardiorespiratory decompensation.
  - Institute measures aimed to improve long term, neurologically intact survival.
- Where necessary, it also includes safe transport of the patient to a tertiary care center/ PICU.
- Meticulous documentation of the following is important: Events leading to arrest (if known), events during CPR, type and doses of drugs, including electrical therapy and finally, time required for *return of spontaneous circulation* (ROSC).
- Time for ROSC has prognostic significance both for immediate survival and long term neurological outcome. In general, the likelihood of good outcome declines with the length of resuscitative efforts.

Meticulous supportive management is the cornerstone of the post arrest intensive care.

ELEMENTS OF POST-RESUSCITATION CARE

A. Respiratory system

- Continue to monitor and support patient airway, oxygenation and ventilation.
- Ensure that the ET is fixed securely.
- Attach the patient to ventilator after selecting appropriate settings and alarms. Obtain an ABG with lactate half an hour after attaching to ventilator.
- Obtain a chest X-ray to identify any significant pulmonary issues and verify placement of endotracheal, gastric and central lines, if present. The radiographic evaluation of heart size should be noted.
- Anticipate and monitor for post arrest acute respiratory distress syndrome (ARDS). Ventilate using lung protective strategies.
- Consider sedation and analgesia for all responsive intubated patients. If the patient's hemodynamics are unstable, use agents with a safe hemodynamic profile.
- Nurse the child with head end up by 30^0 (if out of shock) and neck in midline.

B. Cardiovascular system

- Remove IO access after establishing two secure venous lines. Obtain central venous line and invasive arterial access and initiate arterial blood pressure monitoring. Switch inotropes to central line.

- *Treat hypotension aggressively* to prevent secondary organ dysfunction.
- *Post arrest myocardial dysfunction/myocardial stunning* are common after CPR. It can cause biventricular systolic and/or diastolic dysfunction. This usually resolves in 24-48 hours; however, close hemodynamic monitoring and treatment are necessary. If left untreated it can be the cause of another cardiac arrest. Epinephrine is a preferable inotrope in children with significant circulatory instability.
- Treat uncorrected hypovolemia and low SVR if present.
- Titrate hemodynamic support based on predefined targets and goals (warm extremities, normal mean BP and heart rate for age, urine output, central venous saturation, etc).
- Obtain a bedside echocardiogram to assess heart functions and intravascular volume.
- Start maintenance fluids once intravascular volume is restored.

C. Neurological system

- Priorities are prevention of secondary neuronal injury.
- Maintain high normal MAP in order to optimize *cerebral perfusion pressure* (CPP).
- Seizures: look for convulsive and non-convulsive seizures, as these are common in post-arrest period. Treat them aggressively, consider prophylactic anticonvul sants. Monitor and correct deranged metabolic parameters (glucose, sodium, calcium, magnesium).
- Ventilate to maintain normocarbia (pCO_2 35-40 mmHg).

D. Temperature control

- Both hypo and hyperthermia may occur after cardiac arrest.

  Elevated temperature following cardiac arrest is common and hyperthermia is associated with worse neurological outcomes, both in adults and children. Treat hyperthermia aggressively.
  - *Cooling* to a temperature of 32-34^{0}C for 12 to 24 hours following resuscitation may be neuroprotective.
  - Prevent shivering by providing deep sedation and, if needed, neuromuscular blockade. Closely watch for signs of infection.
  - Other complications of hypothermia include diminished cardiac output, arrhythmia, pancreatitis, coagulopathy, thrombocytopenia, hypophosphatemia, and hypomagnesemia. Neuromuscular blockade can mask seizures.

E. Metabolic and glycemic control

- Both hyperglycemia and hypoglycemia are common; and both are associated with poor neurological outcome. Therefore maintaining euglycemia (blood sugar 120-180 mg%) may be prudent.
- Monitor sodium, other electrolytes closely.

F. Renal system

- Monitor urine output with an indwelling catheter.
- Decreased urine output (< 1 ml/kg per hour in infants and children or < 30 mL/hr in adolescents) may be caused by prerenal failure (e.g., dehydration, inadequate systemic perfusion), renal ischemic damage, or a combination of factors.
- Consider fluid boluses if oliguria persists. Consider dialysis if established renal failure occurs.
- Avoid nephrotoxic medications and adjust the dose of medications excreted by the kidneys until normal renal functions are achieved.
- Monitor for increased urine output (> 4 ml/kg/hour) as a result of osmotic diuresis (glycosuria, mannitol), tubular dysfunction and neurogenic diabetes insipidus (which is an ominous finding).

G. Gastrointestinal system

- Monitor quantity/color of gastric aspirates.
- Institute stress ulcer prophylaxis with H_2 blocker or proton pump inhibitor. Critically ill children can have delayed gastric emptying and ileus.
- Enteral feeds should be commenced once perfusion indices improve and pressor requirements have reduced. In a poorly perfused, acidotic patient with steep pressor requirements, enteral feeds may exacerbate mesenteric ischemia.
- Watch for *abdominal compartment syndrome (ACS)*. It may present with a triad of decreasing urine output, worsening acidosis and increasing ventilator requirements. It is confirmed by an intra-abdominal pressure (IAP) $\geq$ 20 cm H_2O, in association with any two of the above features. Consider early abdominal decompression.
- *Ischemic hepatitis* with elevation of liver transaminases and normal bilirubin levels may occur 24-36 hours after hypoperfusion/shock/arrest. No specific therapy is indicated and prognosis for recovery is generally good provided no further deterioration of the circulatory status occurs.

H. Hematologic system

- Excessive bleeding may occur due to platelet and coagulation defects, superadded sepsis. Consider blood component therapy as clinically indicated.
- Restore adequate oxygen carrying capacity by maintaining a Hb> 7-8 gm%.

I. *Counseling of family*

- This is an important aspect of supportive care; honesty and sensitivity during counseling are essential.

REFERENCES

1. Pediatric basic life support. Circulation 2005;112:IV, 156-166
2. Pediatric advanced life support. Circulation 2005; 112: IV, 167-187
3. Recognition and management of cardiac arrest. Pediatric Advanced Life Support Provider's Manual (Professional) 2006
4. Post-resuscitation management. Pediatric Advanced Life Support Provider's Manual (professional) 2006

5

Anaphylaxis

DEFINITION

A severe, life threatening, IgE mediated immediate hypersensitivity, often dominated by severe bronchospasm and hypotension.

ETIOLOGY

- Drugs: Any drug may be responsible, notably penicillins, cephalosporins, anesthetic agents, aspirin, other NSAIDs, ACE inhibitors etc.
- Foods: Notably, nuts, milk, egg, seafoods, fish.
- Insect bite
- Latex allergy
- Idiopathic
- Others: IV fluids, colloids, IV contrast, antivenoms, blood products.

CLINICAL FEATURES

- Urticaria
- Flushing
- Wheezing
- Abdominal cramps
- Hypotension
- Unconsciousness
- Angio-edema
- Laryngeal edema
- Bradycardia
- Neurocardiogenic syncope.

Anaphylaxis results from complex immunologic mechanism from IgE mediated sudden systemic release of mast cells and basophil mediators.

Anaphylactoid reaction is not mediated through IgE, but has an identical clinical picture as a result of degranulation of mast cells and basophils.

The treatment for both conditions is identical but anaphylactoid reactions do not recur with re-exposure of the etiological agent. Misinterpretation of the reaction as anaphylactoid has resulted in fatal re-exposure of the patient to the allergen concerned.

TIME COURSE OF ANAPHYLAXIS

- Onset may immediate or delayed. Early onset occurs within minutes of exposure. Delayed onset is seen after 30 minutes. Late phase or biphasic reactions may occur after 8-12 hr of exposure.
- Duration: Usually lasts for few minutes. Severe/protracted forms can last up to 32 hr.
- Following resolution of the initial event, an overnight or 24 hour waiting period before discharge is recommended.
- Concomitant asthma, food related anaphylaxis and reactions to insect stings needs PICU admission as fatal reactions are more likely.

TREATMENT

Immediate first line therapies

- Assess airway, breathing, circulation, and level of consciousness (altered mentation suggests the presence of hypoxia).

- *Immediate intubation is essential* in the presence of significant respiratory signs such as stridor, tachypnea, dyspnea or difficulty swallowing as delay may increase difficulty due to progressive airway edema. Cricothyroidotomy may be necessary for established severe edema.
- Head end low if hypotensive.
- Provide 100% oxygen by non-rebreathing mask. Check blood sugar.
- In severe attack, epinephrine (adrenaline) 1:1000 dilution (1 mg/ml), 0.01 mg/kg, maximum 0.3 mg (0.5 mg for >12 yr) *intramuscularly* repeated as necessary every 5 minutes, should be used to control symptoms and increase blood pressure.

  Note: Adrenaline has to be given only by IM route. SQ route is not recommended as absorption may be delayed in shock states. IV adrenaline is recommended for subsequent doses or if the patient is in cardiopulmonary arrest.
- Establish two sites of venous access. Administer fluid boluses of 20 mL/kg of normal saline if hypotensive. If blood pressure does not improve, start an epinephrine infusion.
- Start pressor (dopamine or vasopressin) infusion if patient still hypotensive despite epinephrine infusion (as anaphylaxis leads to profound vasodilatation).
- Systemic glucocorticosteroids such as hydrocortisone 1 mg/kg every 6th hourly or methyl prednisolone, although not helpful in the acute phase, will prevent recurrent or protracted anaphylaxis. Oral administration may suffice for less critical anaphylactic episodes.

Second line therapies with slower onset of action

- H_1 antihistamines: Diphenhydramine, 1 to 2 mg/kg or 25 to 50 mg per dose (parenterally).
- H_2 antagonists: Ranitidine 1 mg/kg diluted in 5% dextrose to a total volume of 20 ml and injected intravenously over 5 minutes.

  In the management of anaphylaxis, a combination of diphenhydramine and ranitidine is superior to diphenhydramine alone.
- Bronchospasm resistant to adequate doses of epinephrine: Administer inhaled beta-agonist (e.g., nebulized salbutamol).
- Consider adrenaline as nebulization in addition to systemic route in the presence of severe laryngeal edema.

Cardiopulmonary arrest during anaphylaxis is different from other forms of arrest

- Second and subsequent dosages of adrenaline are higher (0.1 to 0.2 mg/kg; 0.1-0.2 ml/kg of a 1:1000 solution).
- Atropine is useful for unresponsive asystole or pulseless electrical activity.
- Rapid volume expansion is often required.
- More prolonged resuscitation may be necessary.

REFERENCES

1. Project Team of the Resuscitation Council (UK) (Revised May 2005). The emergency medical treatment of anaphylactic reactions for first medical responders and for community nurses. http://www.resus.org.uk/
2. The diagnosis and management of anaphylaxis: an updated practice parameter. J Allergy Clin Immunol 2005 Mar;115(3 Suppl):S483-523.

SECTION 3 : RESPIRATORY SYSTEM

6

Approach to a Child with Respiratory Failure

- When faced with a sick child, the ability to rapidly assess the airway, breathing and circulation along with institution of appropriate interventions to stabilize the disordered parameters are extremely important skills for emergency and intensive care physicians.
- Children with critical illness pose several unique challenges. They have anatomic disadvantages related to their breathing apparatus (large tongue, high floppy epiglottis, narrow airways, lower FRC, higher closing capacity) and physiological disadvantage related to their higher oxygen consumption rates which makes them especially prone to hypoxemia.
- Irrespective of the cause, a systematic approach will aid in the stabilization of the respiratory system in the critically ill child and facilitate a favorable outcome.

ASSESSMENT OF THE AIRWAY AND BREATHING

During the initial assessment, it is important to attempt to assess both the airway and breathing separately, although it may be difficult to clearly demarcate these as two mutually exclusive functions.

Following assessment, the **airway** may be categorized as:

- *Clear* (open and unobstructed for normal breathing).
- *Maintainable* (airway maintained by simple measures such as positioning, suctioning or adjuncts such as oropharyngeal/nasopharyngeal airways).
- *Not maintainable* (needing advanced interventions such as endotracheal tubes, cricothyrotomy or application of CPAP/positive pressure).

Assessment of **breathing** involves evaluation of:

- Respiratory rate (normal, slow, fast) and rhythm (regular or irregular).
- Tidal volumes: Clinically assessed by the chest excursion (normal, excessive, decreased).
- Assessment of work of breathing (WOB), use of accessory muscles of breathing.
- Lung sounds/air entry, presence of added sounds.
- Pulse oximetry: The 5th vital sign

Respiratory rate (RR): Normal respiratory rate (RR) is inversely related to age (Table 6.1). Infants have higher rates compared to older children due to their higher oxygen requirements, lower lung volumes and capacities and higher dead space volumes. However, *a respiratory rate which is consistently > 60 per minute in any age group is abnormal*. Abnormal rates can be broadly categorized as:

- Tachypnea (high RR for age)
- Bradypnea (low RR for age)
- Apnea (central apnea which is associated with complete cessation of respiration)

Table 6.1 Cut-off values for tachypnea for age

Age	Breaths per min
< 2 months	> 60
2–12 months	> 50
1–5 yr	> 40
5–12 yr	> 30
13–18 yr	> 16

Tidal volume

- The tidal volume may be assessed by evaluation of the chest expansion during inspiration (adequate/shallow/excessive), the symmetry of the movement and also by listening to the air entry by auscultation.
- Decreased or asymmetric chest expansion can occur with airway obstruction, parenchymal lung problems causing volume loss (atelectasis) or pleural pathology such as pneumothorax or effusions. These situations are also associated with decreased air entry in the affected lung segments.
- When the tidal volumes decrease, there is compensatory increase in the RR in order to maintain adequate minute ventilation (MV) resulting in rapid shallow breathing (MV = RR x tidal volume).

Assessment of work of breathing (WOB)

- Tachypnea can be effortless or associated with signs of increased work of breathing, when it is called *respiratory distress*.
- *Effortless or quiet tachypnea* may result from increased catabolic states (fever), SIRS (systemic inflammatory response syndrome), pain, metabolic acidosis and in sepsis even without pneumonia or pulmonary edema. Occasionally, quiet tachypnea may also be seen with disordered respiratory drive secondary to central hyperventilation (encephalitis, hepatic encephalopathy).
- Respiratory distress with increased WOB can occur with conditions associated with increased airway resistance or decreased lung parenchymal compliance (Table 6.2).
- Signs of increased WOB include nasal flaring, chest retractions, head bobbing or see-saw breathing, prolonged inspiratory or expiratory efforts, mouth breathing, gasping or use of accessory muscles.
- Chest retractions can be *mild, moderate* (subcostal, substernal or intercostal) or *severe* (supraclavicular, suprasternal and sternal).
- Head bobbing can be an adavanced sign of respiratory failure, especially in infants. See-saw breathing may either be due to weakness of the respiratory muscles (diaphragm or intercostals) or indicate the presence of severe parenchymal lung disease.

Table 6.2 Conditions associated with respiratory distress

Airway disease (upper or lower airways)	Croup, epiglottitis, retropharyngeal abscess, tracheomalacia *(upper airways)* Bronchiolitis, asthma, dynamic compression of the airways, bronchomalacia, extrinsic airway compression *(lower airways)*
Poor lung compliance	Pneumonias, collapsed lung segments, pulmonary edema, ARDS, pleural effusions, pneumothorax
Poor chest wall compliance	Distended abdomen, chest wall or abdominal wall edema, respiratory muscle paralysis

- Upper airway obstruction may be associated with predominant suprasternal, sternal and subcostal retractions with stridor but without marked tachypnea.

☞ REMEMBER

- Some neurological conditions and sedative drugs can result in advanced hypercapnic respiratory failure and yet not be associated with respiratory distress. Careful evaluation may be required to document the slower respiratory rates and diminished chest excursions in these patients who may also exhibit drowsiness due to CO_2 narcosis.
- Conversely, other conditions such as metabolic acidosis can have significant respiratory symptoms in the absence of respiratory disease.

Lung and airway sounds

- Listening for abnormal respiratory sounds may provide clues towards the cause of the respiratory distress, e.g., grunting, gurgling, stridor, wheezing, crackles and bronchial breathing.
- Stridor or wheezing indicates the presence of upper or lower airway disease, respectively. Grunting and crackles are usually associated with parenchymal lung disease.

Pulse oximetry

- This monitoring modality is often called the 5th vital sign.
- It is a useful noninvasive, portable tool that indicates what percentage of the hemoglobin is saturated with oxygen and can detect hypoxemia in a child well before the appearance of cyanosis or bradycardia.
- Oxygen saturations at or above 92% while breathing room air usually indicate adequate oxygenation.
- Limitations: Interpret pulse oximetry readings cautiously in children with:
  - Extremes of oxygenation (less reliable when saturations < 70%), may miss significant hyperoxia.
  - Poor perfusion.
  - Cyanotic congenital heart diseases with baseline saturations < 70%.
  - Anemia (tissue oxygen delivery may be reduced despite a normal oxygen saturation).
  - Abnormal hemoglobins such as methemoglobin, carboxyhemoglobin etc.

Table 6.3 Causes of hypercapnia *(See also hypercapnia equations)*

Increased CO_2 production	Fever, seizures, hyper-metabolism, sepsis, increased carbohydrate consumption
Decreased minute ventilation	Central hypoventilation, neuromuscular paralysis
Increased dead space	Severe parenchymal lung disease with loss of lung volume (collapse, consolidation), severe airway obstruction, hyperinflation, increased pulmonary vascular resistance, pulmonary hypertension, pulmonary embolism, poor pulmonary perfusion

CATEGORIZATION OF RESPIRATORY PROBLEMS BY SEVERITY

- *Respiratory distress*
  - Increased work of breathing.
  - May be accompanied by tachycardia.
  - Oxygenation and CO_2 maintained in 'normal' ranges at great effort.
  - Potential for fatigue and progression to respiratory failure if increased WOB progresses or unrelieved.
- *Respiratory failure*
  - This is a clinical state of inadequate oxygenation, ventilation or both, due to failure of compensatory mechanisms.

- Clinically, respiratory failure may be recognized by one or more of the following:
  - Signs of severe respiratory distress.
  - Altered mental status.
  - Cyanosis or documented hypoxemia/hypercarbia.

☞ REMEMBER

The above categorization may not apply to children with pre-existing abnormalities such as *cyanotic congenital heart disease* with decreased baseline oxygen saturations or *chronic lung disease* with elevated baseline $paCO_2$.

INADEQUATE VENTILATION OR HYPERCAPNIA

Hypercapnic respiratory failure results from inadequate ventilation and consequent increase in the $paCO_2$.

Causes of hyercapnic respiratory failure

- *Central causes:* Here the lungs are usually normal, unless complications have supervened.
  - Inadequate respiratory drive (sedative drugs, CNS/brainstem lesions)
  - Ineffective respiratory pump (Guillain Barre, diaphragmatic weakness)
- *Peripheral causes:*
  - Pathology in the airways (resulting in hyperinflation)
  - Lung parenchymal disorders
  - Diseases of pleura
- *Conditions associated with decreased effective pulmonary blood flow* to the lung with consequent increased dead space, e.g., pulmonary hypertension, cyanotic spell, pulmonary embolism.

The clinical presentation may be highly variable, depending on the cause, and the patient may present with signs of increased WOB or hypoventilation/apnea or hypoperfusion and shock.

☞ REMEMBER

- Even experienced clinicians may often miss features of central hypoventilation as the patient may not have respiratory distress. The suboptimal respiratory rates and excursions may easily be overlooked.
  - Further contributing to the delayed/missed diagnosis of hypoventilation is the fact that the oxygen saturation may be normal until hypoventilation is advanced. Hypoxemia is usually a late event and is typically associated with a normal alveolar-arterial oxygen gradient ($AaDO_2$) as opposed to hypoxemia associated with parenchymal disorders where the $AaDO_2$ is widened.
  - Administration of oxygen to a patient with central hypoventilation can confer a false sense of security to the clinician as, despite rising $paCO_2$ levels, the oxygen saturations may continue to be normal until late in the course of illness.
  - Rising $paCO_2$ levels may manifest as tachycardia, hypertension, drowsiness, stupor, coma (CO_2 narcosis) and pupillary dilatation.
- Patients with heterogeneous lung/airway disease (chronic lung disease, asthma with collapse) may have both hypercarbia and hypoxemia.
- Here, supplemental oxygen administrations will improve hypoxemia but not hypercarbia, and these children may progress from agitation to depressed responsiveness.

☞ REMEMBER

- *Always suspect hypercarbia in a child with hypoxemia who continues to be drowsy despite correction of hypoxemia.*
- Especially in patients with *chronic respiratory failure* where the brainstem may no longer be responsive to abnormally elevated $paCO_2$, it is important to administer oxygen titrated so as to maintain the O_2 saturation in the range of 88 92% so as not to abolish the hypoxic drive which may be an important backup drive for respiration.

HYPOXIA AND HYPOXEMIA

- It is important to distinguish between the two terminologies.
- Hypoxemia implies poor oxygen saturations in the blood (defined by consensus as < 92%).
- Hypoxia denotes inadequate tissue oxygenation.
- *Early clinical signs of hypoxia* include tachypnea, pallor, agitation, altered mental status and tachycardia.
- *Late signs* include bradypnea, apnea, bradycardia and central cyanosis. The various mechanisms of hypoxemia are listed below.

Hypercapnia and hypoxemia equations

Hypercapnia equations

- MV (minute ventilation) = Tidal volume x respiratory rate (MV= TV x RR)
- Tidal volume (TV) = Volume of gas that moves in and out of the lungs during normal breathing. Range 5-12 ml/kg.
- Dead space ventilation
  = Volume of air that does not participate in gas exchange
  = Alveolar ventilation – dead space ventilation
  = Proportion of tidal volume in conducting airways *(anatomical dead space)* + proportion of tidal volume ventilating underperfused alveoli (*alveolar dead space)*

Dead space ventilation = Anatomical dead space + alveolar dead space

Hypoxemia equations

A. *The $AaDO_2$ or alveolar-arterial oxygen difference*

This is the alveolar-arterial gas equation where:

- 'A' denotes the alveolar oxygen tension (pAO_2)
- 'a' denotes the arterial oxygen tension (paO_2)
- DO_2 denotes the difference between the alveolar and arterial oxygen gas tension, an indirect indicator of ventilation perfusion abnormalities.
- Knowledge of the $AaDO_2$ will aid in the interpretation of oxygenation defects.

Step 1: Determine alveolar oxygen tension (pAO_2)

- $pAO_2 = piO_2 - (paCO_2/RQ)$
- Where piO_2 = tension of inspired oxygen and RQ = respiratory quotient (usually 0.8)
- $piO_2 = FiO_2$ x [barometric pressure *(760 mm Hg)* – water vapour pressure in humidified gas *(47 mm Hg)*]
  $= FiO_2 \times (760 - 47)$
- $pAO_2 = FiO_2\,(760 - 47) - paCO_2/0.8$
  E.g., pAO_2 in room air (where the FiO_2 is assumed to be 0.21) = $150 - paCO_2/0.8$

Step 2: Determine arterial oxygen tension (paO_2) from the arterial blood gas

Step 3: Determine the alveolar-arterial oxygen difference *($pAO_2 - paO_2$) or the $AaDO_2$*
Normal $AaDO_2$ gradient is < 15 mm Hg in patients aged less than 30 yr.
Also note that the normal gradient increases 5–7 mmHg for every 10% rise in FiO_2

B. *The paO_2 / FiO_2 ratio (P/F ratio)*

- The paO_2 / FiO_2 ratio is used as an indirect estimate of the shunt fraction (the fraction of the cardiac output representing the intrapulmonary shunt, i.e., not participating in the gas exchange).
- A paO_2 / FiO_2 ratio of < 200 indicates a shunt fraction of > 20%.
- A paO_2 / FiO_2 ratio of < 200 is indicative of severe lung disease and is one of the defining features of ARDS.
- Hypoxemia of this degree may be refractory to supplemental oxygen and if it perisists, may be reversed only with the application of positive pressure.

Table 6.4 Various mechanisms of hypoxia and their causes

Factor	Mechanism	Treatment	Cause
Low ambient oxygen	Decreased paO_2	Supplemental oxygen	High altitude
Alveolar hypoventilation	Decreased alveolar oxygen content due to higher alveolar $paCO_2$ displacing the alveolar O_2 and thus lowering the arterial oxygen content	Restore normal ventilation. Supplemental oxygen as needed (patients with chronic disease may be dependent on a hypoxic drive). Monitor serial $paCO_2$	Depressant drugs, intracranial infections, space occupying lesions, traumatic brain injury
Ventilation and perfusion mismatch (V/Q mismatch)	Parenchymal disease where alveolar pathology impairs adequate oxygenation.	Supplemental oxygen, PEEP to improve FRC and recruit alveoli, ensure adequate cardiac output	Pneumonia, ARDS, pulmonary edema, asthma or bronchiolitis with areas of atelectasis
Shunt (Intrapulmonary or intracardiac right-to-left shunt)	Deoxygenated blood returning to the left side of the heart, bypassing the oxygenation apparatus	Specific management depending on cause, positive pressure ventilation. Correction of intracardiac shunt	Cyanotic congenital heart disease. Pneumonia, ARDS, asthma or bronchiolitis with areas of atelectasis
Diffusion defect	Impaired movement of O_2 across the alveolar capillary membrane resulting initially in decreased paO_2, $paCO_2$ elevated late	Specific treatment where available. Supplemental oxygen +/- PEEP to increase the mean airway pressures, ensure adequate cardiac output	Interstitial pneumonias

more air will be entrained, decreasing the FiO_2 delivered.

- These masks increase the anatomical dead space and flow rates must be sufficient to prevent CO_2 accumulation.
- Exhaled gases are expelled through the air entrainment ports.

Masks with reservoir bags (partial and non-rebreathing oxygen systems)

- These devices are useful if FiO_2 of greater than 60% required.
- A reservoir bag with a system of valves is attached to the oxygen mask.
- The flow rate should be adjusted to keep the reservoir bag continuously inflated.

Partial rebreathing bags

- These have one-way valves in the exhalation port which permit expulsion of exhaled gases but prevent air entrainment during inspiration.
- There are no valves between the mask and the reservoir bag.
- The initial $^1/_3{}^{rd}$ of the exhaled gases (comprising anatomical dead space which has not participated in gas exchange) flows into the reservoir bag along with fresh gases. The rest of the exhaled gases is forced out through the exhalation ports.
- FiO_2 ranging from 0.6 to 0.8 may be achieved depending on inspiratory flow rate, tidal volume and air leaks.

Non-rebreathing masks

- This device has two systems of one-way valves: between the bag and the mask and also over the exhalation ports.
- During inspiration, the patient has a dual supply of oxygen both from the fresh gas source and from the reservoir bag. Thus the entire inspiratory demand is met by oxygen, thereby permitting up to 100% oxygen to be supplied to the patient.
- This device qualifies as a high flow system as the flow satisfies the patient's inspiratory flow demands.
- Exhalation can occur only via the one way valves between the mask and the atmosphere.
- Gas inlet safety valve allows room air to enter if the oxygen source is accidentally disconnected.
- This device is designed to deliver high FiO_2 at low flow rates of oxygen, but the flow should be sufficient to prevent collapse of the bag during inhalation.

Oxygen hoods / head boxes

- These are clear plexi-glass boxes of various sizes placed over the infant's head and neck to ensure adequate and stable FiO_2.
- Flow rates should be adequate to prevent CO_2 accumulation (> 6 LPM).
- May achieve oxygen concentrations up to 90 – 95%.
- Desirable to monitor delivered oxygen.
- Disadvantage: Patient must be taken out for access and feeds.

HIGH FLOW SYSTEMS

Venturi masks

- Designed to deliver specific O_2 concentration.
- Especially useful in chronic lung disease where control of FiO_2 is crucial, as co-existing problems with hypercapnia may be present.
- Oxygen delivery is based on Bernoulli principle. Oxygen flows through the jet orifice at a set flow rate and room air enters through the entrainment ports.
- FiO_2 depends on size of jet, O_2 flow rate and size of entrainment ports.
- Allows for a predictable O_2 concentration between 24 and 60% if manufacturer's instructions are followed.

Table 7.1 Oxygen delivery techniques

O_2 delivery technique	Flow rate (L/minute)	Concentration delivered (%)	Other
Nasal cannula	1-6	24-44	Inspired O_2 concentration depends on flow rate and patient's tidal volume
Simple face mask	6-10	35-60	May promote CO_2 retention at lower flow rates
Venturi mask	2-12	24-60	Accurately controls proportion of inspired O_2 Use in patients with chronic hypercarbia (i.e., COPD)
Face mask with O_2 reservoir	12-15	60-90	Provides high inspired O_2 concentration
Bag-valve-mask	15	100	Provides the highest inspired O_2 concentration
Blow-by	6-10	Varies	For infant or young child who will not tolerate face mask or cannula

COPD: chronic obstructive pulmonary disease; O_2: oxygen

HAZARDS OF OXYGEN THERAPY

The administration of oxygen is associated with various effects:

- Retinal damage in premature infants.
- Damage to alveolar capillary membrane resulting in increased permeability alveolar edema secondary to free radical damage. Oxygen in concentrations of < 50% may be tolerated for prolonged periods.
- Decreased mucociliary activity and risk of bacterial tracheitis.
- Absorption atelectasis secondary to 'nitrogen washout'.

REFERENCES

1. Wetzel RC. Respiratory failure. In: Textbook of Pediatric Intensive Care. Ed MC Rogers.3rd ed. Baltimore, Williams and Wilkins 1996: 265-368.

8

Endotracheal Intubation

(See also Rapid Sequence Intubation)

- Endotracheal intubation in ICU patients is a high risk but vital procedure.
- Familiarization with the intubation trolleys, equipment and drugs is essential.

> Intubation should ideally ***not*** be done as a sole operator procedure. Skilled assistance should always be sought. If you are alone (i.e., after hours) →***call for help!***

WHAT ARE THE RISKS INVOLVED?

- Usually an emergency procedure, with limited time.
- Optimum positioning is difficult in the ICU bed.
- Patients who have respiratory failure are hypoxic with limited oxygen reserves. Worsening of hypoxia and arrest can occur when sedative/relaxant drugs given.
- Patients may have actual or potential cardiovascular instability that may also be worsened by sedative drugs. Decompensated shock and arrest can occur in peri-intubation period.
- Risk of vomiting and aspiration.
- Visualization of cords may be difficult in small children, especially if the operator is not an expert.
- Visualization of cords may be impossible if oropharyngeal or tracheal hemorrhage present.
- In children, a difficult airway may be unrecognized until laryngoscopy performed. There is a potential for *"Cannot ventilate-Cannot intubate"* situation when muscle relaxants are used without verifying ability to mask ventilate.
- Some trauma patients may need cervical spine precautions, including a collar that may make the procedure difficult.

INDICATIONS FOR INTUBATION

a) *To provide an airway*
  - Airway obstruction: Real (e.g., severe croup, trauma), potential obstruction (e.g., early burns), functional (obstructive sleep apnea)

b) *To protect the airway*
  - Patients at risk of aspiration
  - Altered mental states with loss of patency.
  - Loss of protective glottic reflexes, bulbar dysfunction (GBS)

c) *Tracheal toileting*

d) *Provision of mechanical ventilation*

TECHNIQUES OF INTUBATION

a) *Orotracheal* intubation is the standard method of intubation.

b) *Nasotracheal* intubation may be indicated in:
  - Upper airway obstruction. Once the airway is provided, the patient's symptoms rapidly resolve and they may be more comfortable with nasal tubes, hence require less sedation.
  - Neuromuscular weakness such as GBS.
  - Advantages of nasal tubes are better fixation. Also, as opposed to oral tubes where saliva may loosen tapings, nasal tubes remain secure as the tapes are likely to remain dry. Fewer requirements for sedation, better oral toileting.

- Disadvatanges of nasal tubes in situ for greater than 3-4 days are risk of sinusitis and infectious complications including VAP.
- Nasotracheal intubation is contraindicated in:
  - Head trauma patients who may have base of skull fractures.
  - In patients with retropharyngeal abscess due to risk of perforation and aspiration of pus.

ENDOTRACHEAL TUBES

a) *Cuffed versus uncuffed tubes*

- Tradional teaching emphasized the need to use uncuffed tubes in children < 8 years in view of narrow sub-glottic area (physiologic cuff).
- However, as per the current PALS Guidelines, in the in-hospital setting, a cuffed endotracheal tube is as safe as an uncuffed tube for infants and children.
- In certain circumstances (e.g., poor lung compliance, high airway resistance, or a large glottic air leak), *a cuffed tube may be preferable* provided that attention is paid to endotracheal tube size, position, and cuff inflation pressure.
  - Immediately after intubation, check for a peritubal leak and maintain cuff inflation pressure < 20 cmH_2O.
  - Verify presence of leak and check cuff inflation pressures thrice daily.

b) *Size of endotracheal tubes*

- Uncuffed endotracheal tube size (mm ID) = (age in years/4) + 4.
- Cuffed endotracheal tube size (mm ID) = (age in years/4) + 3.
- Ensure that endotracheal tubes with internal diameters 0.5 mm smaller and 0.5 mm larger are also available.

Protocol for endotracheal intubation in ICU

a) *Personnel*: Intubation is a 3 person procedure (2 doctors and 1 nurse); skilled assistance is mandatory

- "Top end" intubator places the tube and coordinates the procedure.
- Second person administers drugs and monitors the patient.
- Third person to apply *cricoid pressure* once induction commences: Correctly performed cricoid pressure is an important part of emergency intubations as it decreases risk of aspiration and improves visualization of the larynx.
  - The intubator should direct the person who is applying cricoid pressure so that pressure is correctly applied and removed if distortion of the larynx or difficulty in intubation occurs as a result.
- In presence of head or polytrauma where the cervical spine has not been cleared, a 4th person may be required to provide in-line cervical spine immobilization.

b) *Equipment:* Ensure that following equipment is available and functional:

- Adequate light
- Working suction with a rigid (Yankauer) sucker
- Self-inflating (AMBU) device, pediatric anaesthesia (Jackson Rees) circuit with PEEP valve.
- 100% oxygen, i.e., working flowmeter at 15 L/min
- Two working laryngoscopes
- Magill forceps
- FLOVA introducer or gum elastic bougie (preferred to stylet).
- Rapid access to *"difficult intubation"* equipment.

c) *Monitoring*
- ECG
- Pulse oximetry
- Capnography
- Arterial blood pressure: 5-minutely NIBP or continuous invasive arterial monitoring.

d) *Drugs*
- Induction agent: Choose scenario specific agent, see RSI chapter (thiopentone, fentanyl, ketamine or midazolam)
- Muscle relaxant: Vecuronium (0.1-0.2 mg/kg), rocuronium (0.6-1.2 mg/kg) or suxamethonium (1-2 mg/kg) are commonly used.
- Suxamethonium contraindicated in:
  - Burns > 3 days since occurence
  - Chronic spinal injuries, spasticity
  - Chronic neuromuscular disease (e.g., Guillain Barre, myopathies)
  - Hyperkalaemic states. ($K^+ > 5.5$)
- Atropine (1 ml= 0.6 mg), usual dose 10 mcg/kg, minimum 100 mcg.
- Adrenaline. Add 1 ml (=1 mg) to 10 ml water to make up a 1:10,000 solution. Usual dose 0.1 ml/kg.

e) *Procedure*: Rapid sequence induction and orotracheal intubation.
- Pre-oxygenate with 100% oxygen for 3-4 minutes.
- Preload with 20 ml/kg saline or Ringer's lactate (In the presence of cardiogenic shock, give 10 ml/kg colloid slowly with inotrope/pressor)
- Administer induction agent and muscle relaxant.
- Cricoid pressure applied
- Direct visualization of vocal cords and tracheal intubation
- Inflation of cuff until minimal leak present. If no leak with cuff deflated, change ETT to the next size smaller tube.
- Confirmation of end-tidal CO_2 and chest auscultation with manual ventilation.
- Cricoid pressure released
- Secure tube at correct length
- Insertion of nasogastric tube. Insert orogastric tubes if suspected base of skull fracture, risk of bleeding.
- Connect patient to ventilator.
- Ensure administration of post-intubation long acting sedative plus analgesic until infusions ready (so that the patient doesn't awaken and struggle).
- Chest X-ray
- Obtain blood gas analysis and adjust ventilator settings.

f) *Continuous sedative infusion post intubation* (see chapter on sedatives in ICU)
- If hemodynamically unstable: morphine alone +/- oral tricholofos.
- Other patients: Morphine ± midazolam.
  - Fentanyl (ventilation anticipated < 12 hours).

REFERENCES

1. Royal Adelaide Hospital Intensive Care Unit Medical Manual, 2003. http://health.adelaide.edu.au/icu
2. PALS manual 2005. Downloaded from: http://circ.ahajournals.org/cgi/content/full/112/24_suppl/IV-167

(See also chapter on RSI)

9

Rapid Sequence Intubation (RSI)

(Also see chapter on Intubation)

Rapid sequence induction for intubation is a co-ordinated series of procedures that facilitates rapid intubation of a patient without interposed mask ventilation in order to:

- Decrease the risk of aspiration and
- Avoid undesirable physiological responses to intubation such as:
  - Cardiovascular responses to intubation
  - CNS responses to intubation
- RSI also avoids struggling and trauma during intubation, avoids hypoxemia and permits pain control and amnesia.

INDICATIONS FOR RSI

- Risk of pulmonary aspiration
  - Recent oral intake
  - Coma
  - Raised intra-abdominal pressure, distended abdomen.
- Head injury where history of oral intake unknown
- Most intubations performed in Emergency Room and ICU

Use of paralysis may be contraindicated if intubation is anticipated to be difficult due to anatomic abnormality. An anesthesiologist should be consulted.

STEPS IN RSI

Step 1: Preparation including brief history

- Prior to RSI, preparation is essential for successful intubation.

Table 9.1 The 8 P's of rapid sequence induction

Time	Action
Zero minus 10 minutes	Preparation
Zero minus 5 minutes	Pre-oxygenation
Zero minus 3 minutes	Premedication
—Time zero—	Paralysis with induction
Zero plus 20-30 seconds	Protection and positioning
Zero plus 45 seconds	Placement of tube
Zero plus 45 seconds	Proof
Zero plus 1 minute	Post intubation management

- History includes "**AMPLE**" history, i.e., history of **A**llergies, **M**edication history, **P**ast medical history, **L**ast meal history, and **E**vent history with specific reference to previous sedation/anesthesia history.

The steps in preparation may be recalled by the mnemonic SOAP ME (Table 9.2).

Step 2: Pre-oxygenation

Pre-oxygenate with 100% O_2 via a non-rebreathing mask for 2-3 minutes which allows 3-4 minutes

Table 9.2 The steps in preparation (SOAP ME)

Suction	Suction (large-bore Yankauer) should be tested and readily available at the bedside
Oxygen	A high-flow oxygen mask and bag-valve ventilation device should be tested and ready
Airway equipment	At least two functioning laryngoscope handles with appropriately sized and shaped laryngoscope blades should be obtained. An appropriate size endotracheal tube and one smaller size should be prepared as well. The ETT size may be estimated by the formula = 4 + (age in years/4). The ETT cuff should be inflated to test for an air leak. A stylet to facilitate insertion may also be required
Pharmacy	The patient should have at least one patent IV line. The specific RSI medications, proper dosing, and sequence of administration should be determined, and the agents should be drawn up and labeled
Monitoring **E**quipment	Manpower (skilled assistants). Continuous ECG, pulse oximetry

of apnea without hypoxemia. Effective pre-oxygenation leads to nitrogen washout.

Step 3: Premedication

Premedications are administered before laryngoscopy to mitigate the adverse effects such as bronchospasm in reactive airway disease, increased intracranial, intraocular pressure and intragastric pressure, increased sympathetic discharge, and bradycardia.

Premedications: May be recalled by the mnemonic LOAD (Table 9.3).

Step 4: Paralysis with induction

See Tables 9.4 and 9.5

Step 5: Positioning and protection

- Proper positioning of the head before laryngoscopy can help to align oral, pharyngeal, and laryngeal axes, improving visualization of the glottis and greatly increasing the likelihood of a successful intubation.
- Cricoid pressure (Fig. 9.1) should be just sufficient to compress the esophagus so as to minimize aspiration risk. Excessive pressure will impair visualization of the glottis.
- If the glottic aperture is not readily visible, an assistant may elect to perform the BURP maneuver. This involves placement of the right hand on the thyroid cartilage, followed by application of backward, upward, rightward pressure (BURP) to help bring glottis in view.

Step 6: Placement

Endotracheal tube is placed in trachea.

Step 7: Proof of position in trachea

- Clinical examination: Visualizing the ETT passing through the vocal cords during intubation, auscultation of clear and equal breath sounds over both lung fields, observation of symmetrical chest rise during ventilation, observation of "fogging" of the ETT during ventilation.

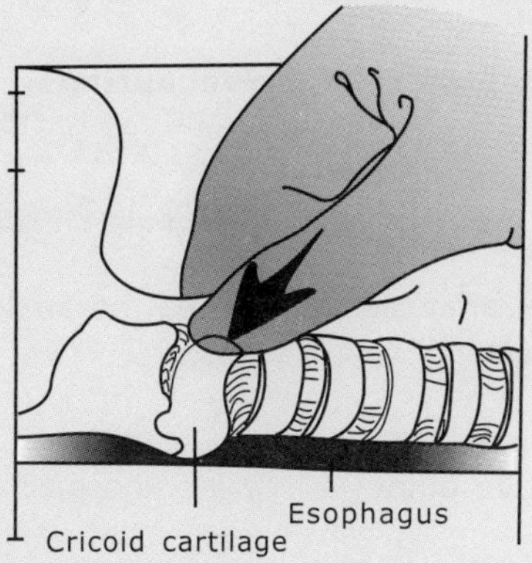

Fig. 9.1 Protection with cricoid pressure applied after inducing sedation and prior to paralysis to prevent aspiration

- These clinical findings are subject to failure and should not be the sole means for confirming ETT placement.
- CXR: ensure that the ETT is between the carina and laryngeal inlet. A CXR cannot differentiate between a tracheal vs oesophageal intubation.
- End-tidal carbon dioxide monitoring: Detection of exhaled CO_2 is the most reliable method for identifying proper placement of the ETT within the trachea provided the patient has a perfusing rhythm.

Step 8: Post-intubation care

- Ensure that the ETT is well secured.
- Pass a gastric tube to decompress the stomach.
- Administer a longer acting sedative agent as the patient may awaken before the muscle relaxant wears off.

Table 9.3 Premedication drugs (LOAD)

Drug	Indication	Mechanism	Dose (IV)
Lidocaine	↑ ICP, reactive airways disease (RAD)	↓ Intracranial response to intubation, mitigates bronchospasm in RAD	1.5 mg/kg
Opioid (fentanyl)	↑ ICP	Blunts sympathetic response to laryngoscopy	1-3 μg/kg
Atropine	Indications: ▪ Administer with 1st dose scoline in patients < 5 yr old ▪ Administer with 2nd dose of scoline at any age ▪ Bradycardia at the time of intubation	Mitigates bradycardic response to scoline and intubation	0.02 mg/kg (minimum dose 0.1 mg)
Defasciculation (pancuronium, vecuronium)	↑ ICP or globe injury	Defasciculates and mitigates ICP response to scoline	0.01 mg/kg

Table 9.4 Induction agents

Induction agents	Induction dose, mg/kg	Duration of action	Benefits	Precautions
Thiopental	1-3 mg/kg	5-10 min	↓ ICP	↓ BP & laryngospasm
Midazolam	0.1-0.2 mg/kg	15-30 min	Sedative, amnesic, anticonvulsant	Apnea, no analgesia
Ketamine	1-2 mg/kg	10-20 min	↑ BP*, bronchodilator. Dissociative amnesia	↑ Secretions, ? laryngospasm
Propofol	1.5-3 mg/kg	5-10 min	Deep hypnosis, airway reflexes abolished	Hypotension, bradycardia, apnea

* Ketamine usually causes tachycardia and hypertension due to centrally mediated catecholamine release. However, in chronically stimulated stress states such as CCF, catecholamine stores are depleted and the BP may fall due to the unopposed negative inotropic effects of ketamine.

Table 9.5 Paralytic agents

Neuromuscular blockers	Intubating dose	Onset	Duration
Depolarizing agents			
Succinylcholine*	2 mg/kg (child) 3 mg/kg (infant)	45-60 sec	6-12 min
Nondepolarizing agents			
Rocuronium	0.60-1.2 mg/kg	50-70 sec	30-60 min
Vecuronium	0.1-0.2 mg/kg	90-120 sec	60-75 min
Pancuronium	0.1 mg/kg	100-150 sec	120-150 min

**Succinylcholine*:

- Bradycardia can occur with 1st dose in infants, and with 2nd and subsequent doses in older children. Premedicate with atropine.
- Increases potassium in patients with muscle injury and burns.
- Can cause fasciculations in children > 5 years, hence if used in children > 5 years of age, a defasciculating dose of a nondepolarizing muscle relaxant (vecuronium 0.01 mg/kg) must precede the depolarizing agent to prevent muscle fasciculations and elevation of intragastric pressure, which may be associated with regurgitation.

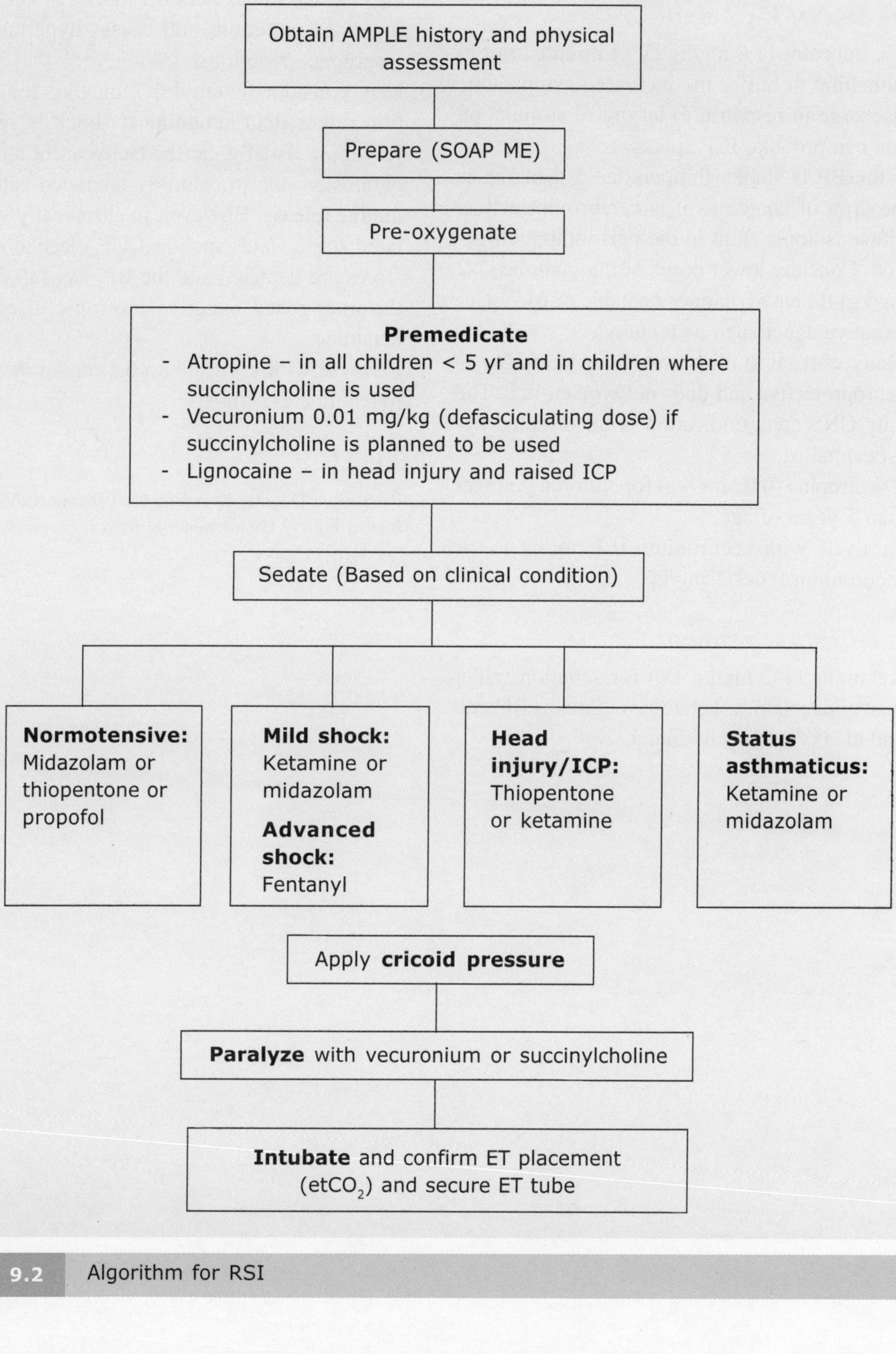

Fig. 9.2 Algorithm for RSI

RSI IN SPECIFIC CASE SCENARIOS

Head injury/ increased ICP

1. Use lidocaine (1.0 mg/kg IV) 1 minute prior to intubation to buffer the increased sympathetic discharge in response to laryngeal stimulation that can provoke ICP spikes.
2. If the BP is stable, thiopentone 3-5 mg/kg is the drug of choice as it is cerebro-protective. Infuse isotonic fluid in the peri-intubation period. Consider lower doses of thiopentone (1-2 mg/kg) if hemodynamics unstable or use an alternative agent such as fentanyl.
3. Many current studies state that ketamine is neuroprotective and does not worsen ICP. The only CNS contraindication is uncorrected hydrocephalus.
4. Use atropine (0.02 mg/kg) for children younger than 5 years of age.
5. Paralysis with vecuronium 0.1 mg/kg IV or rocuronium 0.6-1.2 mg/kg.

Sepsis/ shock/ asthma

1. Ketamine (1-2 mg/kg IV) for sedation rather than midazolam, as ketamine maintains BP well and also is a bronchodilator.
2. Premedicate with atropine 0.02 mg/kg (min 0.1 mg) IV and midazolam 0.1 mg/kg as ketamine increases secretions and causes hypertansion/ emergence reactions.
3. May consider fentanyl 1-2 mcg/kg for sedation rather than ketamine if shock is severe. Ketamine usually causes tachycardia and hypertension due to centrally mediated catecholamine release. However, in chronically stimulated stress states such as CCF, catecholamine stores are depleted and the BP may fall due to the unopposed negative inotropic effects of ketamine.
4. Paralyze with vecuronium 0.1 mg/kg or succinylcholine 1-2 mg/kg.

REFERENCE

1. Revising a Dogma: Ketamine for Patients with Neurological Injury? Himmelseher S, Marcel E. *Anesth Analg* 2005;101:524-34

10

Tracheostomy

- A tracheostomy is the formation of an opening into the trachea usually between the second and third rings of cartilage.
- While an adult with a tracheostomy is fairly commonplace, pediatric caregivers are not completely comfortable or familiar with the care of tracheostomized children.
- However, children with a tracheostomy constitute an important subgroup of patients who are at risk for potentially devastating airway compromise.
- The following outline attempts to acquaint the reader with a brief overview of this important airway device in children.

ADVANTAGES OF TRACHEOSTOMY

- A tracheostomy decreases the anatomic dead-space and resistance and thus the work of breathing.
- Decreases airway resistance and auto-PEEP.
- Improves ventilator synchrony and triggering when compared to endotracheal intubation, hence facilitates weaning.
- Toileting may be facilitated, hence the risk of pneumonia may reduce.
- Improved patient's sense of well being and tolerance of ICU by permitting intake of normal food via mouth (provided swallowing reflexes are intact), phonation (some devices have speaking valves) and improved appearance, including oropharyngeal hygiene.

INDICATIONS AND TIMING

The indications are a logical extension of the advantages above:

- To facilitate weaning from mechanical ventilation in difficult to wean patients on account of decreased muscle strength or incompletely resolved lung pathology.
- To facilitate pulmonary toileting in patients whose cough reflexes are inadequate.
- To bypass acute or chronic upper airway obstruction, either anatomic or functional.

Timing of tracheostomy

- Optimal timing depends on the patient condition and indication, usually considered after 2 weeks.
- Early tracheostomy at 7 days for expected prolonged ventilation improves weaning and quality of life for the patient in ICU.

TRACHEOSTOMY TUBE SELECTION

- The most common type is a surgically placed standard tracheostomy tube.
- Percutaneous dilational tracheostomy is an alternative to surgical tracheostomy with equal safety and low risk of complications. Complications depend on the dilator used. However, experience in smaller children is somewhat limited.
- A permanent tracheostomy is created where the trachea is brought out to the surface of the skin and sutured to the neck wall.

- The size of the tracheostomy in relation to the airway is determined by the underlying problem.
  - The diameter of the tracheostomy tube should be selected to avoid damage to the tracheal wall, minimize work of breathing, and, when possible, to promote translaryngeal airflow.
  - A tracheostomy tube that is relatively large in relation to the diameter of the airway may be required to prevent chronic aspiration.
  - A child who requires nocturnal ventilation, but who plugs the tracheostomy during the day or those with tracheostomy tube inserted for upper airway obstruction, might do well with a much smaller diameter tracheostomy. This will permit some airflow around the tube, and thus avoids damage to the tracheal wall and also permits speech.
- In most cases the selected tracheostomy tube should extend at least 2 cm beyond the stoma, and no closer than 1 to 2 cm to the carina.

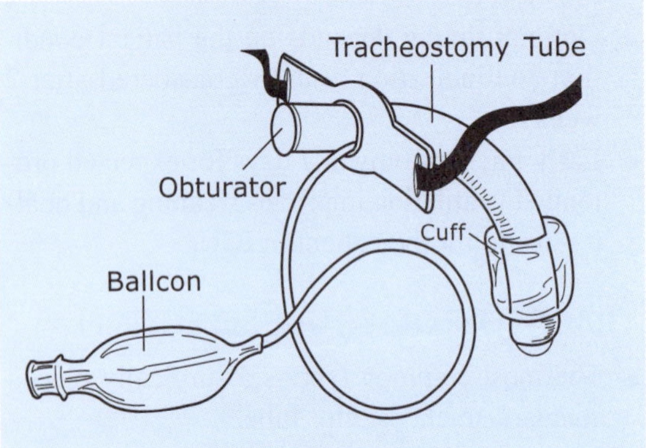

Fig. 10.1 Components of a cuffed tracheostomy tube

Types of tracheostomy tubes

- *Material*: Tracheostomy tubes can be made of metal, PVC or silicone. Silicone tubes are increasingly popular because they are lightweight and there is less crusting of secretions.
  - Polyvinylchloride (PVC): More rigid; tendency for cracks/splits after 3-4 months.
  - Silicone tubes: Do not stiffen, may crack or tear (rare).
  - Metal: Can develop cracks at the soldered joints.
- *Single cannula vs double cannula tracheostomy tube*
  - Single cannula tubes are frequently used in infants and younger children. These are usually uncuffed plastic tracheostomy tubes which do not have an inner tube.
  - A double cannula tracheostomy tube is used in older children and adults. The parts comprise the outer tube, the inner tube (or cannula) and the obturator. The obturator is used only to guide the outer tube during insertion and is removed immediately after the outer tube is in place. The outer tube has ties to secure it around the child's neck. The inner cannula can be withdrawn for brief periods to be cleaned.
- *Uncuffed tubes* vs *cuffed tubes:* Uncuffed tubes are preferred in children under most circumstances.
  - Cuffed tubes are used in children requiring ventilation with high pressures, requiring ventilation only at night, or with chronic translaryngeal aspiration.
  - If a cuffed tube is used, it is preferable to use one with a low pressure, high volume cuff. The lowest pressure that meets the medical needs of the patient should be used to avoid unnecessary injury to the tracheal mucosa. Cuff pressure should be monitored on a regular basis.
- *Fenestrated tubes (Fig. 10.2):*
  - Fenestrated tubes have an opening in the tube that permits breathing through the upper airway when the external opening is blocked, even if the tube is too big to allow airflow around the outer cannula.
  - Fenestrated tracheostomy tubes facilitate

speech by allowing better translaryngeal air flow.
- Fenestrated tubes are not recommended for small children, because they are more prone to granulation tissue that can obstruct the fenestration. The opening of the hole must be at a correct angle to prevent problems.
- These tubes are said to improve swallowing function as restoring normal airflow improves protective mechanism of swallowing.
- In an emergency, a solid non-fenestrated inner cannula must be inserted in order to ventilate the child through the tracheostomy.
- A non-fenestrated inner tube should be inserted for respiratory support or suctioning so that the catheter does not pass through the fenestration instead of into the airway.

- *Speaking valve / tracheostomy button*
  - A speaking valve is a one-way valve that closes during expiration to facilitate speech and swallowing.
  - A button cap may be used to plug the tracheostomy both during inspiration and expiration.

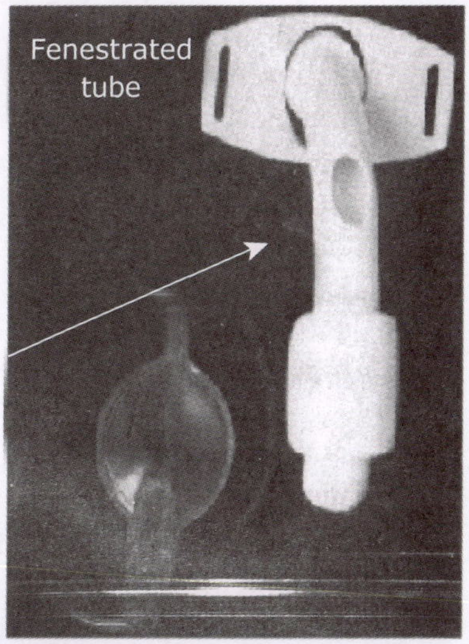

Fig. 10.2 Fenestrated tubes *(Image downloaded from: www.tracheostomy.com/faq/types.htm)*

This is useful to assess the patient's readiness to breathe and protect his own airways prior to planned decannulation.

CARE OF A PATIENT WITH A TRACHEOSTOMY

It is essential at all times to maintain a patent airway, prevent peri-stomal infection, maintain skin integrity and prevent tube displacement.

1. *Immediate post-operative care*

   The initial 4-5 days after a tracheostomy are potentially a hazardous period as the "track" has not matured. The surgical inflammation, bleeding and edema may make re-insertion of a displaced tracheostomy tube extremely difficult and the loss of a patent airway may quickly create a life threatening situation.
   - Great care must be taken to support the tracheostomy tube while the patient coughs or is being turned or suctioned.
   - If the tube gets dislodged, never blindly reinsert the tracheostomy tube. Re-establish airway with an endotracheal tube. If the ETT cannot be inserted via the surgical aperture, initiate BVM ventilation while an assistant occludes the neck orifice with a gauze strip, following which a rapid airway may be established by oral intubation. The tracheostomy may then be electively re-inserted when the patient's vitals are stable.
   - Initial dressing and tapes should remain intact for at least 24 hours.
   - If an inner tube is present, it should be cleaned thrice daily or more frequently if required.

2. *Care of stoma / inner cannula and ties*
   - The tracheostomy stoma should be inspected daily to look for signs of irritation and inflammation. The site should be kept clean and dry by replacing soiled ties and removing any secretions that collect around or under the tracheostomy tube plate. Mild soap and water applied with a cotton bud is usually sufficient to clean the stoma site. Clean secretions

with hydrogen peroxide (1/2 strength with sterile water).

- After the initial 48 hours, avoid dressings that trap moisture (i.e., gauze) or cause pressure necrosis. Avoid routine use of ointment and creams.
- Clean the inner cannula using sterile pipe cleaners and normal saline under sterile precautions.

3. *Suctioning*
   - The general principles of suctioning a tracheostomy tube and ETT are similar.
   - Frequency of suctioning depends on the clinical condition .
   - Ensure that suction catheter is less than half the inner diameter of inner tube.
   - Ensure that a non-fenestrated inner tube is present prior to suctioning to prevent tracheal damage.
   - Clean gloves are as good as sterile gloves. Do not apply suction while introducing the suction catheter.
   - Suctioning time should be less than 15 seconds.
4. *Humidification*
   - Humidification must be provided to keep secretions thin and to avoid mucous plugs. Children with tracheostomies do best in an environment of 50% humidity or higher.
   - Heated humidifiers are preferred in patients with thick tenacious secretions.
   - An HME (heat moisture exchanger) is a humidifying filter that fits onto the end of the tracheostomy tube and comes in several shapes and sizes (all styles fit over the standard trach tube opening). HMEs also help prevent small particles from entering the tracheostomy tube. Change HME daily and as needed if soiled or wet.

COMPLICATIONS OF TRACHEOSTOMY

A. Immediate complications

1. *Tube displacement* is common in the first 5-7 days as the track is not formed. Do not change tube in the first 72 hr.
2. *Tube obstruction*
   - Mucous plugs are the most common cause of respiratory distress in children with tracheostomies.
   - Symptoms of a mucous plug include resistance when trying to suction or bag and/or signs of respiratory distress.
   - Suction tracheostomy or if distress unresolved, consider tracheostomy change. Call for skilled assistance.
3. *Bleeding*
   - Very small amounts of bleeding often occur as a result of routine suctioning that is too frequent, deep or vigorous.
   - The commonest cause is suction pressure that is too high (Suction machine pressure for small children 50-100 mmHg, for older children 100-120 mmHg). Insufficient humidity, infection or granuloma formation are other causes of bleeding.
   - If bleeding persists, a bronchoscopic evaluation may be necessary.
4. *Infection*
   - Children with tracheostomies are at high risk for respiratory infections. The tracheostomy tube bypasses the natural defenses of the upper airway that filter out dust and bacteria.
   - Monitor for local infections at the stoma site. Hand hygiene before any tracheostomy care is one of the best defenses against infection.
   - Signs of infection include thick, large volume secretions that may be yellow/green/blood-tinged.
   - Peristomal infections are indicated by erythematous rash and/or inflammation at stoma site. The patient may be febrile with respiratory distress.
5. *Emphysema and pneumothorax*

B. Delayed complications

1. Stomal infection.
2. Tracheal damage and granuloma formation especially in fenestrated tubes and improper suctioning technique.
3. Tracheal stenosis may result from excessive tracheostomy cuff pressure
4. Catastrophic hemorrhage due to tracheo-innominate fistula.

DECANNULATION

1. *Prerequisites for decannulation*
   - No upper airway obstruction
   - Ability to clear secretions which are neither copious nor thick
   - Presence of effective cough
2. *Bronchoscopic evaluation* of chronic tracheostomies is useful to rule out airway abnormalities such as tracheal granuloma, tracheomalacia, obstruction/stenosis or vocal cord dysfunction.
3. *Techniques of decannulation*
   - Progressive downsizing of tracheal tubes.
   - Progressive capping/blocking of a fenestrated tracheostomy tube or the smaller tracheostomy tube until tolerated for 12, 24, or 48 hours. This can be removed easily if the child shows any signs of breathing difficulties. This stage of the process prepares the child for the next stage when the tracheostomy tube is completely removed, and he or she has to breathe normally. Use of a tracheostomy plug may be particularly useful in patients who have borderline clearance of secretions and require maintenance of the stoma during a prolonged observation period.
   - In some patients in whom the primary indication for tracheostomy has resolved, the airway device may be directly removed and the stoma coversed by gauze.

SECTION 4 : SPECIFIC RESPIRATORY PROBLEMS

11

Upper Airway Obstruction (UAO)

- Airway compromise is a leading cause of cardiac arrest in children.
- Children are at more risk of severe upper airway obstruction as compared to adults due to their unique anatomy (Table 11.1) and higher risk of foreign body aspiration.
- The resistance to airflow is determined by the radius and length of a tube as well as the viscosity of gas flowing through it: Of these, the *radius* of the airway is the most important determinant as resistance is inversely proportional to the fourth power of radius.
- *Stridor* is the hallmark of upper airways obstruction. This is an inspiratory, harsh, high pitched sound caused by partial obstruction of the airway, resulting in turbulent airflow.

CAUSES OF UAO

(Table 11.2)

- Obstruction of the upper airway passages can occur frequently in sick children from a variety of causes, including non-respiratory, e.g., snoring or gurgling can occur in a post ictal patient with falling back of the tongue along with secretions.

Table 11.1 Unique features of the pediatric airway

- A child's airway is already narrow: Further narrowing makes lifethreatening airway obstruction more likely.
- The tongue is relatively large in proportion to oral cavity.
- Infants < 2 months of age are obligate nose breathers.
- The most common cause of upper airway obstruction is loss of muscle tone with the tongue falling back against posterior pharynx.
- Nasal obstruction may result in severe respiratory distress.
- Trachea is smaller and shorter than that of adults, hence marked increase in resistance to air flow occurs when edema or foreign body present. Right main stem intubation and accidental extubation common.
- The cords may be difficult to visualize during laryngoscopy because the larynx is relatively anterior and high: C2 in neonate, C3-C4 in child, C5-C6 in adult.
- The smallest diameter of trachea is at the cricoid ring, below the cords, rather than at the vocal cords themselves, hence ETT size is dictated by caliber of subglottic trachea.
- The chest wall of infants is relatively weak and unstable.
- Immunologic immaturity leads to increased susceptibility to respiratory infections.
- Croup, epiglottitis and bronchiolitis are seen almost exclusively in young children.

Determining the cause/site of UAO

- Ascertain whether onset is acute (infectious, foreign body) or chronic with acute exacerbation (laryngomalacia).
- Determine infectious versus non-infectious cause (history of fever, toxicity, features of viral URI).
- Determine the site of obstruction:
  - *Supraglottic lesions* present with soft inspiratory stridor, prolonged inspiratory phase, muffled cry or voice

    Note the "4 Ds" of supraglottic pathology: ***D***rooling, ***D***yspnoea, ***D***ysphagia and ***D***ysphonia.
  - *Glottic lesions* lead to high-pitched inspiratory stridor and a weak or hoarse voice.
  - *Subglottic lesions* cause stridor with normal voice and brassy cough.

Note: Also look for co-existent lower airway pathology which may be suggested by the presence of prolonged and active expiration, wheeze, use of accessory muscles during expiration, lung signs etc.

GENERAL PRINCIPLES OF MANAGEMENT OF A CHILD WITH UAO

- Most patients will present with partial airway obstruction.

> ☞ **REMEMBER** In upper airway obstruction, the diagnosis and severity of obstruction are determined clinically, not by investigations. Repeated cardiopulmonary assessment is important to determine trends in patient condition (is the child improving or worsening?)

- *Goals of management are:*
  - Support of oxygenation and ventilation by alleviating obstruction wherever possible.

Table 11.2 Causes of UAO in relation to site and symptoms

Supraglottic obstruction

Muffled voice, drooling, soft/absent stridor, no cough

- Retropharyngeal (RPA) or peritonsillar abscess (neck stiffness usually present in RPA)
- Epiglottitis
- Macroglossia ± micrognathia
- Hypertrophic tonsils/adenoids

Glottic pathology

(Stridor, hoarse voice, cough)

- Laryngotracheobronchitis (viral croup): *Commonest acquired cause of stridor*
- Acute spasmodic croup
- Congenital lesions, e.g., laryngomalacia, webs
- Vocal cord paralysis
- Foreign body
- Angioneurotic edema
- Laryngospasm (hypocalcemic tetany)

Infraglottic pathology: Subglottic disease, tracheitis

(Normal voice, stridor, brassy cough +/-)

- Congenital or acquired subglottic stenosis
- Tracheomalacia
- Bacterial tracheitis
- External compression (vascular rings, mediastinal mass)

- Avoid measures that might precipitate complete obstruction

- ☞ **REMEMBER** In the rare event of total obstruction, a multidisciplinary approach is vital. Be prepared for expert intubation by early mobilization of airway specialists (anaesthesia, ENT) and equipment.

- *ABG, oximetry and oxygen requirement*
  - Gases may not help in management. Arterial or venepuncture may precipitate worse obstruction.
  - Oximetry is useful to detect desaturation and determine the need for O_2 (don't wait for cyanosis).
  - Children with UAO have normal lungs and oxygen desaturation is an indication of worsening obstruction.
  - Increasing oxygen requirement should alert the clinician to be prepared for critical obstruction and the need for intubation.

- ☞ **REMEMBER Danger signs of impending near-complete airways obstruction**
  - CNS: Agitation, lethargy, drowsiness (a drowsy child with UAO can go into arrest at any moment!!)
  - Respiratory: Stridor and cough may disappear despite severe retractions, air entry may be decreased/absent, cyanosis may be present.
  - Fatigue, tachycardia, impaired perfusion, pallor.

- *Management of partial airway obstruction:*
  - Specific measures where appropriate (nebulized adrenaline, steroids in croup)
  - Position of comfort (parent's lap)
  - Oxygen in a non-threatening manner (blow-by O_2)
  - Limit agitation as airway obstruction worsens with crying. Defer arterial blood gas sampling, radiography as much as possible.

- ☞ **REMEMBER** Throat examination and laryngoscopy may precipitate complete obstruction and must be performed, if required, by those with expertise in intubation with necessary equipment on standby.

- *Management of near complete airway obstruction*
  - Place child with airway in sniffing position, 100% O_2
  - Initiate bag-valve mask ventilation (may not be successful, two people required)
  - Most expert person to intubate: use a smaller tube than calculated for age and size
- *Intubation*
  - Must be performed by an experienced intubator, preferably anesthesiologist because of possible laryngospasm that may be precipitated by instrumentation of the inflamed larynx.
  - Usually done under deep inhalational anaesthesia which decreases airway reflexes.
  - IV propofol may be an alternative as it produces deep anesthesia, decreases laryngeal reflexes and has an ultra-short duration of action. The patient's spontaneous respiratory effort must be preserved.
  - If anesthetist not available immediately and the patient is deteriorating, the physician at the scene must intubate.

- ☞ **REMEMBER** Never use muscle relaxants in a patient with UAO or abnormal airway anatomy!!

- Endotracheal tube size must be one size smaller than recommended for age.
- Oral intubation best in an emergency. If time permits, nasotracheal intubation preferred, as biting on tube and excess salivation are prevented and the ETT can be better secured. Rarely, if intubation not possible, tracheostomy may be required.

- Once intubated, humidifying device must be attached and oxygen to be given according to oximetry.
- Insert nasogastric tube and apply arm splints while still anesthetized.
- Ventilation generally not difficult as lungs are usually normal. Some patients may not need ventilation at all after intubation.

■ *Post-obstructive pulmonary edema (POPE) / negative pressure pulmonary edema*
- This may be seen in some patients with severe obstruction, either before, or most often after, relief of critical obstruction.
- Management: Single dose frusemide, provision of PEEP till patient improves.

■ *When to extubate:*
- The presence of significant leak suggests edema has resolved and patient is ready to be extubated.
- Usually takes 36-48 hours

COMMON CONDITIONS CAUSING UAO IN CHILDREN

1. Viral croup (Laryngotracheobronchitis, LTB)

■ Viral croup is the commonest cause of upper airways obstruction in children.

■ History: Preceding 2-4 day viral prodrome of low grade fever, nasal discharge. Other family members may also have viral URTI.

■ With increasing airway inflammation, the typical harsh barking cough and stridor appears.

■ Swallowing is usually unaffected. Croup often worsens at night

■ Age: Infants and toddlers (rare after school age).

■ Signs:
- Triad of stridor, barking cough and retractions (sternal and suprasternal)
- Well, mildly febrile child, who is non-toxic, wants to feed.
- Absence of drooling.

■ ***Assessment of Severity:***
Clinical signs are the most useful guide. (Table 11.3)

☞ **REMEMBER** The diagnosis of viral croup cannot be made in the absence of the characteristic barking cough. If cough absent, consider other causes

Management of Croup (Fig. 11.2)

Mild croup

■ Regular observations: Intensity of stridor,

Table 11.3 Croup score

	0	1	2
Stridor	None	Inspiratory	Inspiratory & expiratory
Air entry	Normal	Decreased	Minimal to absent
Retractions	None to minimal	Suprasternal	Suprasternal, sternal, subcostal
Colour	Normal	Cyanosis in room air	Cyanosis in 40% O_2
Consciousness	Alert	Irritable. Consolable by parents	Drowsy

Croup score > 7 needs ICU admission, nebulized adrenaline and steroid.

retractions, alertness, ability to cry/speak/feed.

- Parental comfort to settle child.
- Minimal interference.
- Continue feeds.
- Steroids:
  - Steroids have been shown to reduce the duration and severity of croup.
  - No clear consensus regarding best agent or the number of doses.

The various steroid options are:

- Dexamethasone 0.6 mg/kg IV/oral stat followed by 0.2 mg/kg Q12H. A single dose of dexamethasone may also be effective
- Prednisolone 1-2 mg/kg/day x 24 hrs
- Nebulized budesonide: 2 mg (*not per kg*) in 4 ml NS, single dose.

Moderate obstruction & deteriorating

- Frequent observation and assessment.
- IV fluids, nil by mouth.
- O_2 if saturation < 94%.
- Inhalation of nebulised adrenaline 1:1,000, maximum 5 ml adrenaline, may be repeated as required
- Nebulized adrenaline:
  - The indication for adrenaline is clinical deterioration with severe stridor and retractions at rest.
  - If symptoms are severe, 3 doses of adrenaline given at 20 minutely intervals may provide dramatic relief
  - In moderate croup, nebulised adrenaline can be repeated Q1–2 hourly as clinically indicated; taper frequency as child improves.
  - Review immediately and then everyhour thereafter until stable.
  - Rebound worsening of obstruction may occur after initial improvement. This is because adrenaline gives only temporary relief and is given during a phase of worsening disease.
  - Mechanism of action: topical vasoconstriction (α effect), bronchodilatation (β effect).
- Steroids as above.
- No role for antibiotics in viral croup.

Severe Obstruction

- Avoid instrumentation of throat and excess handling: *Attempts at ABG, throat examination and other noxious stimuli can precipitate complete obstruction secondary to laryngospasm.*
- O_2 according to oximetry.
- Give nebulized adrenaline as above, but stop if there is any worsening of the obstruction.
- Call anesthesiologist immediately and inform admitting consultant.
- Never attempt intubation unless child in impending respiratory arrest.
- IV steroids: Dexamethasone 0.6 mg/kg stat, repeat 0.2 mg/kg/dose Q8H for 48 hr.

Indications for intubation in croup: *If in doubt, seek Consultant advice early*!!

- Severe obstruction with marked respiratory distress.
- Decreased intensity of stridor despite increasing work of breathing (WOB).
- Lethargy/drowsiness
- Need for oxygen/cyanosis despite supportive treatment

Consider other diagnosis if poor response to treatment

- Foreign body, congenital subglottic stenosis, bacterial tracheitis, retropharyngeal abscess, neurogenic stridor, epiglottitis
- Consider evaluation by bronchoscopy, ENT surgeon and anesthesiologist

2. Epiglottitis

- Epiglottitis causes airway obstruction and dysphagia secondary to inflammation of the *supraglottic* structures resulting most commonly from bacterial infections or a non-infectious process (inhalational or caustic burns).

- H. influenzae is best known cause, although relatively rare in India.
- *Age group:* Usually 3-7 yr. Rare in infancy.
- *Clinical features:* Children typically present with a sudden onset of high grade fever with toxicity, soft/muffled cough, dysphagia, drooling of saliva, anxiety, preference to sit in a "tripod" position (leaning forward with weight on outstretched arms). Neck tenderness may be present.
- Progression to complete airway obstruction may be *sudden and rapid.*
- Diagnosis is clinical (Table 11.4).
- Noxious stimuli including positioning for a lateral neck X-ray, IV insertion, throat examination etc., can precipitate complete obstruction, and must be performed if required with equipment and personnel for emergent intubation on standby.
- *Radiology*: X-ray lateral neck (if done) may show the engorged epiglottis: "the thumb sign." (Fig. 11.1 A & B).
- *Management (see general principles, above)*
  - Limit agitation, can be nursed in parent's lap with oxygen in a non-threatening manner (blow-by O_2).
  - Alert expert anesthesia, ENT assistance.
  - Consider intubation *early* with smaller size ET tube if patient not improving.
  - Intubation best accomplished by inhalational anesthesia (sevoflurane/halothane) with a mask held over patient's face while sitting in the parent's lap.
  - Nasotracheal intubation preferred. Tracheostomy rarely required.

3. Bacterial tracheitis

- *Pathology:* Bacterial infection of the trachea, resulting in the formation of copious thick muco-purulent exudates (pseudo-membranes) that may acutely obstruct the upper airway, resulting in a life threatening condition.
- *Organisms:* Staph aureus, H influenzae, Pneumococcus.
- *Clinical features:* High fever, barking cough, stridor, toxic appearance and poor response to epinephrine nebulizations.
- *Diagnosis:* Consider in any child with viral croup that is nonresponsive to conventional therapy. The only definitive way is by direct visualization of the trachea via bronchoscopy; however, this is usually unnecessary. Chest X-ray may show irregular tracheal mucosal wall.

Table 11.4 Comparison of croup vs epiglottitis

	Croup	Epiglottitis
Onset	Slow	Sudden
Duration/intensity	More in evening/night	Same throughout day
Drooling/dysphagia	None	Present
General appearance	Non-toxic	Toxic
Cough	Barking	Minimal, absent
Voice	Hoarse	Muffled
Neck swelling/tenderness	No	Present

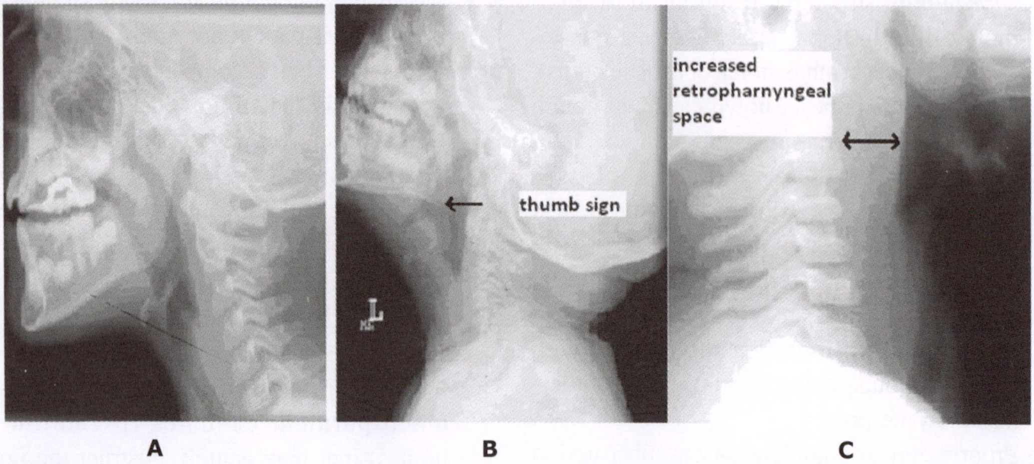

Fig. 11.1 (A): Lateral neck X-ray showing normal epiglottis. (B) Epiglottitis: Thick, rounded epiglottis ("thumb sign"); loss of the vallecular air space; and thickening of the aryepiglottic folds. (C) Retropharyngeal abscess

- *Management:* Close observation and monitoring, early initiation of broad spectrum antibiotics and pain management. The decision to intubate should be individualized based on the severity of symptoms, age of child and ability to clear secretions.
- *Complications:* Pneumonia or progression to ARDS, post obstructive pulmonary edema (POPE).

4. Spasmodic croup

- The term "spasmodic croup" describes a condition clinically similar to LTB.
- Patients with spasmodic croup typically have a barking cough and stridor, but lack fever and a viral prodrome. More common in atopic and asthmatic patients.
- Its onset tends to be abrupt, usually at night, and it often improves within hours either with cool humidified air or without intervention.
- The precise pathogenesis of spasmodic croup is unknown, although it is thought to be allergic or angioneurotic in origin.
- Treatment for severe forms of spasmodic croup is the same as for viral LTB (single-dose steroid, nebulized adrenaline may be needed).

5. Retropharyngeal abscess (RPA)/ retropharyngeal cellulitis

- *Commonest age*: 3-6 years
- Infections of dental or pharyngeal structures, middle ear or sinuses can cause suppuration of draining lymph nodes in the retropharyngeal space with progression to cellulitis or abscess formation.
- *Organisms:* Colonizers of oropharynx such as gram positive cocci and gram positive anaerobes. Staphylococcus aureus, alpha and beta-haemolytic streptococci, haemophilus species. Common anaerobes are bacteroides, peptostreptococci, and fusobacteria.
- *Clinical features:*
  - High fever, neck pain, sore throat are commonest symptoms.
  - Neck stiffness/rigidity and swelling.
  - Dysphagia, drooling, anorexia, hoarse or muffled voice.
  - Frank stridor and obstruction less common.

- Throat exam: Asymmetrical bulging/ fluctuance of the posterior pharyngeal wall.

- *Lateral neck radiograph*:
  - Ideally taken with neck extended (confirm that cervical spine lordosis is visible on the radiograph) and during inspiration.
  - In a patient with RPA, a widened soft tissue shadow anterior to the cervical vertebrae is seen with a normal epiglottis. The diameter of the prevertebral soft tissues will exceeds the width of the vertebral bodies. (FIg. 11.1C)
- *Chest X-ray:* necessary to rule out mediastinal or pulmonary involvement.
- *CT Neck*:
  - Useful to distinguish between abscess (requiring surgical drainage) and a cellulitis (which may be treated with antibiotics without drainage).
  - Provides more precise localization of site and extent of abscess involvement prior to surgical intervention.
- *Management:*
  - Endotracheal intubation may be necessary if significant airway obstruction/respiratory failure. Anticipate difficult intubation. *Oral tubes* preferred in order to avoid soft tissue injury. Use cuffed tube if surgical incision planned to prevent aspiration.
  - Early parenteral antibiotics in maximum doses: 15-50% have cellulitis and may be successfully treated with antibiotics alone. Initial empiric antimicrobial regimen must cover gram-positive aerobic and anaerobic organisms: Cloxacillin/ Clindamycin + Beta-lactamase resistant antibiotic.
  - Definitive treatment of an organized abscess: Surgical drainage/needle aspiration in OT. Obtain aspirate of the pus for gram stain and culture.
- *Complications:*
  - Suppurative mediastinitis and mediastinal abscess
  - Airway obstruction
  - Rupture of the abscess with potential aspiration of pus and pneumonia
  - Systemic sepsis

Foreign body airway obstruction

See Table 11.5

Table 11.5	Signs of FB airway obstruction
Mild	
■ Good air exchange ■ Responsive and can cough forcefully ■ May wheeze between cough	
Severe	
■ Poor or no air exchange ■ Weak, ineffective/absent cough ■ Unable to speak ■ High pitched noise while inhaling or absent air entry ■ Marked respiratory distress ■ Possible cyanosis ■ Universal choking sign (Clutching the neck with thumb and finger)	

Relieving choking in unresponsive infant (See PALS guidelines)

- Back blow, chest thrusts in infants and abdominal thrust in those older than a year.
- Open the airway. If FB visible, remove. Do not perform blind sweep. Give positive pressure breaths with bag-valve mask.
- If bag-valve mask ventilation fails, attempt intubation immediately. Some foreign bodies may be removed by a McGill's forceps.
- If removal not possible, try to push the FB into either right or left main stem bronchus and attempt ventilating one lung.
- Perform standard CPR if patient goes into arrest.

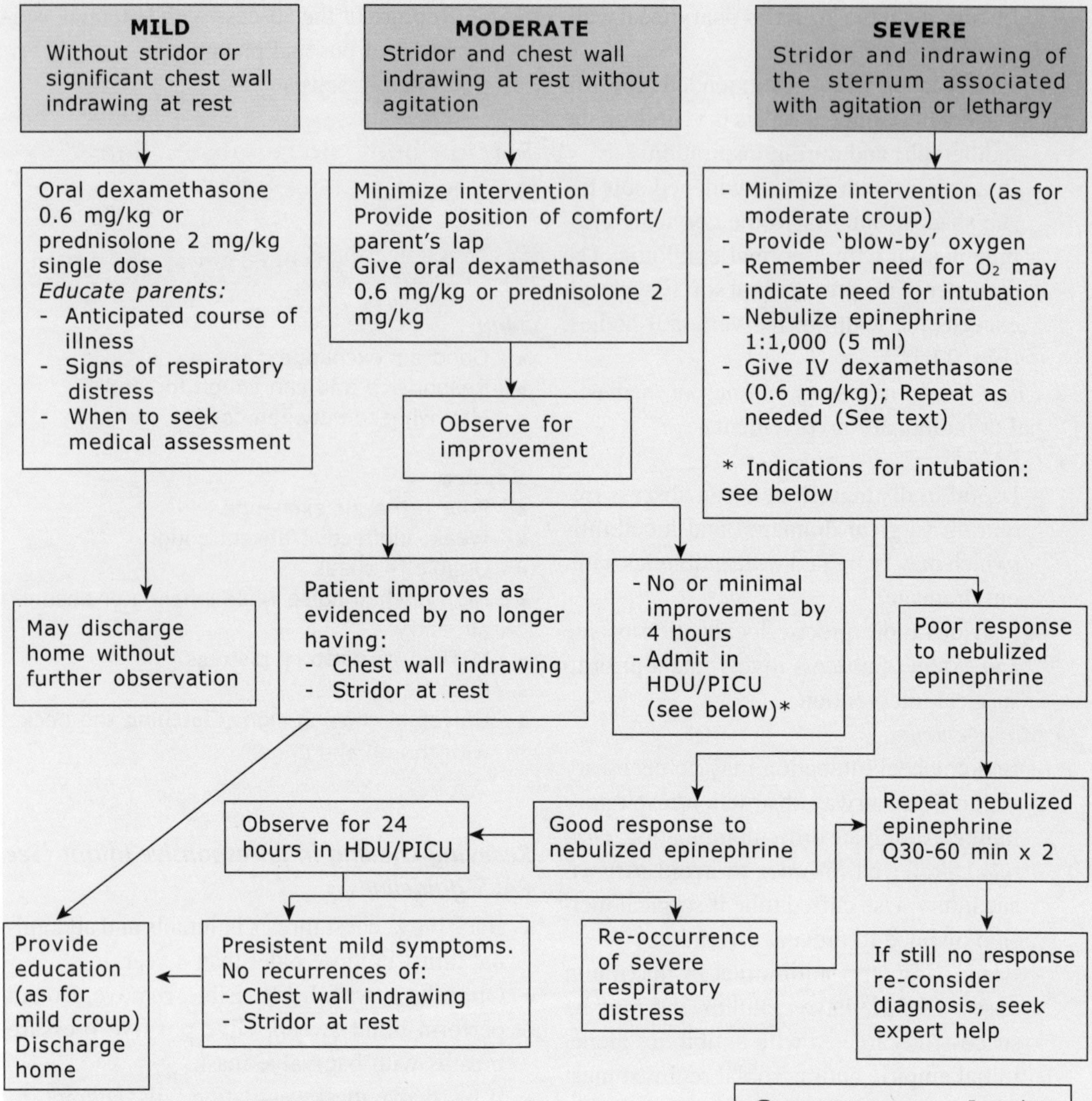

***Indications for intubation**

- Severe obstruction with marked respiratory distress.
- Decreased intensity of stridor despite increased WOB
- Lethargy/drowsiness
- Need for oxygen/cyanosis despite supportive Rx

***Severe croup* - Involve experienced senior consultants early: risk of anoxic brain damage / death if management inappropriat ate/late**

Fig. 11.2 Algorithm for the management of croup in the emergency room

REFERENCES

1. Tunkel DE, Zalzal GH. Stridor in infants and children: ambulatory evaluation and operative diagnosis. Clin Pediatr 1992;31:48-55.
2. Handler SD. Stridor. *In:* Fleisher GR, Ludwig S, eds. Textbook of pediatric emergency medicine. Baltimore: Williams & Wilkins, 1993:474-8.
3. Henning R. Respiratory failure. In: Care of the Critically Ill Infant. New York: Churchill Livingstone; 1999, 53-59
4. Alberta Clinical Practice Guidelines working group. Guidelines for croup. 2005.
5. Wensley D, M South. Respiratory System. In: Macnab AJ, Macrae DJ, and Eds.Care of critically ill Child London: Churchill Livingstone; 1999: 59-186.
6. BLS for Health Care Providers 2005-2006. Guidelines CPR ECC 2005. American Heart Association 2006.

12 Bronchiolitis

- Bronchiolitis is an acute inflammatory disease of the lower respiratory tract, resulting from obstruction of small airways.
- It is initiated by infection of the upper respiratory tract by any one of a number of seasonal viruses, the most common of which is respiratory syncytial virus (RSV).

- **Pathology of lower airways obstruction**
  - Inflammatory edema of bronchiolar mucosal lining with consequent narrowing
  - Excess mucus production
  - Older infants may have bronchospasm (infants <5-6 months have less bronchospasm as bronchial smooth muscle has not yet developed)
- Typical bronchiolitis in infants is a self-limited disease, usually due to an acute viral infection for which antibiotics or other therapies are generally ineffective. The duration of illness for children < 2 years with bronchiolitis is 5-12 days. After 21 days approximately 18% will remain ill, and after 28 days 9% will remain ill.
- There is a wide variation in the way patients with bronchiolitis are managed.
- **Risk for severe protracted disease and mortality**:
  - Infants less than three months of age
  - Premature infants (<35 weeks gestation)
  - Congenital heart disease
  - Immunodeficiency
  - Chronic lung disease/previous ventilation (e.g., BPD)
- **"Red flags" suggest alternative diagnosis** – consider the following
  - Toxic infant (sepsis, bacterial infection)
  - Feeding problems: consider reflux
  - Chronic respiratory symptoms ± failure to thrive →consider the following:
    - CCF: Inappropriate tachycardia, hepatomegaly, cardiomegaly
    - Foreign body: Persistent localized hyperinflation
    - Congenital lung anomaly
    - Cystic fibrosis
- Most infants who contract bronchiolitis recover without sequelae; however, up to 2/5th may have subsequent wheezing episodes up to 5 years of age and approximately 1/10th will continue to wheeze in later childhood.

DIAGNOSIS

- The diagnosis of bronchiolitis and its severity is based on the recognition of a combination of characteristic history, clinical findings and radiography: it is not dependent on any specific clinical finding or diagnostic test.
- Infants with acute bronchiolitis may present with a wide range of clinical symptoms and severity, from mild upper respiratory infections (URI) to impending respiratory failure.
- *Diagnostic criteria* for bronchiolitis include:
  - Preceding upper respiratory illness and/or rhinorrhea
  - Normal temperature to low/moderate grade fever

- Wheezing, tachypnea, subcostal retractions, increased work of breathing, low O_2 saturation, nasal flaring
- Dehydration, color change.

- **Radiologic Studies**
  - Hyperinflated lung spaces.

> **REMEMBER** Hyperinflation is essential for diagnosis: Consider other diagnosis if no hyperinflation on CXR.

  - Segmental/lobar atelectasis: the location of which may change rapidly. This is due to mucous plugs and does not indicate the need for antibiotics.
  - Peribronchial cuffing.
- **Indications for hospitalization**
  - Oxygen saturations < 92% (low room air saturation is an important determinant of severity)
  - Increasing respiratory rate and/or work of breathing as indicated by accessory muscle use, persistent RR > 80/min.
  - Feeding < 50% of usual intake
  - Decreased urine output
  - Lethargy/excessive agitation
  - Worsening general appearance.
- The main benefits of hospitalization of infants with acute bronchiolitis are:
  - Careful monitoring of clinical status
  - Maintenance of a patent airway (through positioning, suctioning, and mucus clearance)
  - Maintenance of adequate hydration

MANAGEMENT

- In children with moderate or severe disease, or those with risk factors for severe disease, admit in High Dependency or ICU for monitoring of continuous heart rate, respiratory rate and pulse oximetry.
- Children with bronchiolitis who present with low initial oxygen saturations have more severe progression of disease.
- Repeated, meticulous assessment is essential to detect deteriorating respiratory status. Monitor for signs of *impending* respiratory failure including increased WOB, inability to maintain satisfactory SpO_2 on inspired oxygen of more than 40% or a rising pCO_2. Very young infants are at risk of apnea and require greater vigilance
- *Oxygen therapy*
  - Supplemental oxygen is indicated when the saturation is consistently less than 91% and consider weaning oxygen when consistently higher than 94%
  - Humidified & warmed inhaled gases useful.
  - Avoid agitation: Blow-by oxygen useful
- *Nutrition and fluid therapy*
  - Infants admitted with viral bronchiolitis frequently have poor feeding and are at risk of aspiration.
  - Some may be dehydrated may require an initial fluid bolus to restore an adequate circulating volume.
  - Thereafter, hourly mainatenance rates may be guided by the serum sodium. Patients with bronchiolitis can have SIADH and resultant water retention with dilutional hyponatremia. This can worsen respiratory dynamics.
  - If admission serum sodium ≤ 137mEq/L, restrict fluids to 2/3rd maintenance rates. Use ½ GNS with maintenance potassium. Continue to monitor hydration and sodium levels.
  - Small frequent feeds as tolerated can be allowed in children with moderate respiratory distress. If direct oral feeds worsen distress, initiate nasogastric feeds (as bolus or infusion) with infant nursed at 45° in order to minimize aspiration. Empty stomach between feeds to prevent gastric distention.
- Nebulized 3% saline, 4 ml at 3-4th hourly intervals will decrease symptoms by decreasing airway edema.
- *Nebulized β agonists:* (Salbutamol or adrenaline)
  - In most cases, treatments effective for treat-

ing the bronchospasm of an asthmatic episode will not be efficacious for treating bronchiolitis, particularly as bronchial smooth muscle will not be developed in infants < 6 months of age.
  - Airways obstruction in bronchiolitis is mainly due to small airways obstruction from airway edema.
  - In infants > 6 months of age, a single administration using epinephrine or salbutamol inhalation may be tried, particularly when there is a family history for allergy, asthma, or atopy.
  - *Further doses of β agonists may be continued only* if definite objective signs of improvement are seen, such as decreased work of breathing, improved air entry and saturation after the nebulization.
- *Nebulized adrenaline* (0.5 ml/kg with saline, repeat 2-4th hourly)
  - This was extremely popular in the past, but used less frequently at present as a large prospective study failed to show decrease in hospital days.
  - Mechanism: Adrenaline mediated vasoconstriction shrinks edematous bronchial mucosa with consequent relief of airways obstruction.
  - As with salbutamol above, continue further doses only if clinical improvement seen.
- ***Do not continue further doses of salbutamol/ adrenaline nebulization if:***
  - Worsening desaturation, increased tachycardia and tachypnea with no improvement in WOB. CNS irritability occurs due to β agonist stimulation.
- Consider pulmonary edema with wheeze in the presence of hepatomegaly and cardiomegaly. Early ECHO is useful.
- *Nasal saline drops and gentle suctioning* with a bulb sucker or low pressure wall source suction may improve the infant's symptoms.
- Antibiotics usually not indicated for this viral condition. Consider for infants with:
  - Recurrent apnea and circulatory impairment
  - Clinical or laboratory features suggesting sepsis
  - Progressive infiltrative changes on chest radiograph
- *Indications for positive pressure (CPAP or IPPV): Decision is predominantly clinical*
  - Falling oxygen saturations
  - Marked increase in work of breathing with fatigue
  - Hypotonia, inconsolable cry, drowsiness, poor response to pain
  - Rising pCO_2 (note: ABG not a prerequisite to initiate positive pressure)
  - *Mask or nasopharyngeal CPAP* (ETT inserted nasally up to tragus of ear) may produce dramatic improvement in most patients. Usual requirements are CPAP levels of 5-8 cmH_2O with FiO_2 titrated to maintaining saturation > 92%.
- In drowsy children who are not maintaining airway or those that fail to improve with nasal CPAP, intubation and IPPV may be required.
- *Therapies that are not recommended*
  - Steroids (inhaled, IV or oral)
  - Anti-histaminics
  - Chest physiotherapy
  - Cool mist therapy
- **Discharge criteria**
  - Decreased tachypnea and work of breathing
  - O_2 saturations stable in room air
  - Ability to feed adequately.
  - Cough and CXR infiltrates may persist for 2-3 weeks

REFERENCES

1. AG Kaditis, E R Wald : Viral croup; current diagnosis and treatment. Pediatric Infectious Disease Journal 1998:7:827-34.
2. Chan PWK, Go h AYT, Lum LCS. Severe bronchiolitis in Malaysian children. J Trop Pediatr 2000;46:234-6

13

Acute Severe Asthma

DEFINITION

Acute severe asthma is a condition of progressively worsening bronchospasm and respiratory dysfunction which fails to respond to conventional therapy (inhaled beta agonists, oral or IV steroids, and O_2) and that which requires admission to the hospital for treatment.

PATHOPHYSIOLOGY

- Asthma is a chronic inflammatory disorder characterized by airflow obstruction due to airway hyper-responsiveness. Lower airways obstruction results from bronchospasm, mucosal edema and mucous plugging of the small airways.
- Decreased airway diameter increases airflow resistance.
- In a normal individual, negative pleural pressure during inspiration causes physiologic intrathoracic airway dilatation. During expiration, pleural pressures become zero, causing physiologic narrowing.
- In status asthmaticus, the above is exaggerated, and there is easier air entry during inspiration but airflow obstruction during expiration.
- Expiration, which is normally passive, becomes an active process resulting in high energy expenditure and increased work of breathing.
- Diaphragmatic flattening from hyperinflation causes additional mechanical disadvantage.

Gas exchange in asthma

- Hypoxemia occurs early and worsens as the disease progresses. Hypoxemia results from airflow obstruction as well as ventilation-perfusion (V/Q) mismatch.
- Hypoxemia causes reflex tachypnea resulting in initial hypocarbia. CO_2 levels rise as the airways obstruction worsens. Even normal pCO_2 levels indicate significant obstruction.
- Hypercarbia occurs due to increased dead-space effect of hyper-inflated alveoli and, as the disease progresses, respiratory muscle fatigue also contributes to high pCO_2.

Cardiopulmonary interactions

- Hemodynamics are compromised in severe airways obstruction because:
  - Fluctuations in pleural pressures decrease venous return.
  - Left ventricular afterload is dramatically increased by the large negative intathoracic pressure during inspiration resulting in decreased systolic blood pressure.
  - High lung volumes increase pulmonary vascular resistance (PVR) and right ventricular afterload.
- Exaggerated variation in SBP during inspiration is termed *pulsus paradoxus*.

DIFFERENTIAL DIAGNOSIS

☞ **REMEMBER** All that wheezes is not asthma; all asthmatics may not wheeze.

Wheeze/prolonged expiration can occur from many causes of lower airways obstruction apart from bronchospasm (see below).

- Differential diagnosis: Consider other causes of wheeze in children with no previous episodes, poor response to nebulized beta-agonists, no hyperinflation on CXR
  - Foreign body, vocal cord dysfunction.
  - Myocarditis/cardiomyopathy with pulmonary edema (H/O of previous episodes that partially improve with beta-agonists may be present).
  - Central hyperventilation (secondary to CNS disorders).
  - Aspiration syndromes.
- High dose nebulization may be toxic and result in marked tachycardia, worsening tachypnea, significant hypokalemia and agitation and should be avoided in wheezy patients who do not have asthma.

ASSESSMENT OF SEVERITY (TABLE 13.1)

- History should include number of previous exacerbations, medications, possible allergen exposure, upper respiratory infection symptoms (which are often triggers), and family history of atopy/asthma.
- Low grade fever and elevated WBC counts may be part of the inflammatory response in severe asthma.
- Fever > 101.5°F suggests lower respiratory infection; asthma and pneumonia can coexist.
- A rapid 30 second cardiopulmonary examination will determine general appearance, airway patency, respiratory effort and adequacy of circulation.

Risk factors for severe exacerbation

- *Current exacerbation:*
  - Rapid onset and progress of symptoms
  - Frequent ER visits in preceding few days
  - Over- reliance on inhaled medications, delay in institution of systemic steroids.
- *Previous exacerbations / Interval treatment*
  - Poorly controlled asthmatics, poor compliance with therapy.
  - Chronic steroid dependency.
  - Adolescents tend to underestimate severity of attack and are particularly at risk.
  - Prior history of ICU admissions, need for assisted ventilation.

LABORATORY EVALUATION

Tests usually obtained are CBC, CXR, electrolytes and arterial or venous blood gas.

- Leucocytosis may suggest respiratory infection, represent a stress response or steroid effect. (Interpret in conjunction with presence or absence of fever > 101.5°F and CXR findings for need of antibiotics.)
- Serum sodium level will help to assess degree of dehydration/presence of dilutional hyponatremia. Hypokalemia may result from intracellular shift of potassium due to beta agonists.
- Lactic acidosis results from dehydration and/or respiratory muscle fatigue. This is significant and indicates impending respiratory arrest. Elevated lactates may also occur due to low cardiac output associated with increased ventricular afterload.
- *Radiology:* CXR is indicated in children with first time wheeze, severe exacerbation or those requiring PICU admission (look for infectious infiltrates, cardiomegaly, pneumothorax, pulmonary edema or masses).

MANAGEMENT OF ACUTE ASTHMA IN THE EMERGENCY ROOM

Aims of management

- Treat to break the cycle of bronchoconstriction and impaired ventilation.
- Reduce inflammation in the airway with steroids.
- Offer supportive ventilation as necessary.
- Treat precipitating factors.

Table 13.1 Assessment of severity / danger signs

	Mild/moderate *(May need hospital admission)*	**Severe exacerbation *(ICU admission)***	**Danger signs *(May need intubation)***
Neurological status	Alert	Alert	Drowsy, responds only to pain, sweating, hypotonic
Physical exhaustion	No	No	Yes
Talks in	Sentences	Phrases (7-10 words)	1-2 words, ill sustained cry
Oxygenation /cyanosis	Room air sats > 91-93%	O_2 required to maintain saturations >92%	Cyanosis in oxygen
Accessory muscles use, WOB	Absent	Moderate	Marked
Air entry (AE)	Normal	AE present, may be reduced at bases	Silent chest signifying critically reduced tidal volumes
Extent of wheeze	Present	Extensive wheeze	Absent wheeze in face of severe retractions
ABG : pCO_2, metabolic acidosis	pCO_2 low/low normal.	pCO_2 normal or high	pCO_2 high, rate of rise <5 mmHg/hr, significant metabolic acidosis (BE $\geq$ –7-10)

The 3 cornerstones of severe asthma treatment in the Emergency Room are administration of oxygen, beta-agonists and steroids

- *Route of inhaled beta-agonists: Nebulizer vs MDI + Spacer*
  - If tidal volumes and air entry are preserved, the most optimum lower airways deposition of salbutamol with least systemic side effects is achieved with administration of beta-agonist via MDI device with spacer and mask.
  - Disadvantages of nebulizer include less lower airways deposition and more systemic complications (tachycardia, agitation).
- Administer steroids systemically (IV/IM or oral), never by inhalation.

Management of mild and moderate exacerbation of asthma

- *The British Thoracic Society recommends MDI device with spacer as the method of choice for mild and moderate attacks of asthma.*

- *Dose of MDI:* Salbutamol MDI vs nebulizer
  < 6 years old: 6 x 100 mcg puff (= 2.5 mg Salbutamol)
  > 6 years old: 6 x 200 mcg puff (= 5.0 mg Salbutamol)
- Steroids: Oral prednisolone 1 mg/kg Q12H PO/NG (max 60 mg).
- Oxygen as needed to maintain O_2 saturations > 92%.
- Reassess every 20 minutes to see if treatment effective.

Severe exacerbation / life threatening episodes of asthma

- Obtain intravenous access; commence cardio-respiratory and oxygen saturation monitoring.
- Oxygen: High flow oxygen at 10-15 L/min via non rebreathing mask.

Oxygen in asthma

- β-agonists may worsen hypoxia by attenuating the hypoxic pulmonary vasoconstriction, hence oxygen should always be administered along with nebulization.
- Maintain oxygen saturation > 92%.

IV fluids

- Resuscitation for a patient in shock: Give IV boluses of 0.9% saline 20 ml/kg.
- Maintenance fluids: Use 5% GNS with 40-60 mEq of K^+ per litre.
- Avoid overhydration as there is risk of SIADH, pulmonary edema.
- Restrict fluids to 2/3rd maintenance if serum $Na^+ \leq 138$ mEq/litre.
- Potassium infusions may be required if serum $K^+ \leq 3.0$ mEq/litre.

Steroids

- IV Hydrocortisone 2-4 mg/kg stat, 1-2 mg/kg Q6H, switch to oral steroids when better.
  OR methylprednisolone 1 mg/kg Q6H, then Q12 x 24 hr, then OD.
- Gastric acid suppression with H_2 blockers/PPI.

Steroids in asthma

- Steroids directly reduce inflammation in this predominantly inflammatory illness.
- Should be used early in all patients with acute severe asthma; underuse of steroids has been incriminated in fatal cases.
- Oral steroids as effective as IV if not vomiting. Inhaled steroids of no benefit in the acute episode.
- Total duration 7 days, can individualize based on severity of attack; mild-moderate exacerbation requires 3-5 days
- If on IV steroids, change to 1 mg/kg oral prednisolone after 48 hours.

High dose beta-agonists

When tidal volumes are severely reduced, MDI and spacers are ineffective and nebulized beta-agonists are indicated.

- Administer continuous nebulized salbutamol at 0.3 mg/kg/hr *OR*
- 3 doses of back-to-back salbutamol each nebulized over 15-20 minutes with oxygen and ECG monitoring. Add ipratropium to each of the 3 nebulizations (see below).
- 1 ml of 0.5% salbutamol = 5 mg.
- Dose of nebulized salbutamol in severe asthma:
  < 20 kg: 2.5 mg (0.5 ml)
  > 20 kg: 5 mg (1 ml)
- These doses may be toxic for patients with less severe disease: use lower doses (0.15 mg/kg) for mild to moderate exacerbations.
- Reassess clinical condition every 20 minutes.
- If no improvement, consider subcutaneous or intravenous route of beta-agonsit.

Subcutaneous beta-agonists

- Treatment options are subcutaneous terbutaline or adrenaline.
- Adrenaline has superior bronchodilatory properties but may cause more tachycardia.
- SC dose of terbutaline or adrenaline: 0.01 mg/kg/dose, max 0.3 mg, can be repeated every 15-20 min x 3 doses.

Intravenous beta-agonists

- IV β-agonist infusions may be effective for patients with severe air flow limitation that persists despite continuous nebulized salbutamol.
- It is essential to use infusion pumps in order to titrate doses accurately.
- Salbutamol load 5 mcg/kg/hr over 1 hour followed by a continuous infusion 1 mcg/kg/min OR
- Terbutaline infusion: Initial bolus of 5-10 μg/kg over 10 minutes followed by 2-10 μg/kg/hr.
- If severe obstruction persists and tachycardia not a concern, doses as high as 3-5 μg/kg/min over 1 hr followed by 0.4 mcg/kg/minute have been used. 1 ml terbutaline = 0.5 mg (500 mcg)
- All patients on IV ß agonists need ECG and K^+ monitoring; those receiving higher doses must have cardiac enzymes (Trop-T or CPK-MB) monitored.

ß-Agonists in asthma

- Inhaled β-agonists are drugs of choice in asthma and are a bridge to support ventilation and oxygenation till anti-inflammatory effects of steroids take effect.
- Patients with acute severe asthma require and tolerate higher doses.
- Tachycardia in severe asthma is related to respiratory distress due to airways obstruction: relief of obstruction with β-agonists often leads to dramatic resolution of tachycardia.
- An increase in the heart rate by >20 bpm should prompt a decrease in the dose and re-evaluation of diagnosis.
- Total β-agonists dose in an hour (Inhaled + SQ + IV) should not exceed 20 mg/hr.
- Side effects of β-agonists: Sinus tachycardia, palpitations, hypertension, diastolic hypotension, ventricular dysrhythmias, CNS stimulation, nausea, vomiting, hypokalemia and hyperglycemia.
- Patients respond variably to salbutamol and some patients do not respond at all: in these circumstances it is worth trying aminophylline.

Ipratropium nebulization

This is a quaternary atropine derivative, 250 mcg/ml.

- Add 250 mcg of ipratropium to salbutamol in same nebulizer every 20 minutes x 3 doses during initial treatment, then every 4 hours.
- Although ipratropium is long acting, it is synergistic with and enhances the performance and efficiency of salbutamol and hence must be given at a higher frequency during initial treatment of an acute exacerbation.

Magnesium sulphate

(50% solution, 1 ml = 500 mg)

- Mechanism: Smooth muscle relaxation by inhibition of calcium uptake, resulting in decreased acetylcholine and histamine release.
- Side effects: Tachycardia/bradycardia, hypotension, respiratory muscle weakness at higher serum levels (rare in children).
- Dose: 20-50 mg/kg over 20 minutes.
- No evidence for benefit from repeat doses; however, toxicity is a concern.

Aminophylline

- Useful for patients who do not respond well to beta-agonists.
- Dose: Loading dose 5-10 mg/kg/hr followed by 0.5-1.0 mg/kg/hr.
- Avoid loading dose if patient already receiving theophylline.
- Dose of IV terbutaline must be decreased by 50% when concurrently infused with aminophylline.

Aminophylline in asthma

- Possible role in improving diaphragmatic contractility. Inflammatory modulation may confer additional benefit.
- High incidence of side effects (approximately 30-40%): Arrhythmias, hypotension, confusion, disorientation, fits, GI symptoms.
- May break cycle of bronchospasm within 6-12 hours, after which it may be ceased.
- If used > 12 hr, monitor drug levels.

1. **Oxygen** to maintain saturation > 90-95%
2. **Nebulisation salbutamol** 3 doses at 20 min intervals
   Salbutamol respule: 1 respule (0.63 mg) *OR*
   Nebulisation solution: Wt < 20 kgs: 0.5 ml with 3 ml NS
   Wt > 20 kgs: 1 ml with 3 ml NS
3. **Nebulised Ipratropium**: (combine with salbutamol 20 minutely x 3 doses)
   < 1 yr: 0.5 ml, >1 yr: 1 ml
4. **Steroids**: Methylprednisolone 2 mg/kg stat IV followed by 1 mg/kg Q6H.
   Add H_2 blocker/PPI
5. **Treat shock** with 20 mL/kg saline boluses

→ Improved

→ Hourly nebulisation with salbutamol 3-4 doses

→ May increase neb interval to 2-4 hourly. Continue steroids

→ Not improved → ***Reassess Diagnosis!!***

→ Adrenaline 0.1 ml/kg (1:10,000) SC Q20 minutes ×3 times
OR
Terbutaline 0.005 to 0.01 ml/kg SC Q20 minutes ×3 times

→ Not improved

→ Inj Magnesium sulphate
50 mg/kg in 10 ml saline over 30 minutes

→ Not improved

→ **Terbutaline infusion** 0.05-0.1 µg/kg/min infusion,
reduce dose if HR ↑ >20/min over baseline or ST changes occur.
Continue nebulization

→ Not improved

→ **Aminophylline** infusion (reduce terbutaline infusion by 50%)

→ May need to consider mechanical ventilation

→ Anesthetic gases

Fig. 13.1 Acute severe asthma

Antibiotics

- Most acute exacerbations of asthma are triggered by viral infections and do not require antibiotics.
- Cover for community acquired pneumonia if temp >101.5°F / changes on CXR, amox-clav effective.

Life threatening asthma

- Treatment as above for severe asthma.
- Consider pneumothorax
- Obtain CXR if time permits
- Consider facial BiPAP, i.e., noninvasive ventilation if patient alert.
- Prepare for intubation – get experienced help.

Intubation and Ventilation in Asthma

- Absolute indications for intubation and ventilation are:
  - Cardiac or respiratory arrest
  - Severe hypoxia
  - Rapid deterioration in mental state
  - Patient with severe asthma working hard and tiring, with no improvement despite maximal therapy.
  - Elevated CO_2 levels alone in an alert child may not be an indication for intubation.
- Why hesitate to intubate and ventilate an asthmatic?
  - The endotracheal tube is a foreign body which will aggravate the bronchospasm.
  - Positive pressure ventilation increases risk of barotrauma and hypotension.

Intubation Technique: Modified Rapid Sequence Intubation (RSI)

- Preoxygenate with 100% oxygen, decompress stomach.
- Sedation: *Ketamine is drug of choice,* dose 1-2 mg/kg (sedative with bronchodilator action, use with anti-sialogogue such as glycopyrrolate), midazolam 0.1 mg/kg +/- fentanyl 1-2 mcg/kg.
- Neuromuscular blockade (may avoid large swings in airway/pleural pressure). Vecuronium 1 mg/kg, ensure that bag-valve-mask ventilation is possible prior to muscle relaxant use.
- Spray vocal cords with ½ cc 2% lignocaine prior to intubation.
- Rapid orotracheal intubation, apply cricoid pressure, consider a cuffed tube even in younger children.
- Anticipate hypotension; ensure that normal saline bolus on flow during intubation. If patient is hypotensive, consider single dose phenylephrine (5-10 mcg/kg) for immediate effect and follow up with noradrenaline infusion until hemodynamics stable.

Ventilation strategies in asthma

(see chapter on disease specific ventilation)

PREVENTION

- Every acute exacerbation of asthma represents a failure of prevention.
  - Education of the family is important.
  - On discharge, patients must be provided with an *Action Plan* to assist parents patients o prevent/terminate asthma attacks. The plan must include:
    a. How to recognize worsening asthma
    b. How to treat worsening asthma
    c. How and when to seek medical attention

PROGNOSIS

Asthma has an excellent outcome in ICU. Any deaths are now attributable to hypoxic injury, which typically occur pre-hospital.

14

Acute Respiratory Distress Syndrome

INTRODUCTION

- Acute lung injury (ALI)/Acute respiratory distress syndrome (ARDS) occurs in 1 to 4% of PICU admissions. As many as 10% of PICU patients who receive mechanical ventilation may meet diagnostic criteria for ARDS.
- Reported mortality varies between 20% and 75%.
- ALI/ARDS are disorders marked by a significant inflammatory response to an insult that may be local (pulmonary) or remote (systemic) resulting in injury to alveolar epithelial and endothelial barriers of the lung, acute inflammation and protein rich pulmonary edema.
- ARDS is a severe form of ALI that has worse oxygenation defects (Table 14.1), also termed as non-cardiogenic pulmonary edema.

Table 14.1	Definition of ARDS
▪ Onset : Lung disease that is acute and persistent	
▪ Oxygenation criteria: $paO_2/FiO_2 \leq 300$ for ALI; ≤ 200 for ARDS	
▪ Radiographic criteria: Bilateral infiltrates	
▪ Exclusion criteria: Pulmonary artery occlusion pressures $\geq$ 18 mmHg or clinical evidence of left atrial hypertension	

Definition of acute lung injury and acute respiratory distress syndrome:
The most commonly used definition for ALI/ARDS is from the 1994 North American European Consensus Conference (NAECC).

- ALI/ARDS represents the end result of an aggressive inflammatory process in the lungs.
- ARDS may occur due to lung disease such as pneumonia or aspiration (primary or pulmonary ARDS) or as a consequence of inflammatory mediators released by injury to other organs in the body, such as septic shock or pancreatitis (secondary or extra-pulmonary ARDS), Table 14.2.

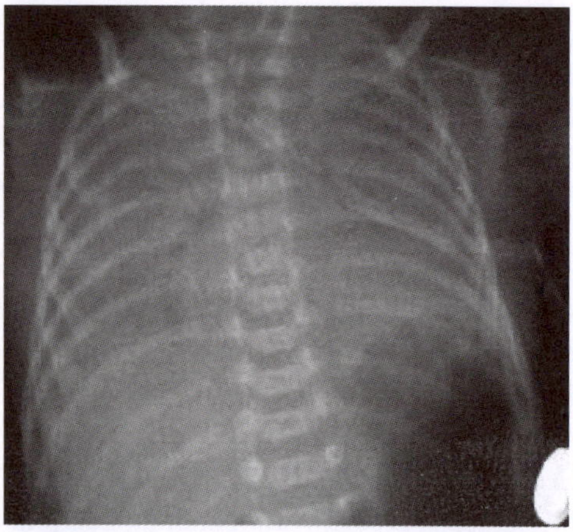

Fig. 14.1 CXR showing typical ARDS

Table 14.2 Causes of ARDS

Pulmonary/Local insult (Primary)	Systemic insult (Secondary)
Pneumonia	Burns
Aspiration event	Sepsis, Shock
Inhalational injury	Major trauma
Fat/Air/Amniotic embolism	Pancreatitis
Radiation injury	Poisoning
Pulmonary contusion	Cardiopulmonary bypass
Drowning	Transfusion-related lung injury (TRALI)

PATHOPHYSIOLOGY

The key pathological events that occur in ARDS/ ALI are dynamic and include:

a. Diffuse alveolar damage

b. Proteinaceous and hemorrhagic interstitial edema.
   The permeability edema in ARDS is not caused by cardiac failure but results from disrupted regulation of alveolar fluid balance.

c. Surfactant dysfunction
   Alveolar epithelial injury results in depleted surfactant and subsequent alveolar flooding.

d. Small airway collapse
   Interstitial edema and airway secretions cause distal airways obstruction.

Lung mechanics in ARDS

- The lung involvement in ARDS is not homogeneous. Posterior, dependent portions of the lungs are more severely affected than anterior, a distribution which is largely governed by gravity.
- Reduced compliance causes the expiratory end lung volume (EELV) to decrease below functional residual capacity (FRC) to a point that approaches closing capacity.
- This favors the development of regional atelectasis, intrapulmonary shunt, alveolar hypoxia and thereby failure of overall oxygenation mechanisms.

Phases of the disease

- Lung disease is a dynamic condition and the pathological features of ARDS are descrbed as passing through three overlapping phases:
  - An inflammatory or exudative phase (0–7 days).
  - A proliferative phase (7–21 days) followed by a fibrotic phase (from day 10), together called the fibro-proliferative phase.
  - Recovery phase after 21 days when lung functions return to normal.

Cardio-pulmonary interactions in ARDS

- The cardiac output is reduced by an acute increase in pulmonary vascular resistance (PVR) and right ventricular afterload that may be exaggerated at extremes of lung volumes. PVR is least when the lung volume is at the FRC, i.e., neither too low or too high.
- The cardiac output may also reduce when the dilated right sided chambers cause interventricular septum to shift towards the left, resulting in decreased left ventricular compliance and poor LV filling.
- Cardiovascular performance may be optimized by adequate preload and also by strategies that maintain an optimal alveolar volume (neither collapsed nor hyperinflated).

CLINICAL FEATURES

- The clinical picture will reflect those of the primary insult as well as respiratory symptoms from ARDS.
- Increased work of breathing, tachypnea and hypoxemia are universal.
- Hypocarbia is often present early in the disease process, when patient is tachypneic. Hypercarbia sets in as patient fatigues or as the physiological dead space increases.

- Auscultation may reveal a combination of rales, decreased air entry and wheeze.

IMAGING STUDIES

Chest radiography (Fig 14.1)

The chest X-ray will show the following changes:-

a) Small volume lungs with diffuse alveolar infiltrates

b) Air bronchograms ± pleural effusion.

c) Widespread atelectasis.

d) Areas of lung injury that are evolving into fibrosis may appear as prominent reticular opacities.

Computed tomography in ARDS (Fig 14.2)

- The CT scans of a patient will show a typically heterogenous distribution of the opacification.
- Increased lung densities are frequently seen in the dependent regions which is caused by consolidation and atelectasis.
- The non-dependent ventral regions are usually well aerated and may appear overdistended.

ARDS MANAGEMENT (TABLE 14.3)

ARDS does not have a specific pharmacological treatment. Supportive measures that aim at minimizing lung and other organ complications offer the best survival advantage.

Mechanical ventilatory strategies

- The goal of mechanical ventilation in ARDS is to maintain adequate gas exchange with minimal ventilator induced lung injury (VILI).
- Mechanisms involved in VILI are:
  - Oxygen toxicity from the use of $FiO_2 > 0.6$.
  - Over-distension of alveoli leading to volutrauma and barotrauma
  - Repetitive opening and closing of alveoli causing shear stress and triggering further release of inflammatory mediators (atelectrauma and biotrauma).

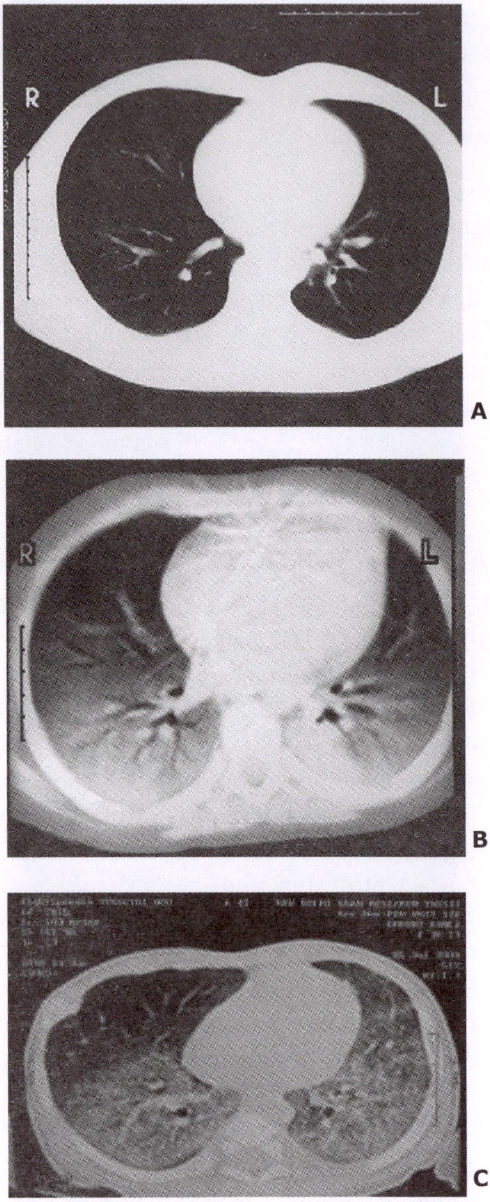

A: CT Chest of Normal patient: Note the fully aerated lung and the absence of any parenchymal densities

B & C: CT chest in ARDS: Note ground-glass opacification, air bronchograms and predominant dependent zone involvement.

Fig. 14.2 CT in ARDS *(Downloaded from www.medscape.com/content/2001/00/41/08/410885)*

Table 14.3 Therapeutic strategies in ARDS

- Control of causative factors (sepsis, shock, etc)
- Mechanical ventilation:
  - Lung protective strategies: Limit VT = 6 ml/kg, plateau pressures = 30 cm H_2O, $FiO_2 < 0.6$, aim for SaO_2 86-90%
  - Recruitment manoeuvres including "optimal PEEP."
- Careful fluid management:
  - Use judicious fluid and inotrope/ pressor to maintain normal cardiac output.
  - Early invasive monitoring lines (CVP, arterial line, Foley's).
  - Serial echocardiograms useful to evaluate left and right heart function, presence of pulmonary hypertension.
- Careful input-output charting
  - Aim to keep lungs "dry" without compromising organ perfusion.
  - Avoid overhydration.
- Consider early High Frequency Oscillatory Ventilation if entry criteria met.
- Positioning: Consider prone ventilation if no contraindications.
- Prevent nosocomial pneumonia (implement VAP bundles)
- Supportive therapy
  - Adequate analgesia and sedation.
  - Nutrition: Early enteral feeds preferred. Keep head end elevated to prevent aspiration.
  - Psychosocial support.
- Drug-based therapies: In selected cases, consider nitric oxide, surfactant, corticosteroids.
- Rescue therapies including extracorporeal membrane oxygenation (ECMO)

- The adoption of "lung protective" strategies is currently the standard of care in ARDS management.
- Lung protective ventilatory strategies include:
  a) Controlled oxygen exposure
  b) Low tidal volume ventilation
  c) Permissive hypercapnia
  d) Optimal PEEP.

a) *Controlled oxygen exposure*

- High FiO_2 should be avoided to minimize the risk of direct cellular injury and absorption atelectasis.
- It is prudent to reduce the FiO_2 to non-toxic levels < 0.6 as soon as possible. Accept oxygen saturations of 86-90% which are adequate to maintain tissue oxygen delivery.

b) *Low tidal volume (VT) ventilation*

- A low VT ventilation strategy is the most important strategy to confer survival benefit.
- Low VT ventilation will limit harmful airway pressures.
- Either pressure control ventilation (PCV) or volume control ventilation (VCV) may be used.
- When using PCV, the PIP should be set to achieve an expired VT of 6 ml/kg while not exceeding 30 cmH_2O.
- When using VCV, set an initial VT of 6 ml/kg and monitor the plateau pressures (Pplat). The Pplat should not exceed 30 cmH_2O. If the Pplat is > 30 cmH_2O, decrease VT further.

c) *Permissive hypercapnia*

- The implementation of a low VT ventilation strategy will cause hypercapnia as well as hypoxemia.
- There are no data to confirm what degree of acidosis is safe. It is probably safe to accept any level of pCO_2 as long as the pH is > 7.15-7.2.
- Practically, a pCO_2 up to 80 mmHg is usually well tolerated, unless pulmonary hypertension is significant.

d) *Optimal PEEP*

- The application of PEEP improves oxygenation by displacement of fluid from the alveolar space into the interstitial space and recruiting (opening up) collapsed alveoli and smaller airways. The end result is improved functional residual capacity (FRC).

- Optimal PEEP will result in the best oxygenation, least hemodynamic compromise and best compliance.

- Initial PEEP is usually set between 8 to 10 cmH_2O; further increments of 1-2 cmH_2O may be required in order to achieve saturations of 86-90% at $FiO_2 < 0.6$.
- With each increment, monitor cardiovascular status/perfusion, oxygenation and compliance.
- In PCV, assess compliance by measuring the generated VT for the delta pressure (ΔP). ΔP is the difference between the PIP and PEEP. While keeping PIP and the ΔP constant, PEEP is increased in increments of 1-2 cmH_2O. The PEEP at which the best expiratory tidal volume is generated with adequate oxygenation and good hemodynamics is considered the "optimal PEEP".
- In VCV, assess compliance by measuring the plateau pressure when PEEP is increased in increments of 1-2 cmH_2O while keeping the set VT constant. The PEEP which results in the lowest Pplat with saturations between 88-92% and stable hemodynamics is considered the "optimal PEEP".
- Limit PEEP to 10-12 cmH_2O in "pulmonary ARDS" as collapsed lungs co-exists with normal and hyperinflated units. Higher PEEPs can result in worse hyperinflation and higher risk of airleak.
- "Extra-pulmonary ARDS" may tolerate higher PEEP of upto even 20 cmH_2O as the lung is more uniformly affected.
- High PEEP requirements suggest bad lung disease. A patient whose PEEP requirement is > 12-15 cmH_2O should be considered for HFOV early rather than wait until further deterioration occurs.

Supportive measures

Fluid management in ARDS

- Many patients with ARDS also have conditions that require early aggressive resuscitation with large volumes of fluid, e.g., septic shock, burns or severe pancreatitis.
- It is important to restore an effective circulating volume in the acute phase. However, after the hemodynamics are stable, a careful "restrictive" fluid strategy is useful, as excess lung water may compromise oxygenation further.
- In our Unit, the policy is initial shock resuscitation (if present) with fluid boluses, then restrict overall fluid input and maintain a negative balance. This is achieved by using furesemide as a continuous infusion over 24 hours at doses of 0.1-0.5 mg/kg /hour while monitoring hemodynamic variables, acid base and serum K^+ levels. Spiranolactone is co-administered to limit K^+ losses.

Sedation & analgesia

- All patients with ARDS should have adequate analgesia and sedation. Muscles relaxation must be avoided as far as possible and only used for a brief period if correctable causes of agitation have been ruled out.
- Longer duration of ventilation means longer sedation and analgesia. Therefore it is essential to prevent withdrawal symptoms when the patient is recovering. This can be prevented by slow wean of the drugs (decrease by 10% each day), use of oral narcotics + benzodiazepines or replacement with drugs such as clonidine which do not cause withdrawal.

Nutrition

- Patients with ARDS should be started on enteral feeds as early as possible in order to maintain integrity of intestinal mucosa and prevent bacterial translocation and systemic infection.
- Early enteral nutrition will reduce also mortality and duration of hospital stay.

Non-invasive ventilation (NIV)

- NIV has no role in florid ARDS.
- NIV may be useful in the management of mild to moderate hypoxemic respiratory failure.
- It is a particularly attractive option in immune-compromised patients with moderate lung disease as tracheal intubation is avoided and VAP rates may be much reduced.

High frequency oscillatory ventilation (See also chapter on HFOV)

- HFOV may easily achieve the desired "lung protective" strategies needed in ARDS.
- Figure 14.3 is a brief outline HFO use in ARDS.

Prone positioning

- Prone positioning is an important therapeutic strategy in ARDS and, in some patients, may result in dramatic improvement in oxygenation and ventilatory requirements.
- Prone positioning improve V/Q mismatch and oxygenation by:
  - Recruitment of the dependent, dorsal regions of the lung that are most affected in ARDS.
  - In the prone position, the heart and mediastinum moves towards the sternum by gravity and relieves pressure on the posterior dependent segments of the lung.
  - It decreases chest wall compliance and therefore transmits airway pressure to alveoli more efficiently, thus allowing previously consolidated alveoli to open and remain open.
- The process of prone positioning is a cumbersome procedure requiring many ICU personnel and also has mechanical problems like tube displacement, bed sores etc. The ETT should be confirmed to be in the lower third of the trachea prior to turning.
- If no deterioration is seen, maintain the prone position for at least 18-20 hours.

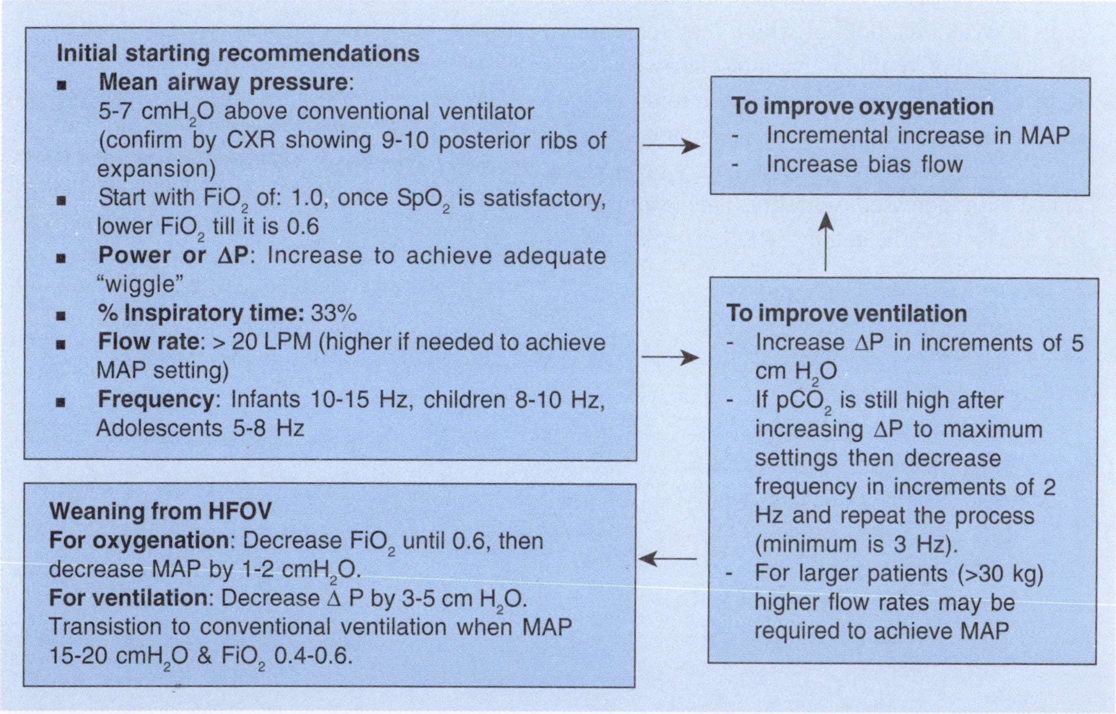

Fig. 14.3 An outline of HFO use in ARDS

- If deterioration occurs or no improvement seen, change back to supine position with care.
- Contradictions include unstable hemodynamics

Drug based therapies

Nitric oxide

- Pulmonary hypertension (PHT) is a common in patients with ARDS. Nitric oxide causes pulmonary vasodilatation. Maximal improvement in oxygenation is achieved at NO levels above 10 ppm (parts per million). If the pulmonary vasculature is very reactive, then the oxygenation improves rapidly, with minutes.

Corticosteroids

- The use of steroids in ARDS is controversial.
- Steroids do not prevent the development of ARDS, nor is it beneficial when employed during the initial phase of the clinical course. Moreover, its use has been associated with a higher incidence of nosocomial infections and muscle weakness, both of which may increase the duration of ventilation and mortality.
- Recent trials suggest that while steroids may result in improved oxygenation, respiratory compliance and blood pressure, they may be associated with increased mortality. Therefore routine use is not indicated in ARDS.

Surfactant

- A few studies have shown oxygenation benefit with surfactant use in patients with primary ARDS and direct lung insults. However, routine use is not recommended. Surfactant use may be considered when oxygenation cannot be achieved with conventional methods, including HFO.

ECMO

- Extracorporeal Membrane Oxygenation (ECMO) is used in some centres as a rescue therapy for refractory hypoxemia.
- An Oxygenation Index (OI) more than 40 is an indication for starting ECMO in children with hypoxemic respiratory failure including ARDS. OI is defined as: MAP x FiO_2/ PaO_2.

REFERENCES

1. Bernard GR, Artigas A, Brigham KL, et al. The American-European Consensus Conference on ARDS. Definitions, mechanisms, relevant outcomes and clinical trial coordination. Am J Respir Crit Care Med 1994; 149: 818-824.
2. Ventilation with lower tidal volumes as compared with traditional tidal volumes for acute lung injury and acute respiratory distress syndrome. The Acute Respiratory Distress Syndrome Network. N Eng J Med 342: 1301-08.
3. Steinberg KP, Hudson LD, Goodman RB, et al. Efficacy and safety of corticosteroids for persistent acute respiratory distress syndrome. N Engl J Med 2006; 354: 1671-84.

15

Empyema

Definitions

- *Empyema* is defined as presence of pus in the pleural cavity.
- *Para-pneumonic effusion* is a reactive pleural fluid collection in association with underlying pneumonia.
- A *complicated para-pneumonic effusion* is the presence of thick pleura with loculations or frank pus. This may be sterile or contaminated and may progress to empyema.
- Suspect para-pneumonic effusion or empyema in any child who has been febrile or remains unwell 48–72 hours after initiation of treatment of pneumonia.

ORGANISMS CAUSING EMPYEMA

- Common: Strep pneumoniae, Staph aureus, H. influenza
- Rare: E.coli, Klebsiella, Pseudomonas, anaerobes.
- Clinical clues to etiology
  - The presence of soft tissue/skin infections suggests staphylococcal infection
  - In chronic aspirators (e.g., cerebral palsy), gram negative rods and anaerobic infection can cause pneumonia.

DIAGNOSIS

- Clinical
- Chest X-ray
- Ultrasound of chest: Is useful for confirmation of pleural fluid or pus, and to guide thoracocentesis or drain placement. It estimates size and density of effusion, differentiates free from loculated pleural fluid, and demonstrates pleural thickening. It is convenient, safe and can be done at bedside.
- CT scan chest: Should not be performed routinely. Useful in non-resolving pneumonia, empyema and in immunocompromised individuals. It is often done prior to surgery to delineate the exact anatomy of the defect and to look for intrapulmonary abscess.

TREATMENT

The aim of empyema treatment is to restore normal lung function. This is achieved by controlling the infection with IV antibiotics, drainage of fluid and expansion of the lung.

A. **Supportive treatment**
- Oxygen as necessary to maintain $SpaO_2$ > 92%.
- Fluid therapy if child is dehydrated or in shock.
- Initiate intravenous antibiotics.
- Analgesia and antipyretics.

B. **Simple drainage for uncomplicated para-pneumonic effusion**
- Effusions which are enlarging and/or compromising respiratory function should not be managed by antibiotics alone.
- *No role for repeated thoracocentesis:* If pleural collections are significant, early tube thoracostomy is preferable to repeated taps.

C. **Antibiotics: Mainstay of treatment**

- All cases should be treated with intravenous antibiotics with coverage against Streptococcus pneumoniae and Staphylococcus.
- A wider spectrum coverage is required for hospital acquired infections, as well as those secondary to surgery, trauma, and aspiration as infection due to resistant and gram negative organisms are more common in such circumstances.
- Critically unwell patients with rapidly spreading necrotizing pneumonia and emphysema will need Staph. cover with drugs that also decrease toxin production such as linezolid or clindamycin (see Table 15.1).
- With appropriate antibiotics, fever should subside by 72 hours in a patient with uncomplicated para-pneumonic effusion. If fever persists > 72 hours, either modify the treatment based on culture reports or rule out empyema formation.
- However, as culture positivity is rare (33%) the initial empiric antibiotic regimen is often continued, especially if clinical improvement is seen. Intravenous antibiotics should be given until the child is afebrile or at least until the chest drain is removed. Change to oral antibiotic at the time of discharge.
- Total duration of antibiotic therapy is 3-6 weeks. In case of cavitatory anaerobic infections, antibiotics are required for 6-12 weeks.

Chest drains

- Thoracostomy tubes should be inserted by trained personnel to reduce the risk of complications.

Table 15.1 Guidelines for antimicrobial therapy of empyema

Infective agent	Drug & dosage	
Aerobic bacteria		
Staphylococcus	Cloxacillin	50 mg/kg/dose Q6H
	Vancomycin*	10 mg/kg/dose Q6H
	Linezolid**	10 mg/kg/dose Q8-12H
	Clindamycin**	10-20 mg/kg/dose Q8H
H. influenza	Cefotaxime	50 mg/kg/dose Q6H
	Ceftriaxone	100 mg/kg/day Q12-24H
Pneumococcus & Streptococcus	Penicillin G	1-4 lakh/kg/day Q6H
Pseudomonas	Ceftazidime	50 mg/kg/dose Q8H
	Ticarcillin	200-300 mg/kg/d Q4-6H
	Tobramycin	5-7 mg/kg/day (once daily)
Anaerobic bacteria Bacteroides fragilis and others	Clindamycin	10-20 mg/kg/dose Q8H IV
		5-7.5 mg/kg/dose Q6H oral
	Metronidazole	7.5 mg/kg/dose Q8H

* *Vancomycin less effective than cloxacillin against methicillin sensitive staphylococcus (MSSA)*

** *Linezolid & clindamycin decrease toxin production in necrotizing staph emphysema/pneumonia*

- Ultrasound should be used to guide thoracocentesis or drain placement.
- Procedural sedation should be administered by anesthesia or ICU personnel.
- Site: Small bore percutaneous drains guided by chest ultrasound, but preferentially placed in the mid-axillary line through the *"safe triangle."* (This is the triangle bordered by the anterior border of latissimus dorsi, the lateral border of the pectoralis major muscle, a line superior to the horizontal level of the nipple, and an apex below the axilla; see chapter on Thoracocentesis.)
- Since there is no evidence that large bore chest drains confer any advantage (see BTS guidelines, Thorax 2005), small drains (including pigtail catheters) should be used whenever possible to minimize patient discomfort. *Neither substantial force nor a trocar should ever be used to insert a drain.*
- A chest radiograph should be performed after insertion of a chest drain. Repeat chest radiograph is done after 12 hours to assess expansion of the lung.
- All chest tubes should be connected to a *unidirectional flow drainage system* (such as an underwater seal bottle) which must be *kept below the level of the patient's chest at all times* with the tube placed in water at a depth of 1-2 cm, has a side vent which allows either escape of air or is connected to a suction pump (at a negative pressure of 5-10 cm H_2O).
- Respiratory swings/oscillation of the fluid in the chest tube is helpful in assessing the tube patency and also for confirming the tube tip position in the pleural space.
- Appropriately trained nursing staff must supervise the use of chest drain suction. If clamped for any reason, unclamp immediately in the event of breathlessness or chest pain. *A bubbling chest drain should never be clamped.*
- The drain should be clamped for 1 hour after the initial 10 ml/kg fluid has been removed to prevent re-expansion pulmonary edema.
- When there is a sudden cessation of fluid draining, the drain must be checked for obstruction (blockage or kinking) by flushing.
- A drain that cannot be unblocked should be removed and replaced if significant pleural fluid remains.
- The drain should be removed once there is clinical resolution of constitutional symptoms with no evidence of air leak and drainage is less than 30 ml per day.

Intrapleural fibrinolytics

- Intrapleural fibrinolysis shortens hospital stay and is recommended for any complicated parapneumonic effusion (thick fluid with loculations) or empyema (overt pus).
- There is no evidence that any of the three fibrinolytics (streptokinase, urokinase, and alteplase) are more effective than the others, but only urokinase has been studied in a randomized controlled trial in children; hence this agent is recommended.
- *Urokinase* should be given twice daily for 3 days (6 doses in total) using 40,000 units in 40 ml 0.9% saline for children weighing 10 kg or above, and 10,000 units in 10 ml 0.9% saline for children weighing less than 10 kg.

Indications for surgery

- Failure of chest tube drainage, antibiotics and fibrinolysis.
- Persisting sepsis in association with a persistent pleural collection, despite chest tube drainage and antibiotics.
- Organized empyema in a symptomatic child.
- Co-existing lung abscess with empyema.

Surgical methods

- *VATS* (Video-assisted thoracoscopic surgery): Attractive minimally invasive technique for debridement of loculations and fibrinous pyogenic material, also facilitates optimal tube placement.

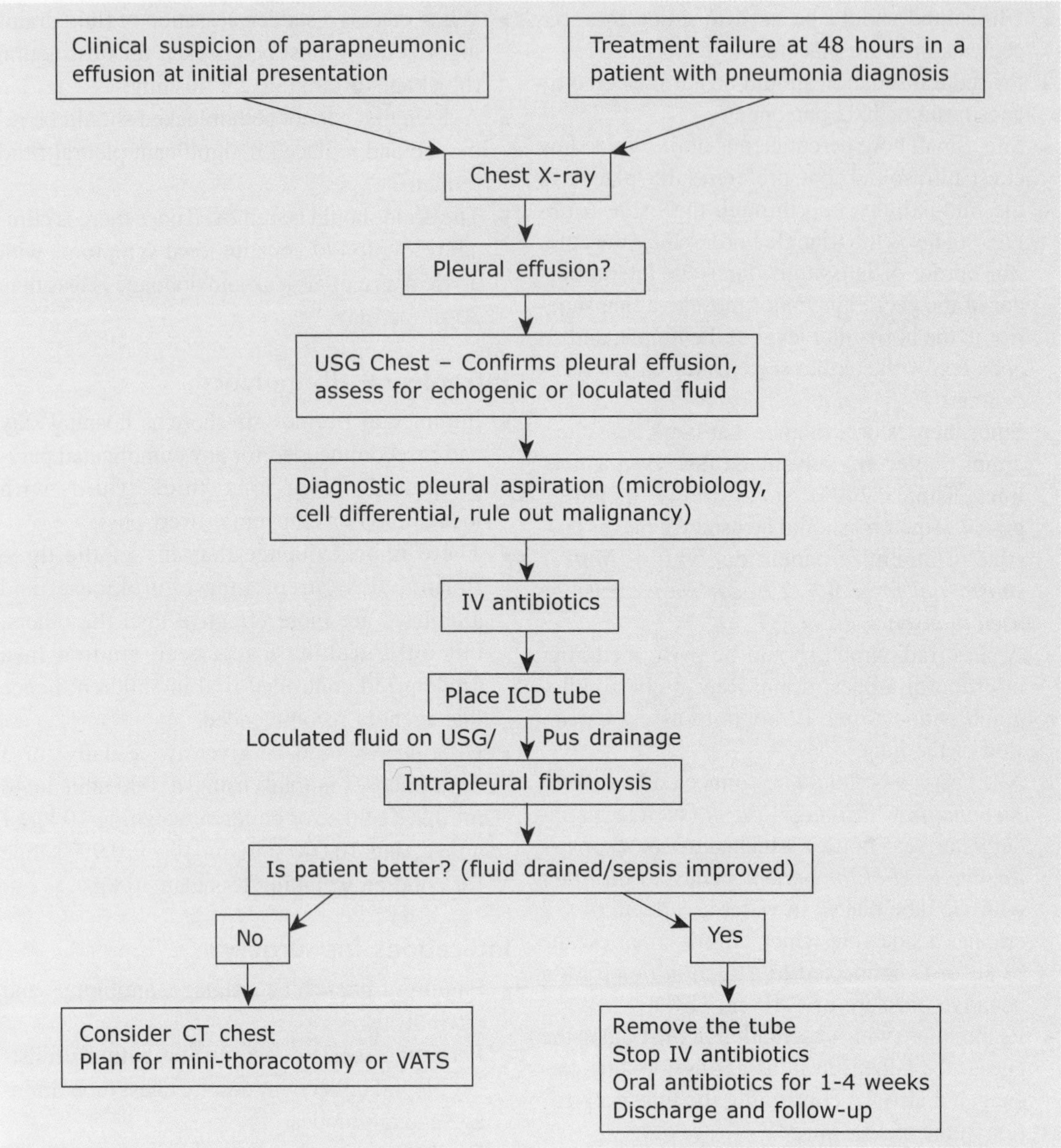

Fig. 15.1 Algorithm for management of pleural infection in children

It is an alternative to decortication and produces only 3 small scars.

- *Decortication*: Multi-loculated and/or thick fibrinous peel entrapping the lung needs decortication.

REFERENCES

1. Pediatric pleural diseases subcommittee of the BTS standards of care committee. BTS guidelines for management of pleural infections in children. Thorax 2005;60 supplement1:i1-21.

16

Pulse Oximetry and Capnometry

While clinical monitoring is the most superior method of monitoring a patient's respiratory status, pulse oximetry and end-tidal CO_2 monitoring are invaluable adjuncts.

PULSE OXIMETRY

- Pulse oximetry is a simple non-invasive method of continuously monitoring the percentage of hemoglobin (Hb) which is saturated with oxygen.
- The popularity of this apparatus stems from various reasons: it is a portable, non-invasive, light-weight, inexpensive monitor which provides real-time data and most importantly, is capable of detecting hypoxia before the patient becomes clinically cyanosed.

How does pulse oximetry work?

- The pulse oximeter consists of a probe attached to the patient's finger or ear lobe which is linked to a computerised unit.
- Within the SpO_2 sensor, light emitting diodes shine red and infrared light (wavelengths 660 nm and 940 nm respectively) through the tissue. Most sensors work on extremities such as a finger, toe or ear.
- The blood, tissue and bone at the application site absorb much of the light.
- However, some light passes through the extremity. A light-sensitive sensor opposite the light source receives it.

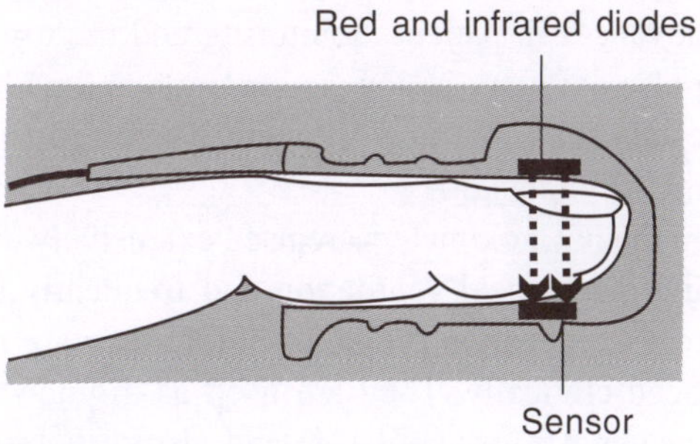

Fig. 16.1 SpO_2 Sensor

- By calculating the absorption at the two wavelengths, the processor can compute the proportion of hemoglobin which is oxygenated.
- The oximeter is dependent on a pulsatile flow and produces a graph of the quality of flow. Where flow is sluggish (e.g., hypovolemia or vasoconstriction) the pulse oximeter may be unable to function.
- The pulse oximetry measures the *functional saturation* which is defined as saturation of hemoglobin capable of carrying oxygen.
- This includes oxygenated hemoglobin (HbO_2) and deoxygenated hemoglobin (Hb).
- Pulse oximeters usually assume there are no non-functioning hemoglobins in the arterial blood and measure the blood oxygen saturation as:

  % saturation = HbO_2 / HbO_2+ Hb
- A co-oximeter measures *fractional saturation* which is determined by:

Fractional saturation = HbO_2 / HbO_2 + Hb + HbCO + MethHb

- When the amount of non-functioning hemoglobin (represented above by HbCO + MethHb + other non-functioning hemoglobins) is very small, both readings are nearly the same.
- When the patient has large amounts of non-functioning hemoglobin, e.g., carbon monoxide poisoning, these measurements vary widely.

Use of pulse oximetry in the ICU

- Pulse oximetry represents one of the greatest advances in patient monitoring and the use of pulse oximetry is now so common and widely established that it is frequently referred to as the 5th vital sign.
- In the ICU, oximeters are used extensively during mechanical ventilation and frequently detect oxygenation problems before they are noticed clinically. They are used as a guide for weaning from ventilation and also to help assess whether a patient's oxygen therapy is adequate.
- Oximetry has been shown to increase safety especially during transport (clinical monitoring difficult) and when patients are sedated for procedures, by alerting the staff to unexpected hypoxia.
- Pulse oximetry will rapidly detect a fall in circulating oxygen in the blood that may occur without immediate clinical signs and symptoms. The alarms usually respond to a slow or fast pulse rate or an oxygen saturation below 90%.
- At this level there is a marked fall in paO_2 representing serious hypoxia.
- Never ignore a reading which suggests the patient is becoming hypoxic.

Limitations of oximetry

- Less accurate when saturation is under 70%.
- The SaO_2 is not linearly related to the paO_2 because of the sigmoid shaped oxyhemoglobin dissociation curve.
  - Hence large changes in the paO_2 occur with small change in SpO_2 on the flat upper part of the dissociation curve.
  - Conversely, on the steep part of curve, large changes in the paO_2 may occur with smaller changes in the SpO_2.
- Oximeters give no information about the level of CO_2 and therefore have limitations in the assessment of patients developing respiratory failure due to CO_2 retention. A reduction in peripheral pulsatile blood flow produced by peripheral vasoconstriction (hypovolemia, severe hypotension, cold extremities, cardiac failure, some cardiac arrhythmias) results in an inadequate signal for analysis.
- Venous congestion of the limb may affect readings as can a badly positioned probe. When readings are lower than expected it is worth repositioning the probe. In general, however, if the waveform on the flow trace is good, then the reading will be accurate.
- Bright overhead lights (theatre, phototherapy) may cause the oximeter to be inaccurate, and the signal may be interrupted by surgical diathermy. Shivering may cause difficulties in picking up an adequate signal.
- Pulse oximetry cannot distinguish between different forms of hemoglobin. Carboxyhemoglobin is registered as 90% oxygenated haemoglobin and 10% desaturated haemoglobin, hence the oximeter will overestimate the saturation. The presence of methemoglobin will prevent the oximeter working accurately and the readings will tend towards 85%, regardless of the true saturation. However the fractional SpO_2 measured by co-oximetry will be accurate.
- Nail varnish may cause falsely low readings. However the readings are not affected by jaundice, dark skin or anemia.
- Motion artifacts result in a poor trace and inaccurate values.

This may be minimized by the use of newer generation pulse oximeters such as:

- *MARS*: Motion artifact rejection system. Here the manufacturers claim improved detection of pulse signal and hence superior analysis in clinical conditions such as low perfusion states and motion artifact
- *Signal extraction technology (SET)*: New algorithm for processing the signal, which measures and subtracts the noise component

Co-Oximetry

- In vitro oximetry
- Transmits four wavelength light through blood sample
- Detects HbCO and meth-HB in addition to oxygenated and reduced hemoglobin.
- Gold standard for the measurement of central venous saturation ($ScvO_2$) for monitoring of hemodynamic status.

CAPNOGRAPHY

- *Capnography* is the measurement of carbon dioxide (CO_2) in each breath of the respiratory cycle. The capnograph displays a waveform as well as the value of the CO_2 at the end of exhalation, which is known as the end-tidal CO_2.
- *Colorimetric* CO_2 *detectors* are not monitors
  - Changes color when exposed to CO_2
  - The color change corresponds to a range of CO_2 values
  - Requires six breaths for accurate determination
- A capnograph display the numeric value of $etCO_2$ as well as the CO_2 waveform while capnometer only measures and displays a numeric value of $etCO_2$.
- Provided the patient has a stable cardiac status, stable body temperature, absence of lung disease and a normal capnograph trace, end-tidal carbon dioxide ($etCO_2$) is slightly lower than the $paCO_2$.
- The normal $paCO_2$ – $etCO_2$ gradient is 3-5 mmHg
- Capnometry reflects 3 major processes in the body (Fig. 16.2 and 16.3)
  - Cellular metabolism (production of CO_2)
  - Cardiac output and circulation (transport of CO_2 from the tissues to the heart, pulmonary perfusion)
  - Ventilation and elimination of CO_2 from the lungs (alveolar ventilation, respiratory pattern).

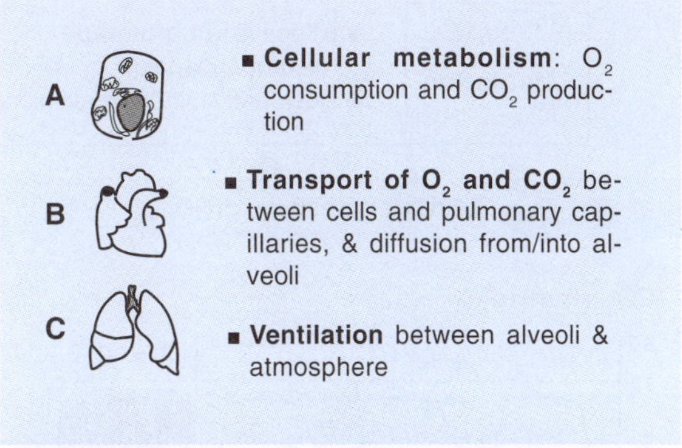

Fig. 16.2 Determinants of CO_2

Parts of the normal capnogram (Fig. 16.4)

- The **first phase** occurs during inspiration.
- The **second phase** is the onset of expiration, which results in a rapid increase in CO_2.
- The **third phase**, the expiratory plateau, occurs as the CO_2 is exhaled from all the alveoli.
- The highest point of the plateau is known as the end-tidal CO_2 ($etCO_2$). This marks the end of expiration.
- **Phase four** is the onset of inspiration.

The $etCO_2$ analyzer: Position of sampling (Table 16.1)

Gas from the breathing system can be sampled either by a sidestream or a mainstream analyzer.

Sidestream: Gas is drawn from the breathing system by a 1.2 mm internal diameter tube. The tube is connected to a lightweight adapter near the patient's end of the breathing system. It delivers the

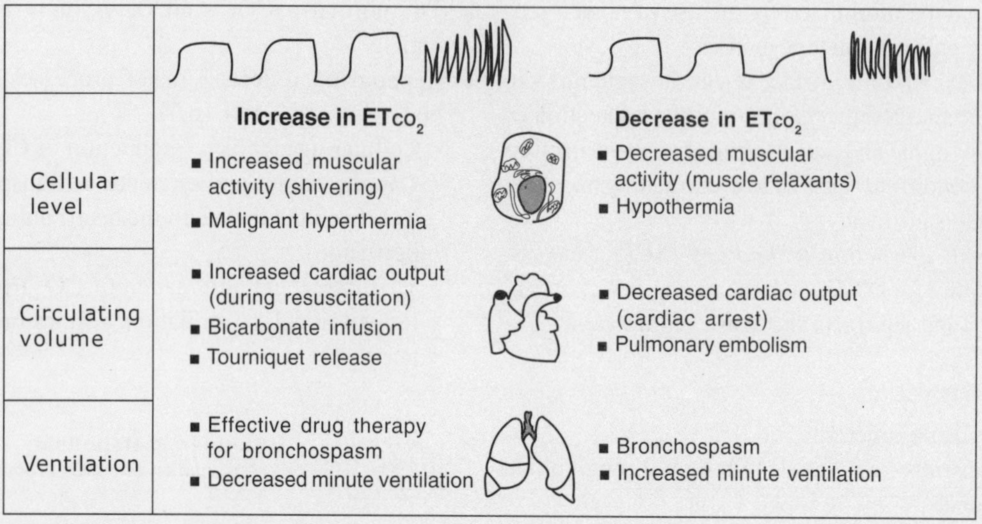

Fig. 16.3 Factors affecting $etCO_2$

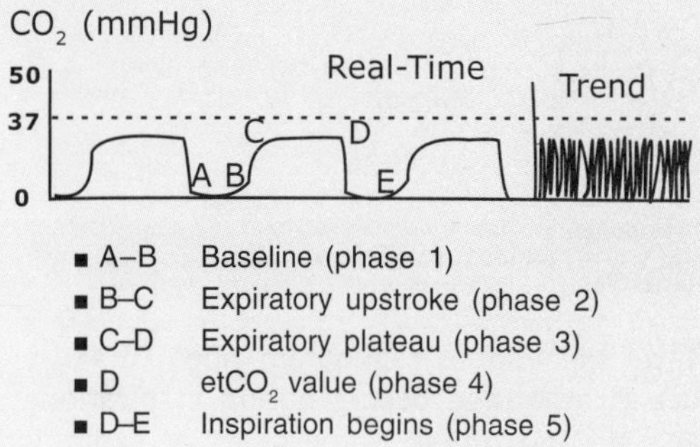

Fig. 16.4 Normal capnogram

gas to the sample chamber. It is made of Teflon so it is impermeable to CO_2 and does not react with anesthetic agents. Only the precise tubing recommended by the manufacturer should be used, and only of the recommended length. Typical infrared instruments sample at a flow rate between 50 and 150 ml/minute. When low fresh gas flows are used the sampled gas may be returned to the breathing circuit. It is important that the tip of the sampling tube should always be as near as possible to the patient's trachea, but the sampled gas mixture must not be contaminated by inspired gas during the expiratory phase.

Table 16.1 Types of $etCO_2$ analyzer

Sampling types	Main stream analyzer	Side stream analyzer
Advantages	Chamber in line at ET adaptor. No time delay in analysis. More accurate.	Aspirates 50-150 ml /min. Less dead space.
Disadvantages	Heavier and more cumbersome. Adds to dead space.	Less accurate. Time delay with slow aspiration/ false low $etCO_2$ with fast aspiration. Aspirates mucus & secretions.

Mainstream: The sample chamber is positioned within the patient's gas stream near the patient's end of the breathing system. Although heavier and more cumbersome, it does have advantages over

Table 16.2 Common abnormal capnograms with causes

Abnormality	Cause	Change in capnogram with trend
Gradual rise of $etCO_2$	Hypoventilation Hyperthermia Partial tube block or Airway obstruction	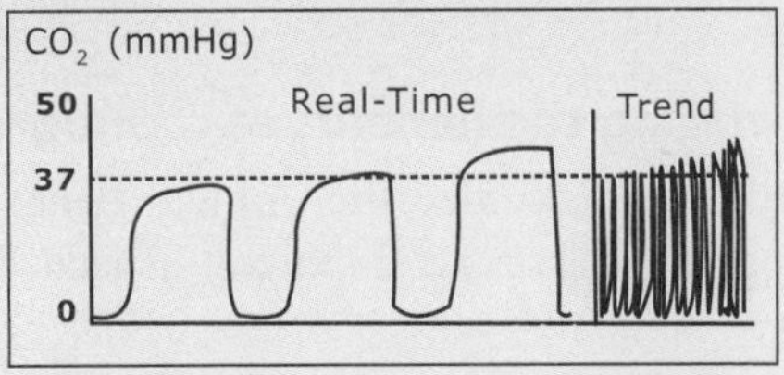
Gradual fall of $etCO_2$	Hyperventilation Hypothermia Low cardiac output states	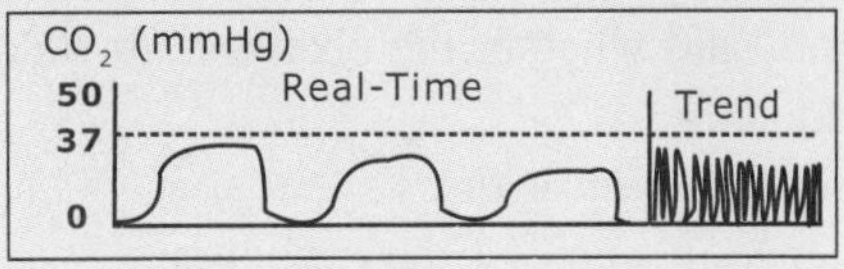
Sudden drop in CO_2	Esophageal intubation Dislodged tube Tube block Ventilator disconnection	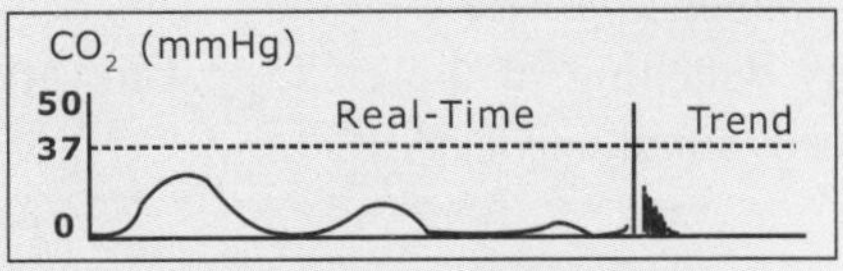
Change in the baseline CO_2	Re-breathing CO_2 absorber saturation Water droplets in CO_2 analyzer	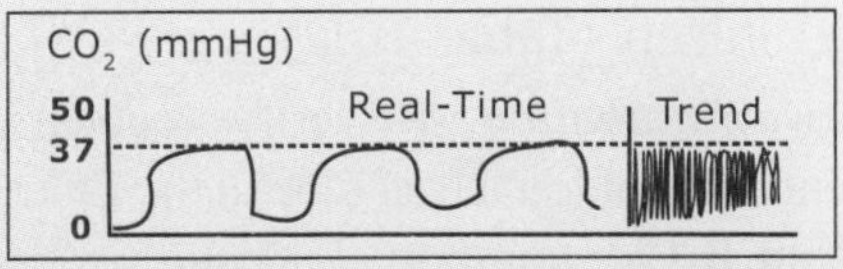
Sudden fall in CO_2 (not to baseline)	Leak in the system Partial tube block	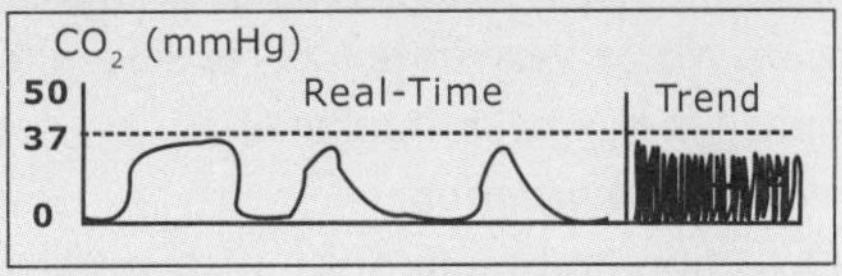
Change in shape (slope)	Lower airways obstruction, bronchoconstriction	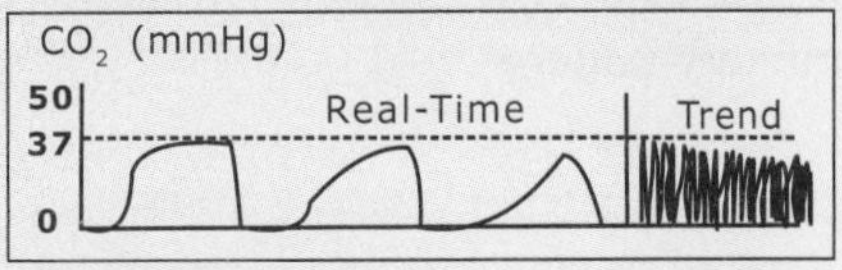
Curare effect	Spontaneous effort in a paralysed patient (muscle relaxant effort wearing off)	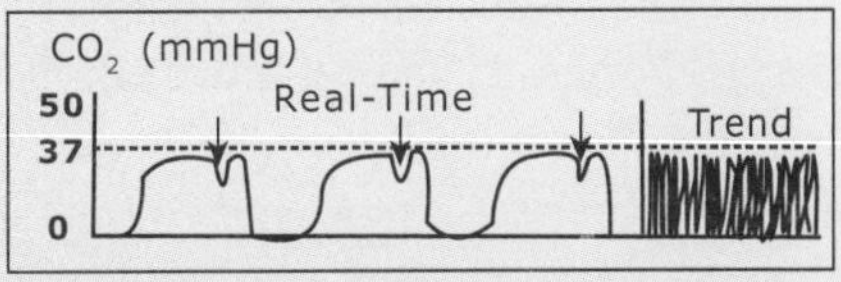

sidestream sampling: there is no delay in the rise and fall times of gas composition changes, no gas is lost from the attachment, no mixing occurs along the capillary tube before analysis, and there are fewer problems with water vapour condensation.

Maximizing the benefits of capnography

In order to maximize the clinical benefits of capnography, assess 3 important aspects of the $etCO_2$:

- Assess for change in actual $etCO_2$ value, the trends and whether the changes are sudden or gradual

  In conjunction with
- Change in shape of the capnogram

  In conjunction with
- Any widening of the $etCO_2$-$paCO_2$ gradient (needs simultaneous ABG for $paCO_2$).

Clinical applications of capnography in sick children (Table 16.2)

- ***Airway/intubation:*** To verify tracheal placement of an endotracheal tube in the Emergency Room, ICU or transport: *The capnograph is the gold standard for detecting esophageal intubation.* No or very little CO_2 is detected if the esophagus has been intubated.
- ***Breathing/Ventilation:***
  - Detection and monitoring of respiratory depression / hypoventilation. Evaluation of respiratory pattern.
  - As a disconnection alarm for a ventilator or a breathing system. There is sudden absence of the capnograph trace.
  - Adjustment of parameter settings in mechanically ventilated patients
- ***Circulation/tissue perfusion:***
  - Widening of the $paCO_2$ and $etCO_2$ gradient is a valuable indicator of inadequate tissue perfusion and shock.
  - Post arrest: The $etCO_2$ is the earliest indicator of return of circulation (ROC) after cardiac arrest and also has prognostic significance (an $etCO_2$ value > 10 mmHg indicates higher chance of survival).
  - May detect air embolism as a sudden decrease in $etCO_2$, assuming that the arterial blood pressure remains stable.
  - Sudden circulatory collapse (tension pneumothorax, cardiac tamponade) may be recognized as a sudden decrease in $etCO_2$.

REFERENCES

1. Downloaded from World Federation of Societies of Anaesthesiologists WWW implementation by the NDA Web Team, Oxford

PEDIATRIC EMERGENCIES & CRITICAL CARE

17

Arterial Line Insertion and Monitoring

Continuous intra-arterial blood pressure monitoring and arterial sampling are essential components of care for many ICU patients; however, this may be associated with significant risks and complications.

INDICATIONS

- Unstable/critically ill patients who need accurate, continuous BP monitoring and
- When noninvasive blood pressure (NIBP) is unreliable: severe edema, extremes of blood pressure, shock states, obesity, burns.
- When accurate measures of BP are crucial: Brain trauma, hypertensive crisis, abdominal compartmental syndromes.
- Following complex surgeries, including post cardiac surgery.
- Monitoring response to vasoactive drugs.
- Frequent blood sampling.

CONTRAINDICATIONS

- A negative Allen test (see below).
- Coagulation abnormalities (may insert after correction).

SITES

- Radial artery
- Femoral artery
- Dorsalis pedis artery
- Posterior tibial artery
- Axillary artery

Note

- The brachial artery should not be used for puncture or cannulation because there is no collateral circulation in this area.
- Axillary artery can be cannulated in desperate situation but should be re-sited as early as possible due to its proximity to heart and risk of embolization.
- Temporal artery cannulation can cause spasm of intracerebral vessels and hence should be avoided.

PRE-PROCEDURE

- Obtain informed written consent.
- The modified Allen's test should be performed to demonstrate collateral flow through the superficial palmar arch prior to cannulation. Compress and clench the hand to squeeze out the blood. Occlude both the radial and ulnar artery with manual pressure. The hand will blanch. Release pressure over the ulnar artery. Return of color in the hand within 5 seconds indicates adequate collateral circulation from the ulnar artery. However, this test is not foolproof, hence continued monitoring of digit perfusion is necessary.

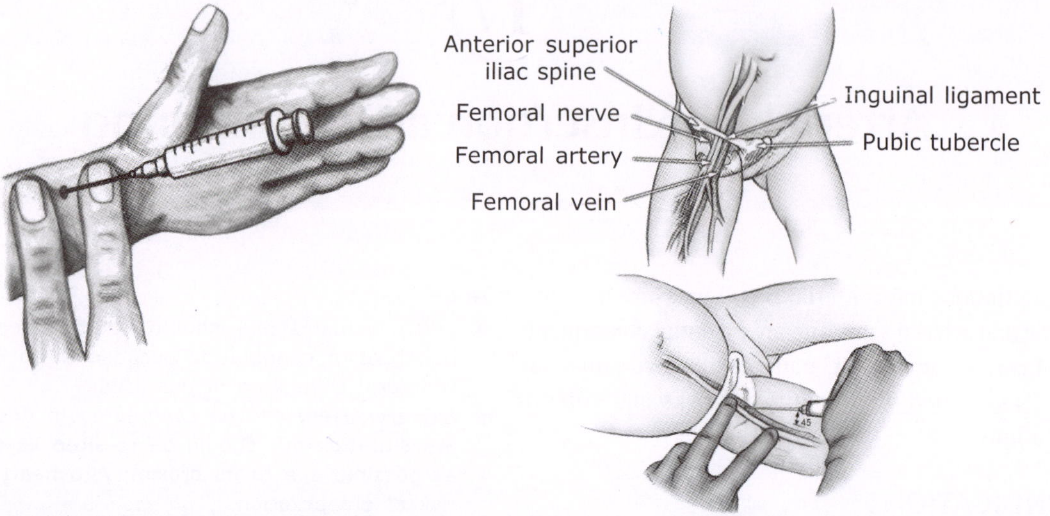

Fig. 17.1 Sites for radial and femoral arteries.

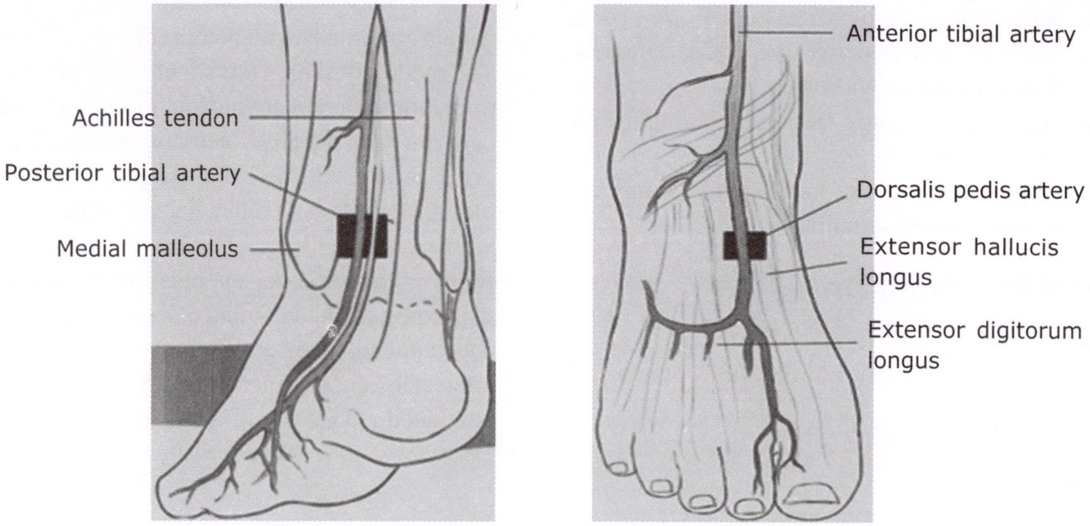

Fig. 17.2 Sites for posterior tibial and dorsalis pedis arteries. (Modified from *Textbook of Pediatric Emergency Procedures*, McGraw-Hill, 2nd Ed, 2007)

PROCEDURE FOR RADIAL ARTERY CANNULATION

- Stabilize the hand and wrist on a firm surface, placing the wrist in approximately 30 to 45 degrees extension over several gauze pads or a bottle.

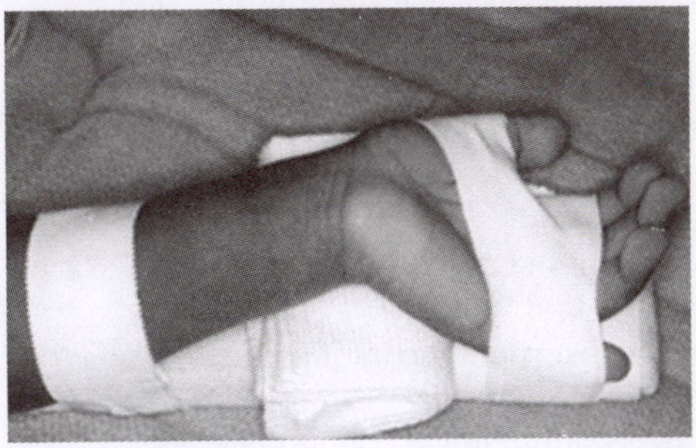

Fig. 17.3 Position for radial artery cannulation. (Modified from *Irwin and Rippe's Intensive Care Medicine*, 6th Ed. Lippincott Williams & Wilkins 2008)

- Prepare wrist with sterile technique and drape the area. Infiltrate skin with 1% lignocaine.
- Once a site is chosen, the most superficial course of the artery is identified by palpation.
- The artery can be directly cannulated using an IV cannula or using the Seldinger technique (catheter over wire). Insert the chosen device at 30^0 angle to the horizontal and advance further until bright red blood appears in the transparent flash chamber of the catheter. Now advance catheter into the artery. Pulsatile blood will appear through the hub of the catheter. A transparent sterile dressing is applied after fixing the line and attaching a 3-way connector with a 10 cm extension/transducer tubing.
- Set up a continuous heparinized saline infusion (1 unit heparin/ml saline) at 1 ml per hour.
- Transducer should be connected and zeroed if invasive monitoring is required.
- Hourly evaluation of digit perfusion should be done by inspection of capillary refill test.

PREVENTION OF COMPLICATIONS AND TROUBLE-SHOOTING (TABLE 17.1)

- Avoid more than two pricks at any one arterial site as there is a risk for spasm, intimal tears.
- Local infiltration of lignocaine improves patient co-operation, increases success rate and also decreases incidence of an arterial spasm.
- If arterial cannulation is unsuccessful, direct pressure should be applied over the site for a full 5 minutes.
- Failure to observe pulsatile blood flow from the catheter may indicate that the posterior wall of the artery has been punctured. When this occurs, the catheter should be slowly withdrawn and, if a flash of blood is seen, advanced again into the artery.
- The catheter should be secured with a transparent dressing so that a window is available to observe any blanching of the skin around the site of the catheter.
- A continuous infusion of heparin (1 U/ml) with or without papaverine (0.12 mg/ml) should be commenced.
- Never "purge"saline into the arterial line via the pig-tail or infusion pump. As the forces are very high, flushing may force air bubbles in a retrograde direction through the radial, brachial, axillary, and subclavian arteries, where they can then travel to the cerebral circulation (retrograde cerebral embolization).
- Flushes are best done with small volume syringes at a slow rate.
- *Ischemic complications*: These are the most dreaded complications as distal ischemia can cause gangrene and loss of digit or extremity.
  - Ischemic complications may be minimized by checking the color, warmth, capillary return and movement if the patient is conscious. By having the limb distal to the cannulae in constant view and placing the pulse oximeter

Table 17.1 Arterial line complications and prevention

	Complications	Prevention
Infection related	- Catheter related infection - Sepsis	- Remove once not needed - Strict asepsis during insertion - Asepsis during sampling - Use disposable tubing - Change system if contaminated - Regular aseptic dressings and frequent inspections of the site for any signs of infection - Use of systems which prevent backflow of blood into the transducer reduces the risk of infection - Transducers should be changed every 72 hr
Procedure related	- Bleeding - Hematoma - Pseudo-aneurysm - Injury to adjacent structures	- Correct insertion techniques - Minimize number of attempts - Check coagulation parameters. - If arterial cannulation is unsuccessful, direct pressure should be applied over the site for 5 minutes after oozing has stopped
Catheter related	- Thrombosis - Distal limb ischemia or gangrene due to thrombus/spasm	- Heparin or saline infusion continuously. Add papavarine (0.12 mg/ml) in flush bag - Check CFT, temperature, color, distal pulses, and saturation 1 hrly. Transparent dressings allow visualization of catheter insertion site for blanching, induration, erythema - Remove catheter immediately if in doubt and inform vascular surgeon immediately
Flush/ Sampling related	- Retrograde cerebral embolization	- Avoid axillary arterial cannulation - Minimize flush rate to 0.5 ml/min - Do not flush if no back flow
Others	- Accidental drug administration - Life threatening exsanguinations in the event of disconnections	- Label prominently as "arterial line" and "No medications"
Technical	- Misinterpretation of values	- Leveling and zeroing with position change and with each shift - Follow MAP if overdamped or underdamped system - Look at the clinical response and don't "treat numbers" - Use non-compliant tubing

probe distal to the insertion site, perfusion may be continually observed.
- Risk factors for ischemic complications: Multiple punctures, protracted hypotension, high dose pressors, acidosis, hypothermia, failure to remove the line at the earliest sign of distal ischemia.

- *Hemorrhage: Having the arterial cannulae itself on view is an important guard against arterial hemorrhage.* Torrential bleeding can occur very rapidly from dislodged arterial catheters or opened circuits. Bulky dressings can mask bleeding. The best way to stop bleeding is manual compression. Pressure dressings will not stop arterial bleeding.

Management of thrombosis with distal ischemia

- Remove the line after instilling intra-arterial tissue plasminogen activator (tPA).
- Systemic thrombolytics (tPA) with anticoagulation (heparin) should be begun if extremity perfusion is compromised.
- Liaise with a vascular surgeon; serial Doppler studies are helpful.

INVASIVE ARTERIAL BLOOD PRESSURE MONITORING

Principle

Conversion of pressure to an electric signal from artery to transducer via fluid filled system and conversion to graphical waveforms by monitor (Fig. 17.4).

Normal arterial waveform (Fig. 17.5)

- A - Rapid upstroke
- B - Peak pressure
- BC - Systolic decline
- C - Dicrotic notch corresponds to aortic valve closure
- CD - Diastolic run off
- D - End-diastolic pressure

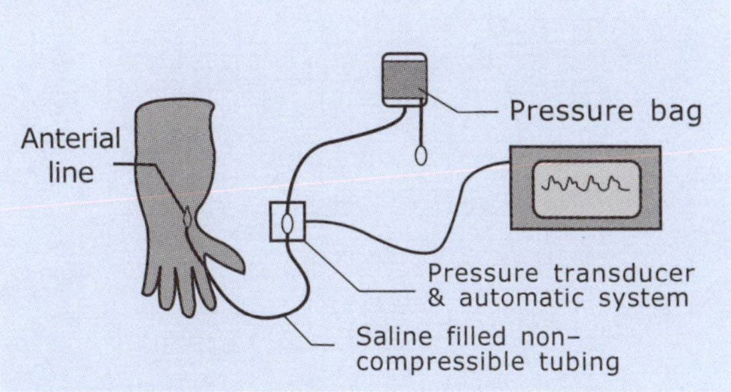

Fig. 17.4 Arterial monitor setup

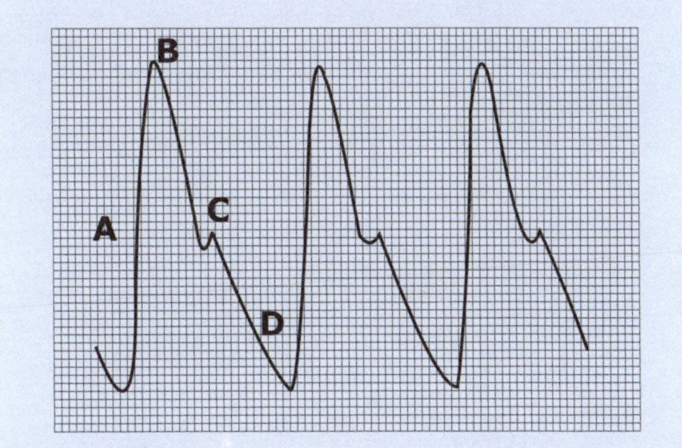

Fig. 17.5 Part of arterial awveform

Arterial blood pressure variations from different arteries (Fig. 17.6)

- Peripheral arterial waveforms have steep rise, higher systolic and lower diastolic values and the dicrotic notch moves away towards base. The mean blood pressure (MAP) is always same.
- Follow the MAP irrespective of the site of cannulation or the systolic and diastolic values.

Parts of the monitoring system (Fig. 17.4)

The transducer is an external, disposable, fluid air interface which detects changes of pressure in the artery. It is able to detect these pressure changes because there is a column of fluid between the blood in the artery and a diaphragm within the transducer.

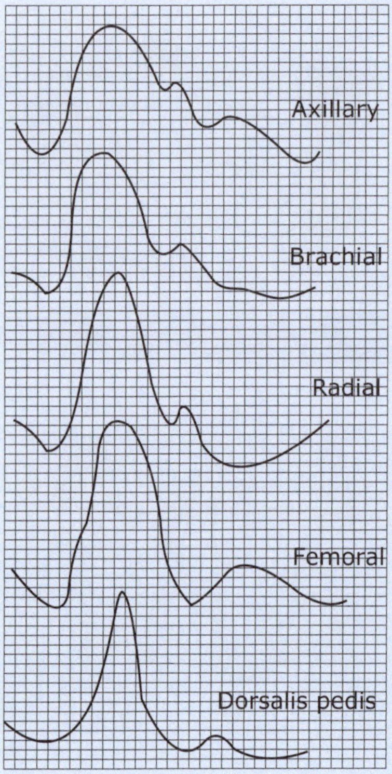

Fig. 17.6 Waveforms vary depending on monitoring site

Air bubbles and blood in the transducer alter this fluid filled column and therefore lead to inaccurate readings. To prevent this, the transducer has a *quick flush mechanism* which is connected to the pressure bag so that air bubbles and blood can be flushed out of the system via an exit port to ensure accurate readings.

Dynamic response testing

- This is done to determine the accuracy of BP representation by the system. The dynamic response of a hemodynamic monitoring system is defined by its natural frequency and the damping coefficient.
- *The natural frequency* indicates how fast the pressure monitoring system vibrates when shock-excited by a signal such as the arterial pressure pulse or the pressure signal caused by a fast flush test.
- *The damping coefficient* of a monitoring system is a measure of how quickly the oscillations of a shock excited system dampens and eventually comes to rest. The system normally is damped to provide correct blood pressure value.

Standardization of the arterial BP measurement

- The precision and accuracy of arterial pressure system depends on meticulous calibration that must be carried out each shift. Three factors have to be considered when using a transducer: (1) zero setting, (2) leveling and (3) the "square wave" or flush test.
- *Why is "zeroing" important?* Zeroing eliminates the effect of atmospheric pressure on measured hemodynamic values. The process of "zeroing" involves opening the fluid column on the measuring device to the atmosphere and setting the system such that atmospheric pressure is the "zero" or starting value.
- Just as important as a proper "zero" is use of the proper "level." The measured pressure is determined by the change in height of the fluid column relative to the transducer. Therefore the accurate position of the transducer level is critical.
- A widely used reference point is the *phlebostatic axis* which corresponds to the midpoint of the right atrium. The phlebostatic axis is determined by the junction of two lines, a transverse line along the fourth intercostal space and a vertical line in the mid-axillary line. The system should be arranged such that the reference stopcock of the transducer must be leveled to the phlebostatic axis.
- *Why is leveling important?* Leveling eliminates the influence of hydrostatic pressure on the transducer. A transducer that is positioned below the patient's heart will produce falsely el-

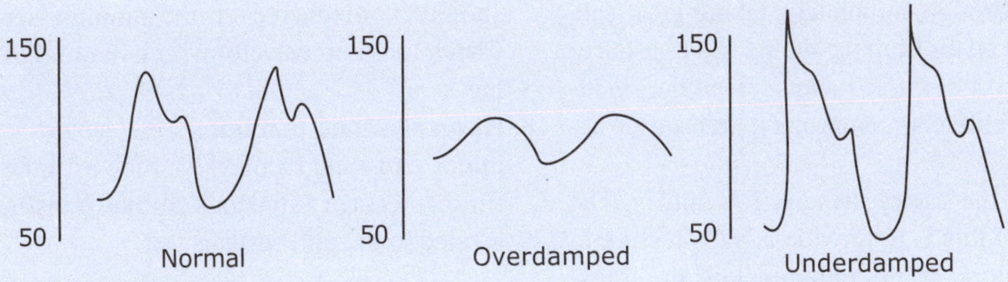

Overdamping
Soft compliant tubing
Blood clot
Air bubbles
Catheter kinks
Numerous connections and stopcocks

Underdamping
Short and stiff tubing
Short and stiff catheter
Transducer with stiff diaphragm

Fig. 17.7

- Overdamped system – Low systolic BP, high diastolic BP, normal MAP
  Slurred upstroke, absent dicrotic notch
- Underdamped – High systolic BP, low diastolic BP, normal MAP
- Optimally damped (Normal) – Normal systolic BP, normal diastolic BP, normal MAP

Note – MAP remains constant in all these conditions

evated pressures and a transducer positioned above the patient's heart will produce falsely low pressures.

- The length of the *tubing* between the transducer and the cannula directly affects the accuracy of the measured values. The tubing must be stiff, non-compliant, less than 120 cm in length and of a sufficient diameter to conduct the pulsatile fluid movement from the tip of the cannula to the transducer without being compressed. If tubing is too long or too short, or if the tubing is soft and pliable, the accuracy of the readings will be compromised (overdamped or underdamped, discussed below).
- *Square Wave Test (Flush Test):* This will determine whether the system is optimally damped.
  - Flush system briefly from pressurized bag by opening pigtail.
  - Pressure increases abruptly and then falls.
  - Watch response at end of test.
  - Look for signal distortion of oscillations.
- *Normal flush test (Fig. 17.8):*
  - Plateau followed by few oscillations (1-2)
  - Width of 1st wave < 1 mm
  - 2nd wave amplitude < $^{1}/_{3}{}^{rd}$ of 1st wave

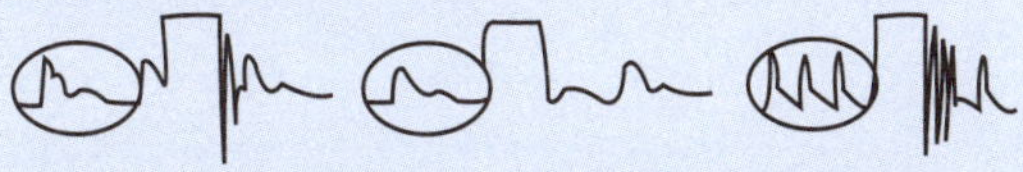

Square waves test – This illustration shows (from left) a normal (optimally damped), a lower and wider wave form (overdamped), and a higher and narrower (underdamped) waveform

Fig. 17.8 The flush test

How to set up an arterial line

1. Prepare a 500 ml bag of heparinized saline (> 30 kg) or 50 ml syringe infusion set with 1 unit heparin per ml. Connect the saline solution and the transducer administration set.

2. Pressurize the bag to 300 mmHg, and flush the solution through completely, taking great care to remove all air from the tubing and transducer set ports. As discussed above, even the smallest air bubble can compromise transducer accuracy.
3. Maintain the bag pressure at 300 mmHg. The purpose of this is to provide a backpressure to prevent blood from contaminating the transducer.
4. With the transducer connected to the monitor, perform a "square wave test" by fast flushing the line and observing a change in the waveform (waveform becomes a flat line at a high pressure, then dips down to a low pressure, before the actual pressure tracing ensues).
5. Zero the transducer and monitor by placing the transducer at the phlebostatic axis of the patient. Close the stopcock to the patient and open it to air. Press zero on the monitor. To monitor pressure, close the stopcock to air and open it to the patient.
6. Connect the patient catheter and fast flush to clear the catheter of blood.
7. An arterial waveform and pressure readings should be displayed on the monitor screen. Check for good waveform with optimal damping.
8. Haemodynamic transducers are zeroed at ach initial setup and then every shift, with the air-fluid interface (stopcock above transducer) leveled to the phlebostatic axis.

REFERENCES

1. Torrey SB, Saladino RA. Arterial Puncture and Catheterization. In: Textbook of Pediatric Emergency Procedures, 2nd ed. Eds: Christopher K, Henretig FM. Lippincott Williams & Wilkins 2008;716-25.
2. Noah Z. Arterial Puncture. In: Current Procedures: Pediatrics. Eds: Goodman DM, Green TP, Unti SM, et al. The McGraw-Hill Companies, Inc. 2007; 54-7.
3. Celinski SA, Seneff MG. Arterial Line Placement and Care. In: Irwin and Rippe's Intensive Care Medicine, 6th ed. Eds: Irwin RS, Rippe JM. Lippincott Williams & Wilkins 2008;39-47.

18

Central Venous Lines and Central Venous Pressure Monitoring

Central lines are long catheters inserted into large veins and threaded in so that the tip lies either in the IVC, SVC or the right atrium.

CLINICAL INDICATIONS

- Measurement of central venous pressure (CVP) in order to assess fluid status. Can also measure central venous saturation ($ScvO_2$).
- Placement of venous access line when other peripheral sites are unavailable
- Administration of fluids or medications which require reliable drug delivery, such as vasoactive drugs. However, rapid fluid boluses are preferably given through short, large bore peripheral lines as central lines are long and narrow and have high resistance resulting in a greater time for delivery to the circulation.
- Administration of hypertonic/irritant/sclerosing agents that can cause phlebitis of peripheral veins such as TPN, high concentration dextrose, potassium chloride, calcium gluconate, amiodarone.
- Long term vascular access, as an alternative to repetitive venous cannulations when long term medications required.
- Access for hemodialysis or plasmapheresis.

☞ **REMEMBER** Blood and platelets may block the catheter unless the CVC is large bore device.

RELATIVE CONTRAINDICATIONS

- Infection over the insertion site
- Distortion of landmarks from any reason
- Suspected injury to the superior vena cava (e.g., SVC syndrome)
- Coagulopathies including anticoagulation therapy
- Pneumothorax or hemothorax on the contralateral side, inability to tolerate pneumothorax on the ipsilateral side.
- Patients unable to tolerate a Trendelenberg position (for IJV/SV)
- Patients receiving ventilatory support with high PEEP (temporarily reduce the pressures)
- Patients with vigorous, ongoing cardiopulmonary resuscitation
- Operator inexperience

INSERTION TECHNIQUE

- **Femoral Vein (FV)**: The needle is inserted at a 45° angle to the skin surface 1 to 2 cm *below the inguinal ligament* and advanced in the direction of the umbilicus. At no time should the tip of the needle pass beyond the inguinal ligament, because, if a retroperitoneal hematoma occurs, application of external pressure is difficult.
- **IJV**: Three approaches are possible: median, anterior and lateral. The median approach is commonly followed. The site of entry is midway on a line joining the sternoclavicular joint and mastoid process just lateral to the sterno-

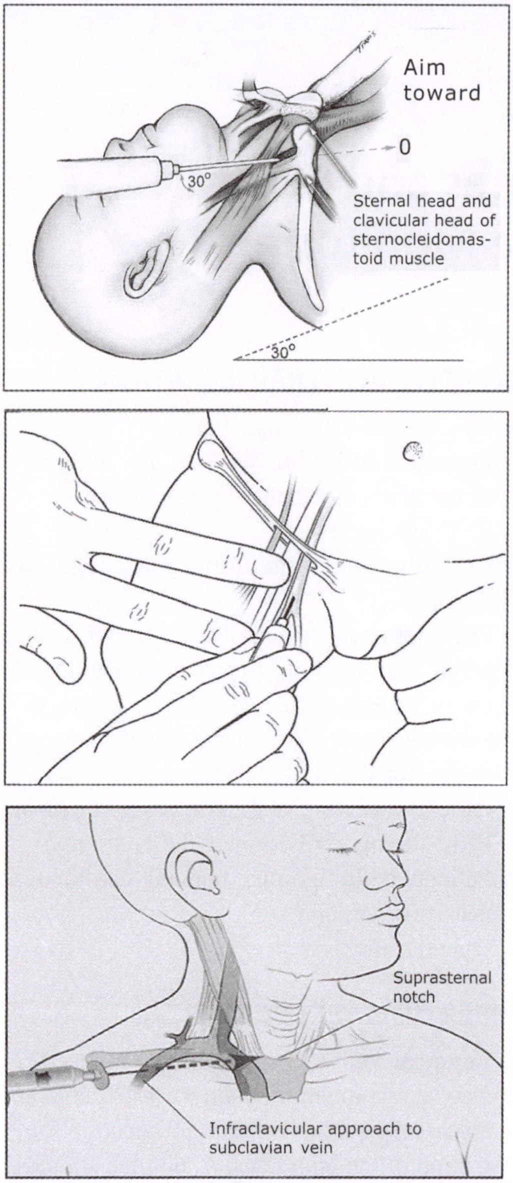

Fig. 18.1 Insertion sites for subclavian, femoral and internal jugular lines. (Modified from *Textbook of Pediatric Emergency Procedures*, 2nd Ed)

mastoid muscle. The carotid pulsation is felt and the carotid artery is moved just medially before entry. The needle is inserted at a 30° angle to the skin and directed toward the ipsilateral nipple. This reduces the chance of causing a pneumothorax.

- **Subclavian Vein**: Two approaches are possible: infraclavicular and supraclavicular. The infraclavicular approach is popular. The needle is advanced slowly just beneath the inferior surface of the clavicle at the junction of middle and lateral thirds, aimed toward the sternal notch and kept as nearly parallel to the horizontal plane of the chest as possible. If the first prick is unsuccessful, the needle is withdrawn and only minimally redirected inferiorly.

Procedure (Fig. 18.1)

- Select a catheter of desired size, length and number of lumens.
- *Size of catheter*
  - 1 month to 1 year: 4-4.5 Fr;
  - 1 year to 8 years: 5-5.5 Fr;
  - >8 yr: 7 Fr.
- The length of the catheter is decided by measuring the landmarks from the site of entry to xiphisternum (for femoral lines) and from the site of entry to 2nd costal cartilage at the sternum for IJV and SV.
- Obtain consent after explaining the risks and benefits of the procedure.
- Ensure availability of a second skilled assistant, sedative drugs and monitoring equipment.
- *Position of the patient.*
  - **FV:** Abduction and external rotation at the hip. A folded towel placed beneath the patient's gluteal region facilitates success.
  - **IJV:** Head is turned 30° away. A small towel can be positioned longitudinally between the child's shoulder blades to help accentuate anatomic landmarks. The head of the bed is tilted down 15° to 30° (Trendelenburg) to promote venous distention.
  - **SV:** The patient is placed in a supine Trendelenburg position with the head turned slightly away from the planned cannulation site. A

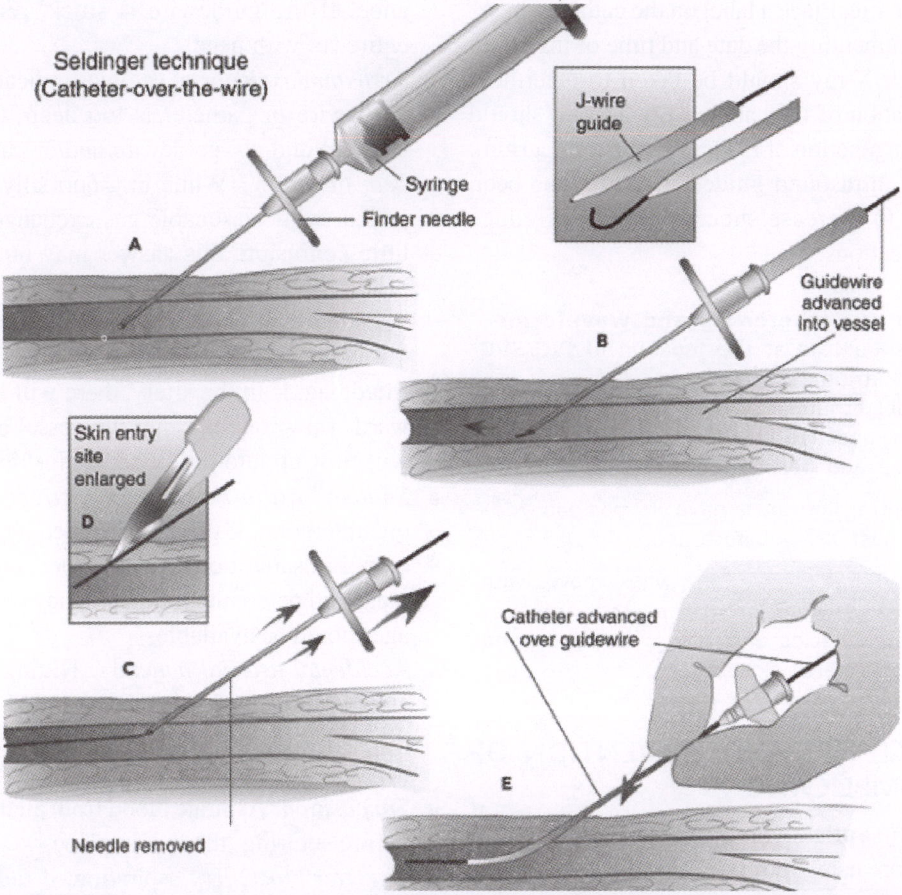

Fig. 18.2 Steps of Seldinger technique. (Modified from *Textbook of Pediatric Emergency Procedures*, 2nd Ed, Christopher and Henretig, 2008)

rolled towel may be positioned longitudinally between the shoulder blades will so that the child's shoulders fall posteriorly away from the chest. The ipsilateral arm should be at the child's side. Gentle downward traction of the ipsilateral arm may also be helpful.

- Prepare area with sterile technique and place drapes covering a large area to avoid guide wire contamination.
- Reduce airway pressures, including PEEP, if possible.
- Infiltrate local anesthetic.
- Introduce catheter by 'Seldinger techinque'.
- When there is blood return, insert the ' J ' tipped end of the guide wire (Fig. 18.2B).
- Remove needle, holding the guidewire firmly (Fig. 18.2C).
- The insertion site may need to be enlarged with a small skin incision and dilator (Fig. 18.2D).
- Insert the catheter that has been pre-flushed with saline over the wire into the vein in a twisting motion up to the predetermined length. (Fig. 18.2E)
- Remove guidewire, suture catheter in place and apply sterile transparent polyurethane dressing

over the site. Place a label on the catheter dressing documenting the date and time of insertion.

- A check X-ray should be taken to determine the location of the catheter tip. The tip should lie at the junction of IVC/SVC and right atrium.
- Use of ultrasound guided insertion has been shown to increase success rates and reduce complications.

Position of Catheter tip and waveforms

The tip should lie at the junction of IVC/SVC and right atrium.

Tip in right atrium may result in flat CVP trace (catheter impacting on the atrial wall), emboli, arrhythmia and perforation of the atrium.

Every central line must have its position verified by chest X-ray before use.

Normal CVP has a wave form which moves with respiration. a-waves from the atria, v-waves from the ventricles and c-waves correspond to tricuspid valve closure.

CLINICAL TIPS AND PREVENTION OF CVC COMPLICATIONS

- Make first prick with a smaller "locator" needle before using introducer needle to assess direction and depth.
- Use small volume syringe to prevent vein collapse while aspirating.
- Minimize number of attempts to a maximum of 3. If unsuccessful, a 2nd preferably more skilled person should attempt the procedure.
- After insertion of the entry needle, withdraw the needle slowly maintaining negative pressure.
- The operator must always ensure that the proximal end of the guidewire is visible at all times.
- *Air embolization*: Occlude introducer needle hub by a finger to prevent air embolus and/or blood loss before guidewire insertion.
- *Stuck guidewire:* If the needle is in position, the guidewire should slide smoothly into the vessel. Never force the guidewire against resistance. If the guidewire is stuck, remove the entire set with needle.
- *Arrhythmias:* Runs of ectopics indicate that the guidewire or catheter is too deep within the heart. Withdraw guidewire and/or catheter.
- *Vein or artery?* While in a normally perfused patient with reasonable gas exchange there is little confusion, this answer may not be clear in a hypoxic hypotensive patient. If in doubt, transduce the tip and check actual pressures OR connect one end of the catheter to a saline filled bag. If in the artery, there will be no forward flow of fluid into the vessel and blood will flow up into the IV set against gravity.
- *Sudden cardio-respiratory distress:* Suspect pneumothorax if there is a sudden hypotension or fall in saturations during procedure. Equipment and personnel for emergency chest drainage should be available.
- *Accidental arterial puncture:* Hitting a central artery can result in significant blood loss. Apply local pressure for 10-15 minutes. Treat underlying coagulopathy, if present.
- *Tip position:* Aspirate blood from all three ports before suturing the line in place.
- *Catheter block:* Try aspirating; if fails, do not flush. Label as "Not In Use". Thrombolytic agents such as streptokinase can be used locally to dissolve the clots.

Complications

- Thrombosis: Can be prevented by running heparin infusion (1 unit/ml)
- Local bleeding at the insertion site: Control with local pressure.
- Vascular laceration: Minimize multiple attempts
- Catheter fragment embolism
- Infection (see central line bundle below): Aseptic handling and remove ASAP when not required.

Table 18.1 Comparison of various sites for CVC insertion

Site	Landmarks	Advantages	Disadvantages	Complications
FV	1–2 cm medial to the femoral artery and 1–2 cm below inguinal ligament	Simple Does not interfere with airway management or chest compressions In the event of bleeding, external pressure possible	Higher risk of contamination Success is position dependent	Infection, bleeding, thrombosis
IJV	Midway of the sternomastoid muscle just lateral to carotid pulsations	Out of resuscitation field Available for direct compression	Requires operator experience Difficult in infants with short, fat neck	Pneumothorax, injury to carotid artery, thoracic duct, stellate ganglion; thrombosis, infection
SV	Beneath junction of middle and lateral thirds of the clavicle	Least infection risk	Requires operator experience Difficult in infants External pressure not possible in the event of arterial puncture	Pneumothorax, artery puncture, dysrhythmias, thoracic duct injury, air embolism

CVP MONITORING

(See also Chapter on Arterial Pressure Monitoring)

What determines the central venous pressure?

- The CVP reflects multiple factors:
  - Preload
  - Afterload
  - Contractility and compliance of the ventricle and
  - External pressures such as positive pressure ventilation (PPV) and high intra-abdominal pressures.
- CVP is not reliable in conditions with right ventricular pathology and pulmonary hypertension.
- *An isolated CVP reading is of limited value;* a trend of readings is much more significant and should be viewed in conjunction with other parameters, e.g., perfusion indices, BP and urine output.

How to interpret the CVP in a patient with shock: Performing a bedside Frank-Starling test

Volume load the patient with 10-20 ml/kg of normal saline or sufficient to increase CVP by >3 mmHg but <8 mmHg. Monitor perfusion and respiratory status and liver span for improvement or deterioration (fluid overload).

Three things can happen:

1. No change in CVP, patient still in shock, no deterioration: *Keep filling*
2. CVP goes up to target and comes down slowly with some improvement in perfusion, no signs

of fluid overload (clinical improvement): *Keep filling at gradual rates*

3. CVP rises to target and stays up ± signs of fluid overload: *Stop filling (The tank is full)*

When is the CVP unreliable?
Right ventricular dysfunction
Pulmonary hypertension
High external PEEP
High systemic vascular resistance
Tense abdominal distension

Determination of preload responsiveness

Does a patient in shock need more fluids?

1. Fluid challenge and see the response of CVP and clinical parameters (see above)
2. Passive leg raising test
3. Hepatojugular reflex
4. Hypovolemic trace on arterial wave form

Always assess above in conjunction with trends in patient clinical status

CVP interpretation in shock

- A low CVP in patient with shock always means hypovolemia
- A high CVP in a patient with shock usually indicates hypervolemia; however, hypovolemia cannot be ruled out if patient on positive pressure ventilation or has RV dysfunction.
- Always follow the CVP trends and clinical response to fluids (especially in ventilated children)

Prevention of Central line Related Blood Stream Infection (CR-BSI)

The single most important complication of central line is catheter associated sepsis.

The central line bundles

Grouping interventions together can decrease the infection rates more effectively compared to implementing a single intervention alone. This is called the ***sepsis bundle***. It includes insertion precautions and maintenance guidelines.

- *Insertion bundle*
  - Meticulous hand hygiene
  - Maximal barrier precautions with large full body drapes during insertion
  - Chlorhexidine antiseptic skin solution for skin preparation.
  - Optimal catheter site selection. In older children, a subclavian line has the least risk of infection.
  - The assistant should also don cap, mask, gown and gloves.
  - The nurse is empowered to stop the procedure if there is breach in any of the above guidelines.
- *Maintenance bundle*
  - All CVC lines must be assessed every 2 hrs initially. Document any changes.
  - Tubings and caps are changed every 72 hrly except whenTPN on flow when it is changed Q24H.
  - If a new CVL is inserted, a new set of tubings should be used.
  - Use luer lock systems at all times.
  - Do not flush different lumens with the same syringe.
  - Use sterile precautions while sampling through CVL.
  - Daily review of lines necessary with prompt removal if the line is no longer necessary.

Other issues in maintenance of CVC

- *Emergency central access:* If central line is introduced in an emergency under less than perfect aseptic conditions, it should be removed within 24 hours and a new line should be electively placed.
- *Dressing:* Transparent semi-permeable adhesive dressing with date of change. Inspect site of insertion for erythema or purulence. Change when soiled or once in 7 days.
- *Heparin infusion:* A continuous heparin flush OR intermittent heparin lock (1,000 units/ml,

approx 0.8 ml in each lumen) every Q12H is mandatory to prevent occlusion.

- *Antimicrobial ointment:* Application of antibiotic ointment at catheter insertion site is not recommended (skin maceration, superadded infection).
- *Central venous line replacement:* Routine or prophylactic replacement not recommended as it does not reduce risk of infection. Remove once not needed. Suspect CVL infection if sepsis without any other focus. Remove and use a new site. Do not use guide wire exchange for suspected catheter related infection.
- *Antibiotic coated catheters:* Antibiotic coated catheters may be used for short term CVCs likely to remain in place for more than five days. They may be considered in patients with high risk of infection (neutropenia, burns). The use of antibiotic coated catheters should not be a substitute for strict adherence to catheter insertion and maintenance protocols.

REFERENCES

1. Lavelle JM, Costarino AT. Central Venous Cannulation. In: Textbook of Pediatric Emergency Procedures, 2nd Ed. Ed: Christopher K, Henretig FM. Lippincott Williams & Wilkins 2008;248-272.
2. Celinski SA, Seneff MG. Central Venous Catheters. In: Irwin and Rippe's Intensive Care Medicine, 6th Ed. Ed: Irwin RS, Rippe JM. Lippincott Williams & Wilkins 2008;39-47.
3. Michelson K. Femoral Venous Catheterization. In: Current Procedures: Pediatrics. Ed: Goodman DM, Green TP, Unti SM, et al. The McGraw-Hill Companies, Inc. 2007; 48-53.
4. Guidance for prevention of intravascular catheter related infection.CDC 2002.

19

Approach to Arterial Blood Gases

INTRODUCTION

- Analysis of arterial blood gases (ABG) is useful for patients with suspected respiratory or metabolic disease.
- Serial blood gases can monitor progression or response to treatment of underlying disease.
- It is important to remember that the measured values are those of the extracellular compartment which do not reflect the values of the intracellular compartment.

Terminology

- An *Acid* is a compound that forms hydrogen ions in solution, also referred to as a "proton donor". Strong acids dissociate completely in solution, whereas weak acids ionize incompletely.
- A *Base* is a compound that combines with hydrogen ions in solution, also referred to as a "proton acceptor".
- *Buffers* are substances that limit change in hydrogen ion concentration (and so the pH) when hydrogen ions are added or removed from a solution. Buffers cannot eliminate H^+ from the body, but temper sudden changes in pH and buy time until the problem is corrected or a new balance is reached.
- Buffers may be thought of as sponges: when hydrogen ions are in excess, the sponge mops up the extra ions. When in short supply, the sponge can be squeezed to release more hydrogen ions.
- Bicarbonate/carbonic acid (HCO_3/H_2CO_3) buffering system (ECF and within RBC) is the most important and abundant buffer in the body.
- Whole body pH can be regulated at 2 sites by bicarbonate, i.e., bicarbonate regulation by the kidney and CO_2 by the lungs.
- Examples of non bicarbonate buffers are hemoglobin, oxyhemoglobin, organic and inorganic phosphates, plasma proteins.
- *Standard base excess (deficit):* Amount of strong acid or base required to titrate 1 litre of blood back to a pH of 7.4 at a temperature of 37°C and pCO_2 of 40 mmHg.
- The BE is another measure of the metabolic (renal) component. The normal range of BE is -2 to +2.

APPLIED PHYSIOLOGY

- Each day, there is a constant production of acid by the body's metabolic processes and in order to maintain acid base balance, the excretion (or metabolism) of these acids must equal the amount produced.
- The various acids produced by the body are classified as respiratory (volatile) acids or as metabolic (fixed) acids.
- *Volatile acids* are produced during oxidative metabolism and can leave a solution and enter the atmosphere (e.g., carbonic acid).
- *Non-volatile (fixed) acids* cannot leave a solution until eliminated by the kidney.

- Fixed acids are produced due to incomplete metabolism of carbohydrate (lactate), fats (ketones), and proteins (sulphates, phosphates).
- The organs involved in the regulation of acid base are the lungs and the kidney.
- The lungs are important for excretion of the huge amounts of CO_2 produced (≅ 12,000 mmol/ each day).
- The kidneys are responsible for the excretion of a smaller amount of fixed acid (70-100 mmol/day).
- The critical role of the kidneys stem from 2 reasons: firstly, although smaller, there is no other method to excrete the fixed acids. Secondly, the kidneys maintain the plasma concentration of bicarbonate, the major extracellular buffer, both by resorption of filtered bicarbonate and regeneration of bicarbonate. The kidneys also regulate acid base balance by increasing the secretion of ammonium (NH_4) by the proximal convoluted tubules in the face of systemic acidosis.
- Response to acid-base perturbation by the body has 3 components
  - First defense: Buffering (immediate).
  - Second defense: Respiratory alteration in arterial pCO_2 (minutes to hours).
  - Third defense: Renal alteration in HCO_3 excretion (hours to days).
- These components work together to maintain a fine balance in order to maintain the extracellular pH around 7.4 (range 7.35-7.45).
- The pH has a widespread effect on cell function: most cell enzymes work best at physiological pH. An abnormal pH can result in disturbances in a many body systems.

APPLIED PHYSICS

- The acidity of the solution is a measure of the hydrogen ion activity
- The normal concentration of H^+ is in nanomole range (nmol/L). 1 nmol/L = 10^{-6} milliequivalents/L, compared to H^+ concentration, serum sodium concentration is 3 million times.
- The pH scale was developed in order to simplify the confusion of handling a large range of numbers, figures and units. The p refers to the German word *'potenz'* (power), so pH means 'power of hydrogen'.
- The pH is calculated by taking the negative logarithm of the hydrogen ion concentration in nmol/l.
- pH = - log [H^+]. Because of the log function, a small change in pH represents a significant change in the H^+ concentration. A change in pH of one point results in a 10-fold change in the hydrogen ion concentration.
- Although the physiological pH of the extracellular fluid is 7.4 (and the intracellular pH is 6.9), a pH of 7.0 is neutral because the H^+ and OH^+ concentration is the same.

Henderson-Hasselbalch equation

- The Henderson-Hasselbalch equation provides the basis for the relationship between the blood pH, $paCO_2$ and HCO_3^-, and it is shown below. The calculation, however, has no practical value.
  $pH = pK + \log [HCO_3^-/paCO_2]$

APPROACH TO DISORDERS

- The usual format of a blood gas result that is obtained from most analyzers world wide will have the following format

7.40/40/98/24/2, or $pH/paCO_2/paO_2/HCO_3^-/BE$

Approach to diagnosing acid-base and gas exchange disorders

First, although not strictly an acid base disorder, important information about the patient's **oxygenation status** must be assessed from an ABG report.

Parameter	Expanded form	Normal range	Units
pH	Arterial blood pH	7.35-7.45	
$paCO_2$	Arterial CO_2 tension	35-45	mmHg
paO_2	Arterial O_2 tension	70-100	mmHg
HCO_3	Serum bicarbonate concentration	22-26	mEq/liter
SBE	Standard base excess	-2 to +2	mEq/liter

Is hypoxemia present?

- *Hypoxia* refers to reduced oxygen pressure in the alveolus. By convention, alveolar oxygen notation is pAO_2 (note the capital "A").
- *Hypoxemia* refers to low arterial oxygen tension. Arterial oxygen tension is notated as paO_2 (note the small "a").
- *Quantification/objective assessment of hypoxemia* may be facilitated by:
  - Calculating the alveolar-arterial oxygen gradient
  - Calculating the ratio between the arterial oxygen pressure (paO_2) and the inspired oxygen tension (FiO_2), also known as the paO_2/FiO_2 ratio or p/F ratio
  - The normal paO_2/FiO_2 ratio is > 450-500.
  - As a rough estimation, the expected paO_2 is 5 times the concentration of the inspired oxygen expressed as a percentage.
- How can we calculate the gradient between the alveolar oxygen and measured arterial oxygen tension? (Generally expressed as the alveolar-arterial oxygen gradient, the $AaDO_2$)
- A normal gradient of about 10 mmHg exists between alveolar oxygen pressure (pAO_2) and the arterial oxygen pressure (paO_2).
- Generally, there is no gradient between the alveolar carbon dioxide pressure ($pACO_2$) and the arterial $paCO_2$.
- In the alveolus, a reciprocal relationship exists between oxygen and carbon dioxide. Carbon dioxide accumulation as a result of inadequate ventilation displaces oxygen from the alveolus and decreases the oxygen available for gas exchange.
- The reciprocal relationship between the pAO_2 and $pACO_2$ is illustrated by the Alveolar Gas Equation shown below.

Alveolar oxygen (pAO_2) = FiO_2 (760–46) - ($paCO_2$ x 1.25) *where*

- FiO_2 = fraction of inspired oxygen which is 0.21 for ambient air,
- 46 stands for the water vapour pressure.
- The correction factor for pCO_2 is derived by dividing by R (respiratory quotient, which is estimated to be 0.8) OR multiplying by 1.25
- The $pACO_2$ is equivalent to $paCO_2$ because there is no gradient.

- Alveolar arterial oxygen gradient ($AaDO_2$) = $pAO_2 - paO_2$. Where pAO_2 is calculated as above and paO_2 is read off from the blood gas.
- These relationships are most pertinent in cases of hypercarbia or elevated $paCO_2$.
- In patients with central hypoventilation, the $AaDO_2$ may be normal despite hypoxemia provided the lungs are normal. In patients with intrinsic airway or parenchymal disease, the $AaDO_2$ will be increased with concomitant hypoxemia.

Following assessment of oxygenation, one can proceed to the following:

Stepwise approach to diagnosing acid-base disorders

Acidemia and **alkalemia** refer to the alterations

in the blood pH. Both respiratory and metabolic disorders can contribute to alterations in pH and are referred to as a respiratory acidosis or respiratory alkalosis, and a metabolic acidosis or metabolic alkalosis. A single disorder may account for the observed acidemia or alkalemia, but often more than one disorder occurs concurrently. These are referred to as mixed or complex acid base disorders. Identifying the simple as well as the complex acid base disorders will be possible by applying the stepwise approach outlined in the following sections.

Step 1: Acidemic or alkalemic?

- The pH of the arterial blood gas measurement identifies the disorder as alkalemic or acidemic.
- Normal arterial blood pH = 7.40 ± 0.05
- Acidemic: pH < 7.35
- Alkalemic: pH > 7.45

Step 2: Is the primary disturbance respiratory or metabolic?

- This step requires one to determine whether the disturbance affects primarily the arterial $paCO_2$ or the serum HCO_3^-
- A respiratory disturbance alters the arterial $paCO_2$ (normal value 40, range 35-45). →*Go to step 3.*
- A metabolic disturbance alters the serum HCO_3^- (normal value 24, range 20-26).
- If HCO_3^- < 20, metabolic acidosis is present. →*Go to step 5.*
- If HCO_3^- > 26, metabolic alkalosis is present, determine if respiratory compensation is adequate? →*Go to step 6.*

Step 3: For a respiratory disturbance, determine whether it is acute or chronic.

- A respiratory acidosis results from accumulation of $paCO_2$ and a respiratory alkalosis results from hyperventilation or a low $paCO_2$ (specific causes of respiratory acidosis and alkalosis are listed in following section).
- For acute disturbances, a $paCO_2$ variation from normal by 10 mmHg is accompanied by a pH shift of approximately 0.08 units.
- A chronic disturbance reflects renal mediated HCO_3^- shifts. Renal compensation requires several hours to develop and is maximal after 4 days.
- Therefore, during chronic disturbances, a $PaCO_2$ variation from normal of 10 is accompanied by a smaller pH shift of only 0.03 units.
- Also, the renal correction brings the pH back towards normal, but not completely. These relationships are detailed in the following equations:

  Acute respiratory acidosis: pH decrease $= 0.08 \times (paCO_2 - 40)/10$

  Chronic respiratory acidosis: pH decrease $= 0.03 \times (paCO_2 - 40)/10$

  Acute respiratory alkalosis: pH increase $= 0.08 \times (40 - paCO_2)/10$

  Chronic respiratory alkalosis: pH increase $= 0.03 \times (40 - paCO_2)/10$

Step 4: For a respiratory disorder, is metabolic compensation adequate?

- Knowledge of the empirical limits of compensation is essential to evaluate if the change in HCO_3^- is appropriate for the change in pCO_2.
- The limits of compensation are dictated not only by the nature of the disorder (respiratory acidosis vs alkalosis), but also by the duration of the disorder (acute vs chronic).
- Thus the upper limits for compensation are:

  Respiratory acidosis:

  <24 hrs: $\Delta [HCO_3] = 1/10\ \Delta\ pCO_2$

  >24 hrs: $\Delta [HCO_3] = 3/10\ \Delta\ pCO_2$

  Respiratory alkalosis:

  1- 2 hrs: $\Delta [HCO_3] = 2/10\ \Delta\ pCO_2$

  >2 days: $\Delta [HCO_3] = 6/10\ \Delta\ pCO_2$

Step 5: Assess the normal compensation by the respiratory system for a metabolic disturbance.

- The respiratory system responds quickly to a

metabolic disturbance and most predictably to a metabolic acidosis.

- The change in $paCO_2$ exhibits a linear correlation with the change in HCO_3^-.
- The equation that predicts the respiratory response to a metabolic acidosis is called Winter's formula:
  Expected $paCO_2 = (1.5 \times HCO_3^-) + (8 \pm 2)$
- In the setting of a simple metabolic acidosis, the measured $paCO_2$ will fall within the range predicted by Winter's formula.
- If a respiratory disturbance is occurring concurrently with the metabolic acidosis, it would be defined by the direction the $paCO_2$ varies outside the range predicted by Winter's formula, not by the $paCO_2$ variation from the normal value of 40.
- Working through the following example illustrates how to utilize Winter's formula to assess the respiratory response to metabolic acidosis.

If the serum HCO_3^- is 10 mEq/L, the $paCO_2$ should be between 21 and 25 according to Winter's formula. If the measured $paCO_2$ falls outside of this range, then an additional respiratory disturbance must be occurring concurrently. If the measured $paCO_2$ is less than 21, then the additional disturbance is a respiratory alkalosis. If the measured $paCO_2$ is greater than 25, then the additional disturbance is a respiratory acidosis.

- Winter's formula does not predict the respiratory response to a metabolic alkalosis.
- The magnitude of respiratory response to metabolic alkalosis is not easily predictable. When present, the respiratory response to metabolic alkalosis is hypoventilation, but the degree of $paCO_2$ increase does not exhibit a linear relationship with the HCO_3^-.
- Two general rules hold up for the respiratory response to a metabolic alkalosis:
  - A patient will increase $paCO_2$ above 40 but not greater than 50-55 to compensate for a metabolic alkalosis.
  - A patient will be alkalemic (pH > 7.42) if the $paCO_2$ is elevated to compensate for a metabolic alkalosis (If the patient is acidemic, pH < 7.38, then an additional respiratory acidosis is present).

Step 6: For a metabolic acidosis, determine whether an anion gap is present.

- The anion gap calculation simplifies the diagnosis of the cause for a metabolic acidosis.
- What is the anion gap? The normal anion gap is 12 mEq/L.
- The anion gap is the calculated difference between negatively charged (anion) and positively charged (cation) electrolytes, which are measured in routine serum assays.
- The total of measured cations represented by sodium (Na^+), is greater than the total measured anions, HCO_3^- and chloride (Cl^-).
- Turned around, that difference or gap also can be viewed as the unmeasured anion concentration. The unmeasured anion concentration dominates the balance between the unmeasured serum anions (albumin, organic acids, phosphates, sulpates) and cations (calcium, potassium, magnesium).
- The causes of an anion gap acidosis differ from those of a normal or non-anion gap acidosis (see causes of metabolic acidosis below).
- The anion gap determination is an excellent tool for narrowing the list of potential causes of a metabolic acidosis.
- The simple calculation is shown below.

The anion gap calculation requires values for the serum Na^+, Cl^-, and HCO_3^-:
Anion gap = $Na^+ - (Cl^- + HCO_3^-)$,

- Anion gap metabolic acidosis, anion gap > 12. Normal or non-anion gap acidosis, anion gap <12
- The calculation of the anion gap provides reliable data with the following rare exceptions: Patients with *a low serum albumin* (e.g., cir-

rhosis, nephrotic syndrome, malnutrition) have an anion gap acidosis, but the measured anion gap is normal or < 12. The reason is that albumin has many negative charges on its surface and accounts for a significant proportion of the unmeasured anions.

Step 7: Determine whether other metabolic disturbances co-exist with an anion gap acidosis.

- A non-anion gap acidosis or a metabolic alkalosis may exist concurrently with an anion gap acidosis.
- This determination requires one to account for the increase in the anion gap and determine whether additional variation in HCO_3^- exists. If no other metabolic disturbance exists, then the following calculation would result in 24: Corrected HCO_3^- = Measured HCO_3^- + (anion gap – 12)
- If the corrected HCO_3^- varies significantly above or below 24, then a mixed or more complex metabolic disturbance exists.
- To be more specific, if the corrected HCO_3^- is greater than 24, a metabolic alkalosis co-exists. If the corrected HCO_3^- is less than 24 then a non-gap acidosis co-exists.
- The following examples help one understand how this step works. A patient with an anion gap metabolic acidosis has a HCO_3^- of 10 mEq/L and an anion gap of 26. By calculating the corrected HCO_3^- one finds the result to be 24 and can conclude that no other metabolic disturbance co-exists. If this patient had a HCO_3^- of 15 and an anion gap of 26, then the corrected HCO_3^- would be calculated to 29, a value significantly greater than 24. One would then conclude that metabolic alkalosis co-exists with the gap acidosis.

SPECIFIC ACID-BASE DISORDERS AND DIAGNOSES

1. **Respiratory acidosis**

   Respiratory acidosis results from ypoventilation which is manifested by the accumulation of CO_2 in the blood and a drop in blood pH. Examples of specific causes can be categorized as follows:
   - Central nervous system depression (sedatives, CNS disease, obesity hypoventilation syndrome)
   - Pleural disease (pneumothorax, effusion)
   - Lung disease (bronchiolitis, pneumonia)
   - Musculo-skeletal disorders (kyphoscoliosis, Guillain Barre, myasthenia gravis, polio)

2. **Respiratory alkalosis**

   Respiratory alkalosis results from hyperventilation which is manifested by excess elimination of CO_2 from the blood and a rise in the blood pH. Examples of specific causes are listed below:
   - Catastrophic CNS event (CNS hemorrhage)
   - Drugs (salicylates)
   - Decreased lung compliance (interstitial lung disease)
   - Liver cirrhosis
   - Anxiety

3. **Anion gap metabolic acidosis**

   Anion gap acidosis results from accumulation of acidic metabolites and is manifested by a low HCO_3^- and an anion gap > 12 (anion gap calculation discussed in step 3). Examples of specific causes:
   - Uremia
   - Ketoacidosis, diabetic hyperglycemia.
   - Alcohol poisons or drug intoxication (methanol, ethylene glycol, paraldehyde, salicylates)
   - Lactic acidosis (sepsis, left ventricular failure)

One may use a mnemonic device to remember these items. MULEPAK is a mnemonic commonly used (methanol, uremia, lactic acidosis, ethylene glycol intoxication, paraldehyde intoxication, aspirin, ketoacidosis). (Also KUSMAL & MUDPIES)

4. **Non-anion gap metabolic acidosis**
   - Non-anion gap acidosis results from loss of bicarbonate or external acid infusion and is manifested by a low HCO_3^-, but the anion gap is <12.
   - Examples of specific causes:
     - GI loss of HCO_3^- (diarrhea)
     - Renal loss of $HCO3^-$
     - Compensation for respiratory alkalosis
     - Carbonic anhydrase inhibitor (Diamox)
     - Renal tubular acidosis

Table. 19.1 7 Steps to your ABG

Step 1	Is it Acidosis (pH < 7.35) Or Alkalosis (pH > 7.45)
Step 2	If it is Acidosis is it – Respiratory (pCO_2 > 45) or – Metabolic (HCO_3 < 20) If it is Alkalosis is it – Respiratory (pCO_2 < 35) Or – Metabolic (HCO_3 > 28)
Step 3	If it is a Respiratory problem – **Is it Acute?** Calculate Δ pH Δ pH = 0.08 x Δ pCO2 /10 Expected pH = 7.4 – Δ pH If the pH in the ABG is = to the expected pH then it is acute If the pH in the ABG is > the expected pH then it is chronic
Step 4	If it is a Respiratory problem – **Is the renal compensation OK?** In Resp Acidosis - < 24 hours - Δ HCO_3 = 1/10 x Δ pCO_2 > 24 hours - Δ HCO_3 = 3/10 x Δ pCO_2 In Resp Alkalosis- < 2 hours - Δ HCO_3 = 2/10 x Δ pCO_2 > 2 days - Δ HCO_3 = 6/10 x Δ pCO_2
Step 5	If it is a Metabolic problem – **Is the respiratory compensation OK?** In metabolic acidosis - Expected PCO_2 = (1.5x HCO_3) +8 ± 2 In metabolic alkalosis Expected pCO_2 = (0.7x HCO_3) + 21± 1.5
Step 6	If Metabolic Acidosis – **Look for anion gap (AG)** AG = Na – (Cl + HCO_3) If AG > 12 Look for causes – MUDPIE
Step 7	In Metabolic acidosis – **Does the AG account for the change in HCO_3?** Usually Δ AG = Δ HCO_3 If AG is > Consider additional metabolic alkalosis If AG is < Consider non AG metabolic acidosis

- Ureteral diversion
- Other causes: Hyperalimentation

A mnemonic device may be used to remember this list of causes. The commonly used mnemonic is ACCRUED (acid infusion, compensation for respiratory alkalosis, carbonic anhydrase inhibitor, renal tubular acidosis, ureteral diversion, "extra" alimentation or hyperalimentation, diarrhea).

5. **Metabolic alkalosis**

Metabolic alkalosis results from elevation of serum bicarbonate. Examples of specific causes:
- Volume contraction (vomiting, overdiuresis, ascites)
- Hypokalemia
- Alkali ingestion (bicarbonate)
- Excess gluco- or mineralocorticoids
- Bartter's syndrome.

REFERENCES

1. Ram E Rajagopalan. An Approach to the Analysis of Arterial Blood Gases and Acid-Base Disorders. Modified from Teaching Resource of the ICU Refresher course, Chennai

SECTION 6 : MECHANICAL VENTILATION

20 Assisted Ventilation in Children: Basic Physiology and Terminology

INTRODUCTION

- **Respiration** is defined as the process of gas exchange within the lungs (external) or at the tissue level (internal).
- **Ventilation** may be defined as the movement of air in and out of the lungs.
- It may be spontaneous (patient breathing for himself) or assisted.
- *Assisted ventilation* involves an external device connected directly to the patient that generates a controlled flow of gas into a patient's airway. This device may be a resuscitative bag or a mechanical ventilator.
- Ventilation requires the development of a *pressure gradient* between the mouth and the alveoli.
  - During *spontaneous breathing,* this gradient is achieved by contraction of the respiratory muscles that enlarge the pleural cavity and lower pleural and intra-alveolar pressure to sub-atmospheric. This pressure gradient causes air to move into the lungs.
  - During *positive pressure ventilation (PPV),* a higher pressure is generated by the ventilator and gases flow from the ventilator down the pressure gradient into the alveoli.
  - Expiration is usually passive. The natural elastic recoil of the lung tissue causes an increase in intra-alveolar pressure which reverses the pressure gradient and allows air to flow out of the lungs.
- **Positive pressure ventilators**: The central premise of positive pressure ventilation is that gas flows along a pressure gradient between the upper airway and the alveoli. The magnitude, rate and duration of flow are determined by the operator.
- Most ICUs use conventional ventilators which provide breathing patterns that attempt to replicate physiological breathing. The tidal volumes will be greater than the anatomical dead space and the set breathing frequency will be the same or slightly less than age appropriate rates for the patient.
- These are opposed to High Frequency Oscillation Ventilators (HFOV) that employ tidal volumes < dead space at extremely high frequencies. HFOV are employed for a special set of extremely sick patients.
- Pressure, volume, and flow are functions of time and are called *variables.* More will be described in the following sections.
- Oxygen and air are received from cylinders or wall outlets, the gas is pressure reduced and blended according to the prescribed inspired oxygen tension (FiO_2), accumulated in a receptacle within the machine, and delivered to the patient using one of many available modes of ventilation.
- Flow is either *volume targeted (volume controlled)* and pressure variable, or *pressure limited (pressure controlled)* and volume variable.

- The pattern of flow may be either sinusoidal (which is normal), decelerating or constant. Flow is controlled by an array of sensors and microprocessors.

PHYSIOLOGY OF NORMAL VENTILATION

1. **Functional residual capacity (FRC)**
   - This is the volume of gas remaining in the lungs at the end of normal expiration.
   - The FRC is a balance of the forces causing outward recoil of the chest wall (maintains alveolar inflation) vs those causing elastic inward recoil of the lungs (promotes alveolar closure).
   - Disease states that decrease FRC can cause hypoxemia (pneumonia, ARDS).
   - This can often be overcome by restoring FRC by increasing baseline airway pressure using CPAP/PEEP.
2. **Closing capacity (CC) / Closing volume**
   - *Closing capacity (CC)* or Closing volume is the volume of lung that is still inflated when small airways in the dependent parts of the lung begin to collapse during expiration.
   - In normal health, closing volume is less than FRC and accounts for the residual volume (RV) of the lung at the end of expiration.
   - Which conditions can cause CC to become greater than FRC?
   - In yonger children (< 6 years), certain restrictive lung diseases and post-thoracic surgical states result in reduction of FRC below the CC.
   - This is because the outward recoil of the chest wall is insufficient to balance the alveolar closure at these volumes.
   - These patients have a greater tendency for atelectasis of dependent lung regions, even during tidal breathing.
   - Application of PEEP can result in restoration of FRC to greater than the CC levels by opening up collapsed regions of the lung.
3. **Applied pulmonary mechanics**

   The predominant factors which influence distribution of inspired gases are:

   a) Compliance

   b) Resistance

   c) Time constants

   a) *Compliance*
   - Compliance of the lung is defined as the change in volume per unit change in pressure and is expressed in ml/cmH_2O.

     Compliance (ml/cmH_2O) = Change in volume/unit change in pressure

   - It is a measure of the *'stiffness'* of the chest and is determined by elastic forces of the lung, chest wall as well as surface tension generated within the alveoli.
   - Total lung compliance is the summation of both lung and chest wall compliance.
   - Chest wall compliance is a function of the elastic recoil of the chest wall and may decrease in edematous states.
   - Normal lungs are highly compliant *(less stiff)*.
   - *Static compliance* is measured by the change in tidal volume that occurs with a change in trans-pulmonary pressure or "delta P" (ΔP) = (plateau pressure – PEEP) in a sedated/muscle relaxed patient. It is measured when flow into the airways and lungs has ceased.

     Static compliance =Tidal volume/ (plateau pressure – PEEP)

   - *Dynamic compliance* is the compliance measured during spontaneous breathing when flow into the lungs is continuing. This better reflects the elastic recoil of the lungs.

Dynamic compliance =Tidal volume/PIP–PEEP.

- Diseased lungs may have reduced compliance *(increased stiffness)* requiring higher pressures to produce lung expansion, e.g., *restrictive lung diseases,* such as ARDS, pneumonia, Hyaline Membrane Disease (HMD), pulmonary edema.
- It is often forgotten that decreased lung compliance may also be seen in patients with *over-distended lungs/high lung volumes* (severe bronchiolitis, asthma, high PEEP).
- Normal compliance ranges from 5 ml/cmH_2O in smaller infants to 50-100 ml/cmH_2O in adults.

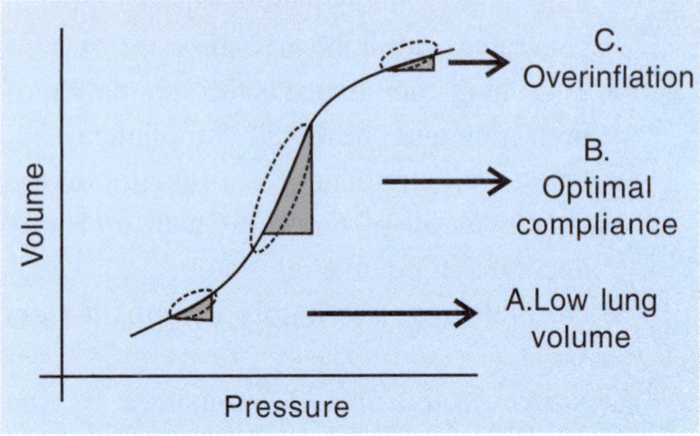

Fig. 20.1 The pressure-volume curve

Figure 20.1 describes the lung compliance curve where

- The most favorable portion of the curve is loop B where a small change in pressure produces a large change in volume *(optimal compliance).*
- Both loops A and C demonstrate small changes in volume despite the same changes in pressure *(reduced compliance).*
- Loop A states may be seen in diseases with low lung volumes and that require application of PEEP to open alveoli/lung units.
- Loop C, conversely, may be seen in over-distended lungs where further increments of distending pressure produce only minimal rise in volumes.
- When ventilating a patient, the practitioner may try to ventilate the patient on the most favorable part of the pressure volume curve (loop B) by application of PEEP in order to keep diseased alveoli open while simultaneously attempting to minimize lung over-distension by limiting distending volumes and pressures.

b) *Airway resistance*

- Airway resistance is the pressure difference between the mouth and alveoli and is expressed in cmH_2O/litre/second.
- The determinants of airway resistance during laminar flow are the viscosity of the gas and length of tube divided by the fourth power of the radius of the airways (trachea, bronchi, bronchioles).
- The *radius of the airways is the most important contributor to airway resistance.*
- Even minor degrees of narrowing of the airway from bronchospasm, edema or mucus accumulation can cause significant increase in airway resistance.
- Total pulmonary resistance is determined by both airway resistance (major contributor) and tissue resistance (viscous resistance of lung tissue).
- Expiratory resistance is greater than inspiratory resistance and clinically more significant as expiration is passive (as opposed to inspiratory effort that is active).
- Excessive expiratory resistance may result in air-trapping that may also result in mechanical disadvantage with greater imposed inspiratory loads to the spontaneously breathing patient.

c) *Time constant (TC)*

- The time constant of a person's lungs is a measure of how quickly the lungs can inhale or exhale or how long it takes for pressures delivered in the proximal airways to reach the alveoli.

- The time constant is the product of airway resistance and compliance and is measured in seconds.
- Three to five time constants are required for complete filling or emptying of an alveolar unit.
- In a normal infant, one time constant equals 0.15 seconds and three time constants equal 0.45 seconds.
- Various disease states can alter the time constants and understanding the concept of time constants aids greatly in choosing the safest and most effective ventilator setting for an individual patient.
- The TC will be prolonged in disease states associated with increased resistance (bronchiolitis, asthma): a longer time is required for emptying of the lungs.
  However, these patients are clinically tachypneic, with less than normal expiratory times. Thus, a significant fraction of the tidal volume remains trapped in the lungs with each breath: this results in *air-trapping* or *intrinsic PEEP.*
- Ventilatory strategies in such diseases must cater to the prolonged TC by providing greater than normal expiratory time with slow rates.
- Conversely, diseases associated with reduced compliance (ARDS, pneumonia) have reduced TC and can be safely ventilated with higher rates, longer inspiratory and shorter expiratory times. Oxygenation improves but risk of air trapping is less.
- However, it is important to remember that many critically ill patients have heterogeneous lung diseases (areas of hyper-inflation co-existing with atelectasis) and ventilatory strategies must be carefully customized in order to avoid iatrogenic complications.

ASSISTED VENTILATION

Mechanical ventilation may deliver a volume of gas to the patient's lungs in one of two ways.

- Positive pressure ventilation: Positive pressure is applied directly to the airways which forces air down the airways and into the lungs.
- Negative pressure ventilation: Negative pressure is applied externally to the chest cage which changes the pressure dynamics such that gas flows from the relatively positive atmosphere to the relatively negative air spaces.
  - Negative pressure ventilators range from tank ventilators (iron lungs) to abdominal and thoracic cuirasses.
  - Although negative pressure ventilators are more physiological and avoid many of the complications of endotracheal intubation and positive pressure ventilation, the apparatus is more cumbersome and access to the patient is limited.
  - Both techniques may be used in pediatric ventilation although positive pressure ventilation is more common by far.
  - As discussed previously, gas flows along a pressure gradient between the upper airway and the alveoli.
- Flow is controlled within the ventilator by an array of sensors and microprocessors. Additionally, the magnitude, rate and duration of flow are determined by the operator so as to deliver a controlled rate of flow into the patient's airways.

Basic terminology of mechanical ventilation

1. **Flow pattern**

   There are several types of flow patterns depending on the breath type and mode of ventilation. These include constant, accelerating, decelerating or sinusoidal patterns of flow.

   - *Decelerating flow*
     - Decelerating flows may be more physiologic and is seen in pressure targeted

ventilation (pressure control and pressure support).
- Rapid initial flow fills large airways first, flow slows down as alveolar pressure increases and smaller airways then fill with a more laminar flow.
- The flow is *variable* and depends on compliance, resistance and patient effort. The flow can increase if the patient's peak flow requirements are high.
- Since the flow is not limited, it leads to better synchrony.
- This flow pattern results in a *lower peak and higher mean airway pressure* than constant flow.
- Decelerating flows have better distribution characteristics particularly in heterogeneous lung units that have both slow and fast units.

- *Constant flow*
  - Flow waveform is preset and continues at a constant rate until the set tidal volume is delivered.
  - Constant flow pattern is seen in volume targeted ventilation.
  - The generated PIP is higher and mean airway pressures are lower than with decelerating flows.
- *Sinusoidal* = this is the flow pattern seen in spontaneous breathing and CPAP.
- *Continuous flow vs constant flow*
  - Continuous flow needs to be differentiated from constant flow. Constant flow occurs *only during the inspiratory period* at a constant flow rate.
  - Most infant ventilators have a continuous flow of gas into the circuit *throughout the respiratory cycle.*
  - During inspiration, the expiratory valve closes and gas flow is diverted to the patient's lungs. At the end of inspiration, the expiratory valve opens and gas flows out of the lungs.
  - Since there is a continuous flow of gas in the circuit, spontaneous breathing efforts are facilitated.
  - However, there is greater wastage of oxygen and expiratory resistance may increase and contribute to work of breathing and weaning difficulty.

2. **Tidal volume** (VT)
   - This is the volume of gas that flows in and out of the chest during quiet breathing.
   - In adults, the normal tidal volume is 500 ml. In children the tidal volume ranges from 6-12 ml/kg.
   - Current best practice stress the importance of minimizing ventilation induced lung injury (VILI) by limiting tidal volumes to 6 ml/kg for both normal and diseased lung (lung protective ventilation).

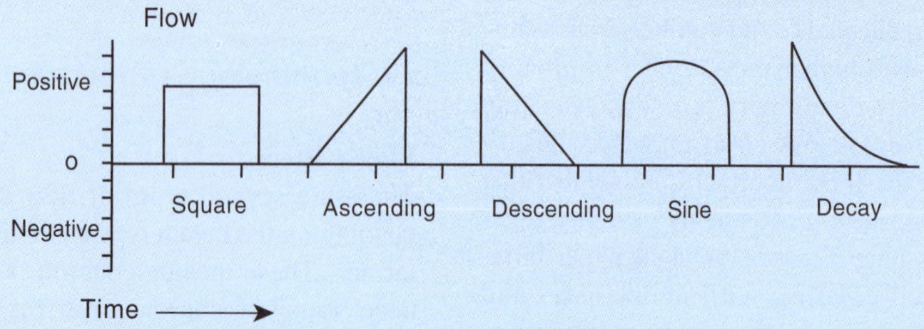

Fig. 20.2 Types of flow patterns

3. **Frequency/ventilatory rate ('f')**
   - The rate that is initially set depends on the indication for ventilation and the physiologic norm for the patient's age.
4. **Minute ventilation (MV)**
   - This is the product of the tidal volume and the ventilatory rate and is expressed in litres/minute.
5. **Peak inspiratory pressure (PIP)**
   - This is the highest pressure that can be met during the inspiratory period.
   - The PIP level is usually kept as low as possible since it has been implicated as one of the causes of barotrauma.
6. **Positive end expiratory pressure (PEEP)**
   - PEEP is usually applied by regulating pressure in the expiratory valve of the ventilator system and is designed to keep alveoli from collapsing at the end of expiration.
   - PEEP improves oxygenation by recruiting (splinting open) diseased alveoli and thus improving FRC.
   - A normal level of PEEP (physiological PEEP) is 3-5 cmH_2O.
   - Higher PEEP (10-15 cm or, on occasion, even greater) may be used with caution in the child with diffusely non-compliant lungs and has become the mainstay of treatment of ARDS and pulmonary edema.

> The **hemodynamic effects of PEEP** depend on the state of cardiac function:
> - PEEP decreases cardiac output by decreasing venous return in a patient with a normal heart.
> - However when cardiac function is impaired, PEEP improves cardiac output by
>   - ↓ LV afterload (positive intra-thoracic pressure helps forward flow of a failing heart)
>   - ↓ LV preload is helpful when heart function is impaired (similar to diuresis).
>   - ↓ Work of breathing by improving compliance
>   - Improved oxygenation.

   - PEEP can also be generated in alveoli if the expiratory time is inadequate for the lung to return to its "rest volume" or if significant flow limitation prevents full lung emptying (intrinsic PEEP, sometimes referred to as "auto-PEEP," "occult PEEP," or "air trapping").
   - *Adverse effects of PEEP*
     - While the most important function of PEEP is improving compliance of atelectatic lungs, excess PEEP can paradoxically decrease compliance by causing overinflation. Excess PEEP also increases dead space (with CO_2 retention).
     - Hyperinflated lungs segments can have decreased perfusion (Q) as the capillaries perfusing these areas are compressed: V/Q mismatch can potentially worsen.
     - This is most likely to occur in heterogeneous lung disease where some areas of collapsed lung co-exist with normal segments. PEEP can preferentially hyperinflate the normal lung with a lesser change of the collapsed areas.
     - PEEP can contribute to barotrauma.
     - PEEP can ↑ intracranial tension by ↓cerebral venous return, this is more of concern when PEEP levels are > 15 cmH_2O.
   - *The optimal PEEP* must be a balance between maintaining adequate oxygenation by recruiting collapsed segments at safe levels of FiO_2 while maintaining adequate tissue perfusion.
7. **Inspiratory time and I:E ratios**
   - The I:E ratio refers to the relationship between inspiratory time (I) and expiratory time (E). The normal I:E ratio is usually 1:1.5 to 1:2.
   - Adjustment of the inspiratory time is the primary method by which the I:E ratio is altered.
   - Normal settings for I-time range from 0.45 to 1.5 seconds depending on the ventilatory rate and underlying lung disease.

- The major consideration when adjusting inspiratory times and I:E ratios should be the specific type and severity of lung disease.
- Expiratory times may be decreased to < 0.5 seconds only in conditions with reduced compliance and short time constants. Here the risk of air-trapping is low.
- Oxygenation can be improved without increasing peak airway pressure by using prolonged inspiratory times. This results in a reversal of the I:E ratio, such that inspiration is as long or longer than expiration *(inverse I:E ratios).*
- Inverse ratio ventilation also results in the development of *auto-PEEP* and is employed as a strategy to improve oxygenation in ARDS. However, It can result in increased dead-space and the consequent rise of pCO_2.

8. **FiO_2**
   - FiO_2 stands for fractional inspired oxygen concentration where 100% oxygen is represented as 1.0, oxygen in room air (21%) as 0.21 and so on.
9. **Mean airway pressure (MAP)**
   - This is not a ventilator setting, but rather the average positive pressure generated in the lung over time.
   - MAP is a critical factor in determining both oxygenation and the potential for barotrauma.
   - It is determined by several factors including PIP, PEEP, inspiratory time, flow rate and respiratory rate.
   - Many ventilators have the ability to continuously monitor and display MAP allowing the clinician to see the effects of ventilatory adjustments on this value.
10. **Variables vs parameters**

    An understanding of the various modes and types of ventilation may be greatly simplified if common definitions are understood.
   - Pressure, volume, and flow are functions of time and are called *variables.*
   - Depending on the mode of ventilation, one of the variables may be pre-determined, making it the *control variable* or *independent variable*, while the other two become the *dependent variables.*
   - Elastance/compliance and resistance are assumed to remain constant (for a given patient with a given disease state) and are called *parameters.*
11. **Phase variables**

    Because ventilation is a periodic event, the ventilator must be able to determine the various *phases* of the respiratory cycle, i.e., how a ventilator knows when to start, sustain and stop an inspiration and what it does between inspirations.

    One of the variables associated with the equation of motion (pressure, volume, flow or time) is used to start, sustain and end each phase. Hence, in this context, these are referred to as *phase variables.*

    A. *Trigger variable:* This is the parameter that controls the initiation of inspiration. Ventilators may be time triggered, pressure triggered or flow triggered.
      - *Time triggered ventilation*: Inspiration is initiated at a pre-determined time that is determined by the set frequency/rate independent of the patient's spontaneous inspiratory effort.
      - Time triggering is the commonest way that ventilator breaths are delivered to a patient on controlled or mandatory mode of ventilation. The patient's effort or co-operation is not required.
      - Synchronized, assisted and pressure supported modes require the ventilator to sense the patient effort so that the ventilator delivered breath is appropriately coordinated and in synchrony with the patient's neural respiratory drive.
      - Pressure and flow triggering are mechanisms that allow the patient's effort to be reliably sensed.

- *Pressure triggered ventilation*: The ventilator senses a drop in the baseline pressure caused by the patient's inspiratory effort and initiates a mechanical breath (Fig. 20.3).
- Lowering the baseline airway pressure in order to trigger the ventilator requires effort by the patient.
- *Flow triggered ventilation*: Modern ventilators deliver a low constant background flow rate in the circuit throughout the respiratory cycle *(flow-by)*. A deflection in this flow by the patient's inspiratory effort is detected by the ventilator resulting in a breath being delivered.
- While flow triggering requires less work by the patient than pressure triggering, system leaks (including that produced by the use of uncuffed tubes) may lead to asynchrony.
- The *response time* determines how quickly the ventilator delivers a breath in response to a patient effort.
- The degree of patient effort required to trigger inspiration determines the *sensitivity* setting.
- Setting the sensitivity too low may increase the work of breathing (the patient must create a higher intra-thoracic negative pressure in order to get assistance from the ventilator).
- Setting the sensitivity too high may lead to over-triggering and the patient being over ventilated.
- Whether flow or pressure triggering is selected, the trigger should be sensitive enough so that all the patient's efforts are sensed but not too sensitive in order to avoid over-triggering.

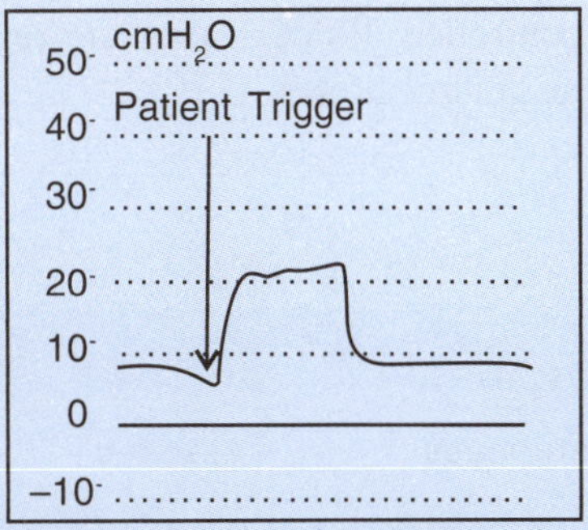

Fig. 20.3 Pressure trigger is a fall in the baseline pressure initiated by the patient's spontaneous effort

B. *Limit variable:* This is the variable that determines the magnitude of inspiration.
   - A limit variable can be reached and maintained at a pre-set value during inspiration, but does not end the inspiratory period.
   - Pressure, volume or time may be limit variables, and more than one can act in a single breath (dual control).
   - The limit variable does not end inspiration: it only sets an upper limit for pressure, volume or flow.

C. *Cycle variable*: This is the variable that determines the end of inspiration and the switch from inspiration to expiration.
   - Pressure, volume, flow or time may be cycle variables
   - Controlled modes and some assisted modes have *time* as the cycling variable, so that at the end of a pre-set inspiratory time, inspiration ends and cycles to expiration.
   - In the pressure support (PS) mode, *flow* is the cycling variable. Inspiration ends in the PS mode when the flow falls to a pre-determined percentage of the peak flow, signaling the end of the patient's spontaneous inspiratory effort.

REFERENCES

1. Venkataraman ST: Mechanical ventilation and Respiratory Care. In: Pediatric Critical Care. Fuhrman and Zimmerman (Eds). 3rd ed. Philadelphia, PA, 2006, Mosby Elsevier, 683-719.
2. Nelligan P. Critical Care forum

PEDIATRIC EMERGENCIES & CRITICAL CARE

21

Modes of Ventilation

- A ventilator mode may have a single or varying combinations of breath types that are delivered in a particular pattern. There is a wide variability in the way ventilatory modes are described amongst physicians and manufacturers. One method is described below.

When describing a particular ventilator mode, attention should be given to the following:
The breath type, control variable, timing of breath delivery or breath pattern.

1. BREATH TYPE

- *Mandatory/controlled breaths:* The ventilator controls the initiation (triggering), limit and the termination (cycling) of each breath.
- *Spontaneous breath:* Patient controls both the triggering and cycling of the breath. The limit may be ventilator or patient determined.

☞ **REMEMBER** Any breath that is terminated/cycled by the patient is always spontaneous.

- *Assisted breath:* These have variable combinations of both mandatory and spontaneous breaths. Breaths may be patient or ventilator triggered, limited and cycled.

2. CONTROL VARIABLE

- Essentially *volume control* or *pressure control*, newer modes have dual control.
- This is the key variable that the clinician controls when ventilating a patient. The chosen variable (pressure/volume) becomes the *independent variable* while the other becomes the *dependent variable.*
- The control variable decides what determines gas flow to the patient's lungs. Thus the breaths may be pressure controlled breaths or volume controlled/targeted breaths.
- A more recent type of controlled breath is dual controlled: PRVC – pressure regulated volume control breath.

Table 21.1 Determinants of a ventilator mode

1.	Breath type	Mandatory	Spontaneous	Assisted
2.	Control variable	Pressure control	Volume control	Dual control
3.	Timing of breath delivery/breath pattern	CMV	Spontaneous	Assisted

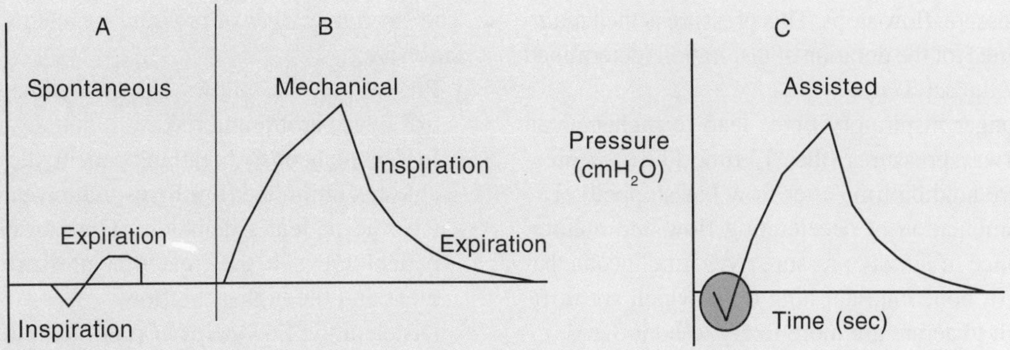

Fig. 21.1 Pressure scalars for spontaneous (A), mandatory/mechanical (B) and assisted breaths (C). *Note that inspiration is negative and expiration is positive for spontaneous breaths and vice versa for mechanical breaths: this is the fundamental difference between spontaneous ventilation and PPV.*

What are the differences between pressure control and volume control breaths?

A. Pressure controlled (PC) breaths

In PC breaths, pressure is the independent variable that remains constant whereas volume delivery is the dependent variable that can change. Here, the clinician has control over the set pressures and thus risk of barotrauma is less.

- In pressure control, a pressure limited, time cycled breath is delivered at a set rate.
- The resultant tidal volume is determined by the ΔP (difference between the PEEP and pre-set pressure limit, PIP), along with the compliance and resistance properties of the lung, airways and circuit and also patient effort.
- The inspiratory time (Ti) is also set by the operator.
- The flow waveform is *always decelerating* in pressure control: the high initial peak flow rate is *variable* (greater the pressure difference, the greater the flow).
- *Gas flows into the chest along the pressure gradient.* As the alveoli fill during inspiration the airway pressure rises, the pressure gradient decreases and the flow slows down. When the delivered pressure equals the pre-set airway

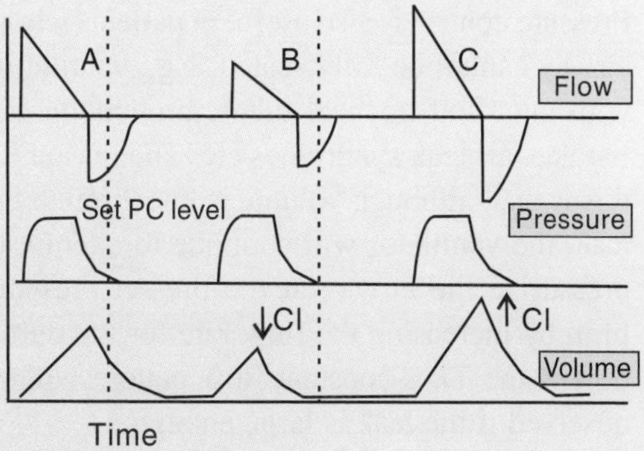

Fig. 21.2 Waveforms in pressure control ventilation in normal lung, and situations with decreased (↓) and increased (↑) compliance. Cl–lung compliance.

A: Normal compliance.
B: Decreased compliance: Note decreased flows and volumes although set pressures are same
C: Increased compliance: Note increased flows and volumes although set pressures are same

pressure, flow stops. This pressure is then maintained for the duration of inspiration (determined by the set Ti).

- Longer inspiratory times lead to higher mean airway pressures (the "I" time [Ti] is a pressure holding time after flow has stopped). The combination of decelerating flow and maintenance of airway pressure over time means that stiff, noncompliant lung units which are difficult to aerate are more likely to be inflated.
- *Gas distribution in pressure control is like dropping a glass of water on the floor: the water trickles into every nook and cranny.*
- Decelerating flow patterns improve the distribution of ventilation in a lung with heterogeneous mechanical properties (as in acute lung injury).
- Pressure control is also useful in patients whose airway cannot be fully sealed; e.g., ventilation with uncuffed tracheal tubes, bronchopleural fistulae, air leak syndromes etc. The reason for this is that, although volume is lost through the leak, the ventilator will continue to attempt to pressurize the airway at the pre-set pressure limit by increasing the flow rate for the duration of the Ti: a constant flow pattern will be observed if the leak is large enough.
- The *key advantages* of pressure targeted ventilation are:
  - Pre-set pressure allows clinician some control over barotrauma risk.
  - In a spontaneously breathing patient, the variable and unlimited flow in inspiration can satisfy the patient's demands. The harder the patient draws in, the greater the pressure gradient and the higher the flow.
  - Decelerating flow helps in ventilation of heterogeneous lungs with varying time constants.
- *Disadvantages of PC*
  - PC does not guarantee minute ventilation, hence tidal volumes are variable when pulmonary mechanics change. If there is a rapid decrease in the compliance and the lung becomes stiff, then the patient will receive lower tidal volumes for the same pressure. Hypercapnia/hypoxemia may ensue.
  - With improvement of the lung compliance/airway resistance, potentially excessive VT can occur, with paradoxical higher incidence of volutrauma/air leaks during recovery. Therefore, close clinical monitoring by the operator is required to adjust the set PIP

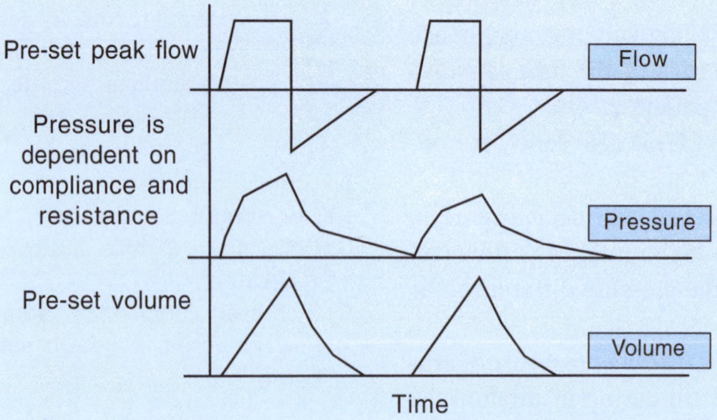

Fig. 21.3 Waveforms showing volume-control ventilation. Note that the volume is pre-set, hence remains constant. The generated pressure varies with compliance and resistance changes.

to prevent both hypoventilation and hyperventilation.

B. Volume controlled (VC) breaths (Fig. 21.3)

- VC breaths are chosen when the clinician desires constancy over the volumes delivered. VC is popular in older children.
- Volume control breaths may be part of a mandatory controlled mode (CMV) or SIMV.
- Volume controlled or regulated ventilation can be delivered by volume limited/regulated breath where the tidal volume delivered is regulated by adjusting the inspiratory flow rate. The cycling mechanism is inspiratory time which is pre-set.
- Some adult ventilators deliver VC breaths by delivering a *volume cycled breath*, where inspiration is terminated after a preset volume is delivered and Ti is allowed to vary.
- Thus, in volume control breaths, the cycling mechanism may be either time or volume.
- Both PIP and plateau pressures (Pplat = alveolar pressure) can be measured in volume control mode, unlike just PIP in PC.
- The flow waveform in VC is usually a constant flow. However, some ventilators have the option for decelerating flow in volume control.
- The *main advantage* of volume controlled ventilators is:
  - *Guaranteed (constant)* tidal volume (VT) and minute ventilation even with variable compliance and resistance. This is particularly important in patients with airway diseases (bronchial asthma) where pre-set volumes will be delivered despite narrow airways.
- *Drawbacks*
  - Although tidal volumes are guaranteed, *VC breaths do not have control of the pressure generated.* When compliance decreases or resistance increases, the same volume can generate higher pressures with the attendant risk of barotrauma.
  - The constant flow pattern is fixed and cannot increase in response to the patient's desired inspiratory flow demand (unlike the high variable decelerating flows in PC ventilation), thus there is a potential for asynchrony due to flow starvation and increases work of breathing (WOB).
  - Since the pre-set tidal volume is divided between the ventilator circuit, airways and the patient's lungs, the *effective tidal volume* that reaches the patient's lungs may be variable. Altered lung mechanics may result in more gas ventilating the ventilator circuit rather than the patient's lungs. *This is more relevant in infants with smaller tidal volume,* hence PC breaths may be preferred in this age group. Many ventilators have a "System Self Test" that needs to be performed prior to connecting the patient to the ventilator. This calculates and compensates for "compressible volume" of the circuit when measuring the expired VT.

C. PRVC (pressure regulated volume control) breaths

PRVC is a *dual control breath* where the ventilator adjusts the pressure 'breath by breath' to achieve the pre-set or target VT.

- When the PRVC mode is selected, the ventilator initially delivers a few test breaths to measure the generated pressure and calculates the total compliance. The ventilator then aims to deliver the pre-set VT at the lowest possible pressure level.
- If the measured exhaled VT (VTe) is less than the pre-set VT, the ventilator increases the pressure level progressively over several breaths until the pre-set and the monitored VTe are about equal.
- PRVC is a more *subtle* volume control mode that not only strives to maintain the minimum peak pressure required to keep target VT, but also maintains more consistent VT with varying compliance or resistance.

- If the volume generated is too low, the pressure level is increased to achieve the target tidal volumes. If the volume is too high, the pressure level is decreased.
- All patient initiated breaths also receive the same target VT.
- PRVC is thus a patient or time triggered, volume targeted, pressure regulated, time cycled breath.
- Variables that need to be set include the target VT, PEEP, rate, Ti percentage, and upper pressure limit.
- The ventilator does not allow the pressure to rise higher than 5 cmH_2O below the upper pressure limit setting. If the generated pressures are < 5 cmH_2O below the upper pressure limit, further gas flow is vented off, an audible alarm will sound and no further volume will be delivered. This alarm provides the clinician with an indicator of worsening lung (compliance/resistance) or ET status (kinks, secretions).
- If the problem cannot be rectified, the clinician may have to either increase the upper pressure limit in order to assure pre-set volume delivery or decrease the target VT if the delivered pressures are already too high.
- As the patient improves, less pressure is required to deliver the set volume.
- *Disadvantages of PRVC*
  When the patient's demand increases because of worsening disease, the tidal volumes may increase because of more patient effort. The ventilator responds by re-setting the pressure to a lower level, thus giving less ventilator support at a time when the patient may in fact be needing more.

3. TIMING OF BREATH DELIVERY, BREATH PATTERN OR MODE OF VENTILATION

As described earlier, the term **mode** includes 3 parts: the breath type, the control variable and the timing of breath delivery (breath pattern). There are 3 well described breath delivery techniques or modes.

- **CMV** = Controlled mechanical ventilation, without allowances for spontaneous breathing. **Assist-Control** = Where assisted breaths are facsimiles of controlled breaths.
- **Assisted Modes** = e.g., Intermittent Mandatory Ventilation **(IMV)** which mixes controlled breaths and spontaneous breaths. Breaths may also be ***synchronized*** to prevent "stacking" **(SIMV)**.
- **Spontaneous Modes (pressure support and CPAP)** = Here the patient has control over all aspects of his/her breath except the pressure limit.

Controlled mandatory/mechanical ventilation (CMV)

- When the ventilator delivers a tidal breath irrespective of the patient's effort, it is referred to as CMV.
- *CMV may utilize either pressure controlled, volume controlled or PRVC breaths.*
- In this mode, all breaths are initiated, limited (regulated) and cycled by the ventilator with the patient taking no active role in the ventilatory cycle.
- In general, this mode is reserved for patients who have insufficient/absent ventilatory drive (either from the disease process or iatrogenically due to sedative and/or paralytic agents).
- "Locking out" a patient's effort is appropriate only when the clinician desires very tight control of the pCO_2 (controlled hyperventilation for elevated ICP or pulmonary hypertension).

Assist control and assisted modes

- If the patient is making some effort to breathe, then an assist mode of ventilation can be used. **Assist control** ventilation is *essentially identical to the respective controlled modes except that the patient plays a role in initiating the breath.* The breath may be triggered by the pa-

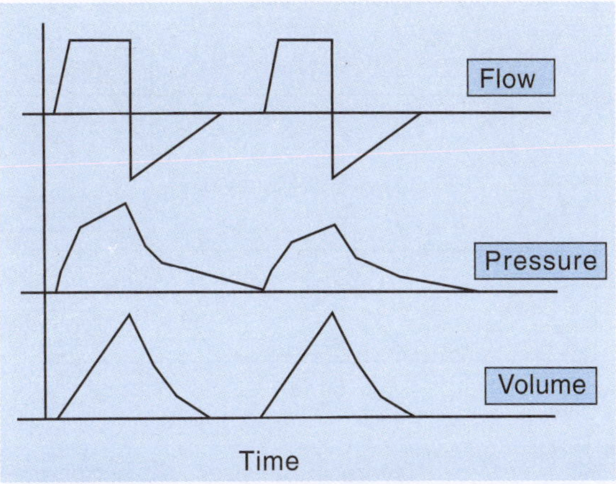

Fig. 21.4 Waveforms in controlled mandatory ventilation

tient or the ventilator (at a pre-set time), whichever comes first. The patient performs only the triggering work, while the ventilator completes the remaining work of limiting and cycling of the ventilated breath.

Assisted modes: Intermittent mandatory ventilation (IMV) and synchronized IMV (SIMV)

- **IMV** was developed as a method of partial ventilatory support to "facilitate liberation" from mechanical ventilation. The goal was to gradually increase the patient's WOB by permitting him/her to actively breathe in order to condition his/her respiratory muscle strength. Concurrently, in order to prevent fatigue, IMV breaths were delivered.
- Thus, periodic IMV breaths (that may be volume or pressure controlled) are delivered at set intervals (time triggered) and in between the IMV breaths, spontaneous breaths are permitted from the baseline pressure (PEEP).
- As the patient's respiratory function improves, the number of IMV may be decreased, with the patient assuming more and more of the WOB until the point that the patient is breathing unassisted on CPAP.

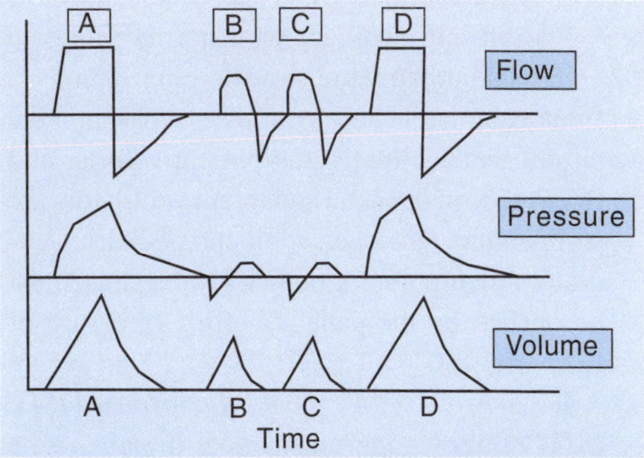

Fig. 21.5 Waveforms in IMV. A&D = IMV breaths, B&C = Spontaneous breaths

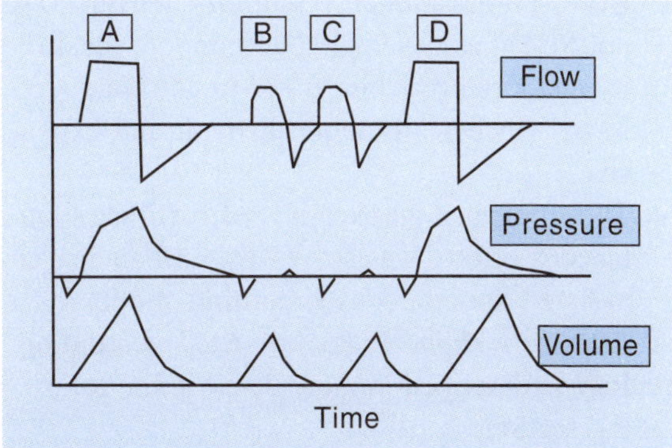

Fig. 21.6 Waveforms in SIMV: Note the negative pressure trigger for the SIMV breaths.
A&D: SIMV breaths
B&C: Unassisted spontaneous breaths

- Unfortunately, there are two problems with this system:
  a) It is possible for the patient and the ventilator to inspire in series, thus "stacking" one breath on top of another, leading to high airway pressures.
  b) The workload of spontaneous breaths remains quite high – remember that the patient still has to inspire without assistance through

an endotracheal tube and open a demand valve – a difficult prospect with normal lungs, a serious burden with an acute lung injury.

- Infant ventilators have continuous flow into the circuit that facilitates the patient efforts, and IMV mode in neonatal and infant ventilators are still popular. However, adult and pediatric ventilators incorporate a demand valve that must be opened by the patient's effort (pressure or flow trigger).
- A variation of the IMV mode, ***synchronized IMV (SIMV)*** allows the mechanical breaths to be given on patient demand. The issue of breath stacking is solved by an in-built sensor that synchronizes the patient's spontaneous breaths to the set rate.
- However, most *infant ventilators* deliver IMV, not SIMV, as developing appropriate sensitivity and rapid response times to an infant's efforts is technically more difficult and expensive.
- The problem of the excessive effort of the spontaneous efforts was solved by introducing an assisted spontaneous breathing mode, viz., *"Pressure support (PSV or PS)"* ventilation. PSV is described in more detail in the following section.
- The combination of SIMV-PS remains a popular weaning mode in paediatrics although its use is infrequent in adult weaning protocols.

Spontaneous modes

- This includes Continuous Positive Airway Pressure (CPAP), Pressure Support Ventilation (PSV) and Volume Support (VS)
- **Pressure support ventilation (PS)**: PSV or PS (and volume support or VS) are also classified as assisted modes.
- In this mode, all of the patient's ventilatory efforts are supported ('boosted') by the ventilator to various degrees determined by the operator.
- PSV is best suited for patients who have a reliable and stable central respiratory drive.

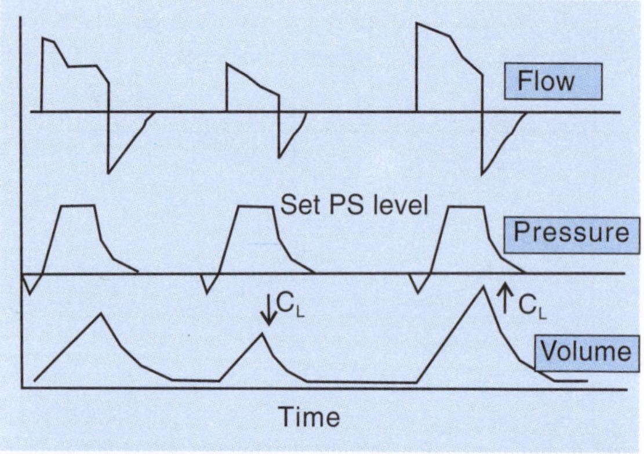

Fig. 21.7 Waveforms in pressure support ventilation (PSV)

- The clinician sets the inspiratory pressure (PS level), PEEP and sensitivity.
- The patient controls the breathing rate, inspiratory flow rate and the length of inspiration and expiration.
- The flow is variable and has a decelerating pattern. When the patient's spontaneous inspiratory effort is sensed, gas flows until a pre-set pressure is reached. This pressure is actively sustained until the end of inspiration.
- *PSV is a prototype of "flow cycled" ventilation:* the ventilation cycles to expiration when the flow decreases to a predetermined value (usually 25%) during inspiration. This drop in flow indicates to the ventilator that the patient's inspiratory effort is slowing and expiration is about to begin.
- Thus, each PS breath is patient triggered (pressure/flow), pressure limited and flow cycled.
- The PS level is PS selected depending on the desired VT that is generated (which depends on the underlying disease state) and the respiratory rate. If the PS level is inadequate, the VT may be low and the rates will be high.
- As the patient's lung mechanics and respiratory muscle strength improve, the levels of PS will have to be reduced as the same level of PS

will produce greater VT (with higher minute ventilation), and the respiratory rates may fall.

- This mode may be used by itself so that all breaths are initiated by the patient and pressure supported by the ventilator or it may be combined with SIMV (SIMV + PSV mode).
  - Breaths A and C (Fig. 21.8) are SIMV volume controlled. Note the constant flow.
  - Breaths B & D are pressure supported.
  - For PSV breaths, note the decelerating flow and cycling to expiration when flow rate decreases to 25% of peak flow rate.
  - Note that both SIMV and PSV breaths are pressure triggered.
- In the SIMV + PS mode, the patient receives some mechanical breaths (SIMV) and some pressure supported spontaneous breaths.
- PSV is useful in difficult to wean patients as it may decrease inspiratory work and abolish diaphragmatic fatigue in patients who have failed conventional weaning attempts. Here, PS overcomes the work of breathing imposed by the resistance of the ETT in spontaneously breathing patient.
- Weaning is also facilitated since the level of pressure support may be adjusted from full to partial to none in a gradual fashion.
- PS may also sometimes be used to provide full ventilatory support. The patient should have a dependable, intact respiratory centre and fairly stable lung mechanics, otherwise the tidal volumes and respiratory rates may vary.
- Large leaks in the ventilator circuit (e.g., due to uncuffed tubes etc) may cause cycling problems in PSV. In order to compensate for the leak, the flow will remain high and may never drop to satisfy the cycling criteria. For the patient, asynchrony and discomfort will result, as inspiratory flow will be continuing and the expiratory valve will remain closed when he desires to exhale.
- Many ventilators have secondary cycling criteria (time cycling) as a safeguard for leaks during PSV so that cycling occurs when the Ti exceeds 80% of the total cycle time.

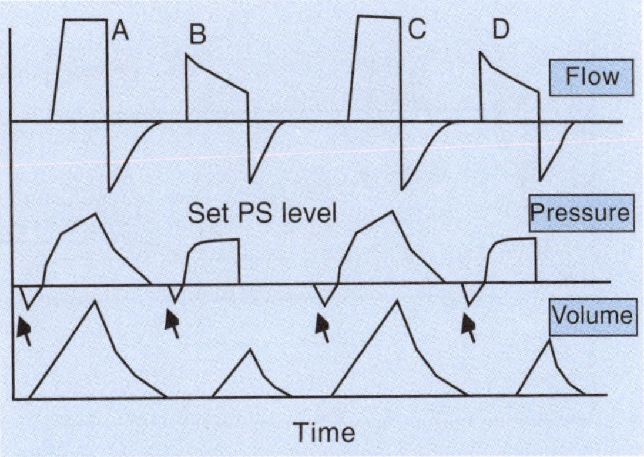

Fig. 21.8 SIMV + PS. Arrowhead represents pressure trigger; A + C = SIMV; B + D = PS

Volume support (VS)

VS is considered a *"smart"* pressure support mode that functions on the same principle as PRVC and is very similar to PSV (patient triggered, pressure targeted and flow cycled) except that the *PS level is automatically adjusted to achieve a pre-set volume target.*

- The two parameters that the operator sets in VS are target VT and PEEP.
- The ventitator performs a 'breath to breath' adjustment of the pressure support (as in PRVC) to achieve the set volume. If the volume generated is too low, the PS level is increased to achieve the target tidal volumes. If the volume is too high, the PS level is decreased.
- Some ventilators have the option of switching from VS to PRVC in the event the patient becomes apneic.

Continuous positive airway pressure (CPAP)

(See also Chapter on "Introduction and terminology" for a more complete discussion on CPAP/PEEP)

- CPAP is defined as positive pressure maintained

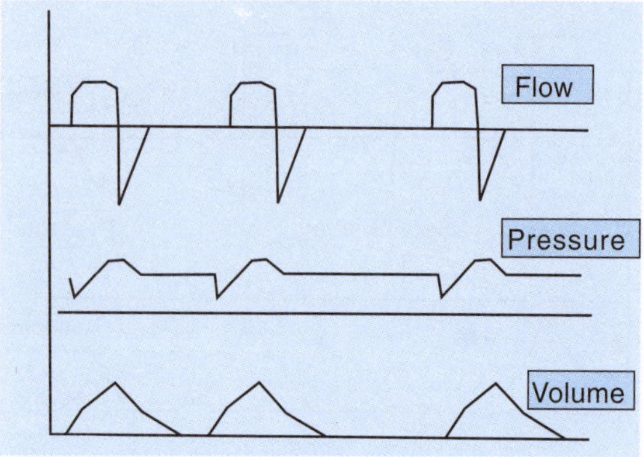

Fig. 21.9 Waveforms in CPAP

in the airways throughout the respiratory cycle during spontaneous respiration.

- CPAP should not be confused with PEEP. PEEP refers to the elevation of baseline pressure during mechanical ventilation (IPPV) whereas CPAP is the elevation in baseline pressure during spontaneous ventilation.
- Gregory et al in 1971 first described the usefulness of CPAP in improving oxygenation in infants with neonatal respiratory distress syndrome and this technique is now widely used in both neonatal and pediatric intensive care units.
- *Pulmonary effects of CPAP*
  - Improvement in arterial oxygenation by opening up collapsed alveoli (*recruitment*) and decreasing intrapulmonary shunting. This allows the clinician to decrease the FiO_2 to non-toxic levels in many cases while maintaining acceptable arterial oxygen levels.
- *Technical considerations*
  - Many devices have been developed to deliver CPAP. All work on the same principle: a continuous gas flow, a valve to maintain positive pressure above atmospheric and a humidification device. A reservoir bag may be incorporated to augment the flow rates when patient's flow demands are high.
  - CPAP is most commonly applied to the patient's airways via an endotracheal tube. Other modes of application include face mask or nasal prongs.
- *Side effects of CPAP*
  - CPAP may cause alveolar overdistention, barotrauma and a paradoxical *decrease in compliance* as the lungs are now ventilated on the upper flat part of the pressure-volume curve.
  - Cardiovascular effects: CPAP induced positive intrathoracic pressure may decrease venous return to the heart and consequently decrease cardiac output. In a failing heart, CPAP decreases LV afterload and is helpful.
  - CNS: In a hypoxic patient with CNS disease, PEEP may be beneficial in preventing secondary brain injury induced by hypoxemia. However PEEP in excess of 15 cmH_2O may decrease venous return from the brain and cause a rise in ICP.
  - Renal: As with other forms of intrathoracic positive pressure, CPAP may stimulate a reflex secretion of antidiuretic hormone (ADH) leading to decreased urine output and significant water retention.
- *Indications and application of CPAP*
  - The primary indication is in acute lung injury (e.g., ARDS and HMD).
  - PEEP improves oxygenation by recruiting alveoli and thus improving FRC.
  - Other conditions in which CPAP is useful include apnea, tracheobronchomalacia and during weaning from mechanical ventilation.

Table 21.2 Modes of Mechanical Ventilation: Summary

Volume control	- Main advantage is *volume guarantee* (remember circuit "compressible volume") - Set VT, PEEP, I:E ratio, rate, FiO_2 - Delivered *pressure is variable*; depends on compliance, resistance. - Constant flow may not satisfy patient demand (some ventilators have option of decelerating flow) - Monitor plateau pressure and patient-ventilator synchrony.
Pressure control	- *Pressure guarantee*, preferred for infants < 8 kg and for patients with leaks in system. - *High, variable, decelerating flow* useful for heterogeneous lungs, satisfies patient's demand - Delivered volumes are variable, depends on compliance, resistance. - Set PIP, PEEP, Ti, rate, FiO_2 - Monitor VTe, respiratory rate, patient-ventilator synchrony and mean airway pressure (MAP).
Pressure support (PS)	- Set inspiratory assist pressure (pressure support) PEEP, FiO_2. - Setting tidal volume, Ti or rate *not required.* - Patient MUST be able to initiate breaths, after which the ventilator delivers a pre-set airway pressure. - Patient triggered (pressure/flow), pressure limited, flow cycled. - Delivered volumes variable, depend on compliance, resistance. - As patient's efforts improve, the pre-set PS levels may be reduced - Monitor respiratory rate, exhaled tidal volume, and patient effort - May be combined with SIMV (SIMV+PS)
Intermittent mandatory ventilation (IMV)	- IMV used in infant ventilators as a weaning mode. - IMV breaths may be PC or VC breaths. - Set IMV rate, PEEP and tidal volume or pressure limit, FiO_2. - Patient allowed to breathe spontaneously between IMV breaths without assistance. - Patient does not receive any assistance when breathing spontaneously. - Tidal volumes will vary between mandatory breaths (IMV) and those initiated by the patient (spontaneous breaths). - Lack of synchrony can result in IMV and spontaneous breath "stacking" resulting in high airway pressures. - As patient's spontaneous efforts improve, the IMV rate may be reduced. - Monitor respiratory rate, exhaled tidal volume, and patient effort.
Synchronized IMV (SIMV)	- Similar to IMV but overcomes issue of stacking by aiming to synchronize with patient effort. - Set SIMV rate, VT/pressure, PEEP, trigger sensitivity, FiO_2. - The ventilator monitors the patient's inspiratory effort. If the patient initiates a breath, the ventilator synchronizes with the patient's effort; if no patient effort detected, an SIMV breath is delivered.

contd.

	- Patient allowed to breathe spontaneously between SIMV breaths without assistance. - Tidal volumes will vary between those breaths initiated by the ventilator and those initiated by the patient. - Monitor respiratory rate, peak inspiratory pressure, and patient ventilator synchrony.
SIMV+PS	- This mode combines SIMV and PS by adding PS to SIMV so that a set amount of pressure is delivered by the ventilator whenever the patient breathes spontaneously. - Set SIMV rate, VT or pressure and pressure support level, PEEP, trigger sensitivity, FiO_2. - Monitor respiratory rate, exhaled tidal volume, and patient effort.
Continuous positive airway pressure (CPAP)	- This mode is only used in patients with adequate spontaneous effort. - A baseline pressure is applied to maintain alveolar stability upon expiration (as in PEEP). - This stabilization serves to increase the PaO_2 by improving the FRC. - The patient receives no other assistance from the ventilator

REFERENCES

1. Pilbeam SP. Selecting the ventilator and the mode. In: Mechanical ventilation. Pilbeam and Cairo (eds). 4th ed. Philadelphia, PA 2006, Mosby Elsevier, 81–105.
2. Venkataraman ST: Mechanical ventilation and Respiratory Care. In: Pediatric Critical Care. Fuhrman and Zimmerman (eds). 3rd ed. Philadelphia, PA, 2006, Mosby Elsevier, 683–719.
3. Restrepo RD, Deshpande VM. Essentials of Ventilator Graphics. RespiMedu 2000.

22

Troubleshooting the Ventilator Using Ventilator Graphics

INTRODUCTION

- Troubleshooting = Systematic identification and resolution of potentially dangerous situations in the patient ventilator system.
- Red flags: Deterioration in patient status, alarm activation on the ventilator or monitor.
- Rapidly assess the patient's ABCs, mental status, colour, HR, BP, perfusion, pulse oximetry reading and respiratory status: WOB, accessory muscle use, breath sounds. Assess ETT for patency and position. See Table 22.1.
- Familiarity with ventilator graphics will aid in early detection and focused troubleshooting even before clinical deterioration occurs.

1. **Acute deterioration with severe cardiopulmonary compromise**
   - Always rule out "*DOPE*" first: D – Displacement, O – Obstruction, P – Pneumothorax, E – Equipment failure
   - If patient's condition is acutely unstable, disconnect from ventilator and initiate manual bag-ventilation with 100% O_2. This also helps to assess the lung characteristics such as compliance and resistance. Decompress gastric tubes, call for assistance.
   - If the patient rapidly improves, the ventilator is likely to have a problem. Check for leaks, kinks, disconnects; check ventilator functioning with a test lung and re-connect the ventilator after rectifying the problem.
   - If the patient's condition remains unstable, check for tube patency by passing a suction catheter, perform vigorous suctioning. If suction catheter cannot pass (deflate cuff to encourage patient effort around a cuffed tube if present) or esophageal displacement suspected, re-intubate the patient.
   - If the clinician cannot determine by clinical examination whether the ETT is in the trachea or esophagus, a definitive method to verify tube position is with the laryngoscope: under direct vision, identify the ETT passing through the vocal cords.
   - Despite a patent ET in good position, if patient is difficult to ventilate and is critically unstable, suspect a tension pneumothorax or acutely worsening underlying lung disease. If air entry is asymmetric, insert a 16 or 18 Fr Venflon in the 2nd intercostal space in the midclavicular line, consider a chest tube. Manually ventilate the patient with a PEEP device. Order an urgent CXR.
   - Suspect massive auto-PEEP as a cause for sudden cardiorespiratory collapse in a patient with underlying airways disease (asthma, bronchiolitis): disconnect the ventilator for 20-30 seconds, may need a brief manual squeeze of chest. Check for auto-PEEP and air-trapping frequently. Re-set ventilator setting to improve alveolar emptying, consider increased sedation.

Table 22.1 Causes for patient-ventilator dysynchrony

A: Patient related problems	B: Ventilator related problems
▪ Airway problems - Bronchospasm - Secretions, biting, kinking of ET - Alterations in head position leading to tube displacement ▪ Pulmonary problems - Pulmonary edema - Pneumothorax - Worsening underlying disease ▪ Abdominal distension ▪ Pain and anxiety	▪ System leak ▪ Circuit malfunction or disconnection ▪ Inadequate FiO_2 ▪ Inappropriate settings - Inappropriate mode - Inappropriate trigger sensitivity - Inappropriate inspiratory flow setting - Inappropriate cycle variable - Inappropriate PEEP setting

2. **Identify patient-ventilator dysynchrony – why is the patient "fighting the ventilator"? (Table 22.1)**
   - A major goal of ventilation is to decrease the patient's work of breathing (WOB). For this to happen, the patient's and ventilated breaths must be coordinated and the ventilator must satisfy the patient's demands.
   - A patient is "out of synch" with the ventilator if he wishes to inspire when inspiratory flow has ceased or is trying to exhale against an incoming mechanical breath.
   - A flow setting that is too low to satisfy the patient's peak inspiratory flow rate will also cause dysynchrony due to "flow starvation" with flow-time graphics exhibiting scalloping of the inspiratory phase (Fig. 22.1).
   - Patients who have asynchrony will be distressed and uncomfortable and may have a combination of the following clinical features: Tachypnea, tachycardia, nasal flaring, use of accessory muscles, increased WOB, paradoxical movements of abdomen and thorax, diaphoresis etc.
   - Pulse oximetry readings, graphics, peak inspired pressures (PIP), plateau pressure (Pplat) and exhaled volumes may help identify the cause of the problem.

☞ **REMEMBER** Patient-ventilator synchrony may have multiple causes: it is always a safe policy to identify the problem prior to the administration of sedatives +/- muscle relaxants. Muscle relaxants will cause rapid cardiac arrest of a patient with a blocked ETT.

3. **ETT related problems**
   - Tube migration (extension and flexion of the head and neck causes movement of the tube; the tube moves in the same direction as the tip of nose). The ET may have migrated either above the vocal cord or into right main bronchus.
   - Patient biting the tube or kinking of tube.
   - Secretions and mucus plugging in the airway or tube.
   - ETT impinging on the carina: This is a very sensitive area and can cause persistent cough, bronchospasm, and high airway pressures.
4. **Air trapping / Auto-PEEP (Fig. 22.2, 22.3)**
   - This is defined as unintentional PEEP that results when a new inspiratory breath is begun before the previous expiratory flow has ended.
   - Causes of auto-PEEP
     - *Without airway obstruction*: Inadequate expiratory time, rapid respiratory rates, high minute ventilation.

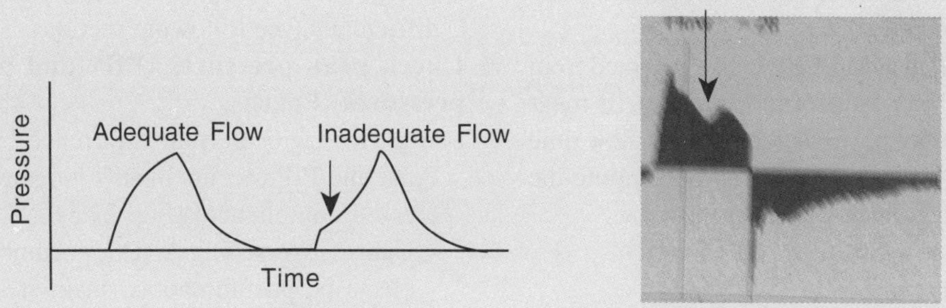

Fig. 22.1 Pressure-time and flow-time scalars showing scalloping of inspiratory flow (Flow starvation)

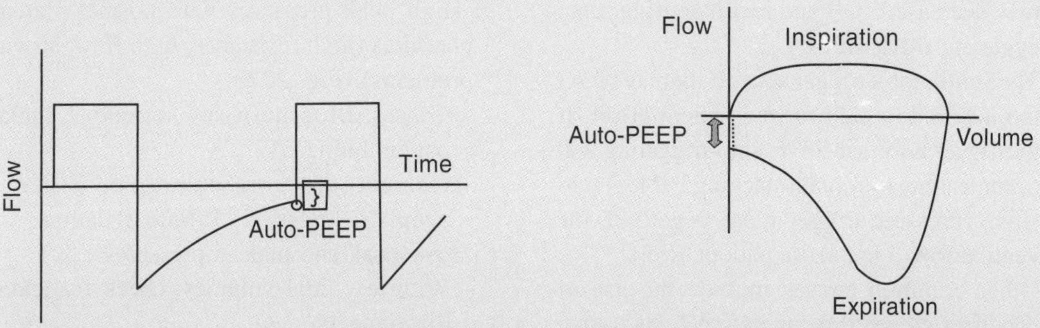

Fig. 22.2 Flow-time and flow-volume waveforms showing air-trapping

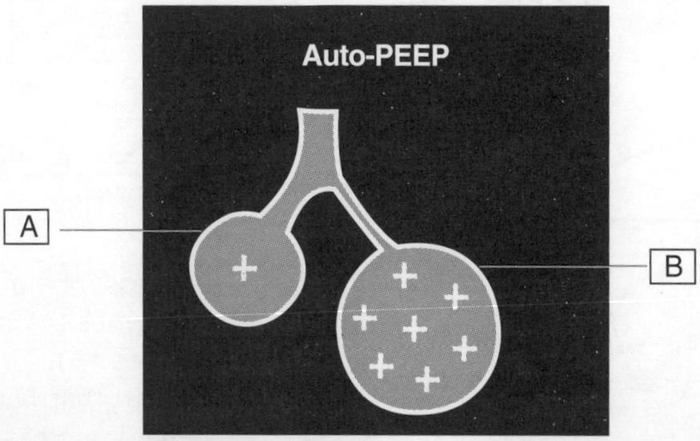

Fig. 22.3 Auto-PEEP: (A) Incomplete emptying of alveolus, (B) resulting in auto-PEEP

- *With airway obstruction*: Bronchospasm, ETT secretions
- Even though auto-PEEP is best detected from the flow time waveform (Fig. 22.2), its magnitude cannot be measured from the flow time scalar. It is best measured by performing the expiratory hold and reading the value.
- Methods to reduce auto-PEEP:
  - Decrease rate
  - Increase expiratory time
  - Reduce VT, if possible
  - Clear secretions; treat bronchospasm.
- If auto-PEEP exists in a spontaneously breathing patient, the set PEEP may be increased to $^2/_3{}^{rd}$ of measured auto-PEEP. This may decrease WOB and facilitate triggering.

5. **Triggering difficulties**
   - The ventilator's trigger sensitivity may be set too low or too high for the patient effort. If the trigger is too sensitive, auto-triggering will occur leading to "breath stacking." If less sensitive (pressure trigger more negative), the ventilator will not sense patient effort.
   - Other common causes include the use of nebulizer powered by an external gas source – this can interfere with triggering.
   - Water in the circuit may also cause triggering problems with the ventilator mistaking water movement as patient effort. Circuits without a heater wire may especially have excessive "rain-out" resulting in auto-triggering.
   - Excess auto-PEEP may also cause triggering difficulties (see following section).
6. **Check peak pressures (PIP) and plateau pressures (Pplat)**

   a) High PIP with normal difference between Pplat and PIP (occurs in stiff lungs with decreased compliance) (Fig. 22.5)
   - Causes: Worsening ARDS, pneumonia, atelectasis, pneumothorax, main stem intubation, decreased chest wall/abdominal compliance.
   - Correct the correctable: CXR, gases may help in identifying the problem.
   - Higher PEEP may be required if the underlying disease is worsening.

   b) High peak pressures with normal plateau pressures (high resistance, high flow, airway problems) (Fig. 22.6)
   - Causes: Bronchospasm, secretions, kinks, patient biting ET.
   - Correct the correctable, consider β agonists, ↓rates, ↑ E-time, sedation.

   c) Low peak and plateau pressures:
   - With low tidal volumes: check for leaks, disconnects
   - With normal tidal volumes: could patient be improving?

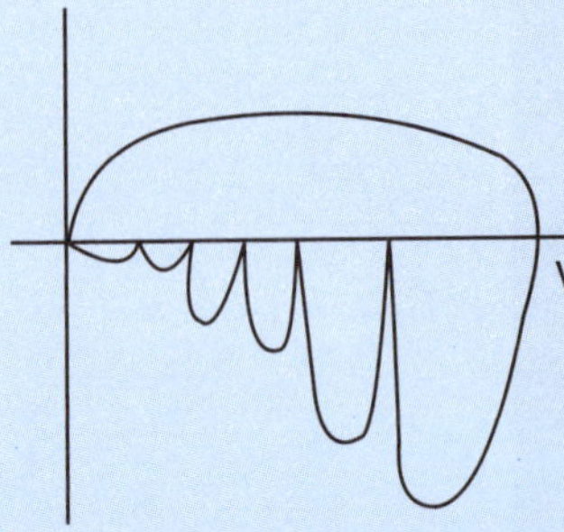

Fig. 22.4 Airway secretions / pooling of the condensate in the circuit

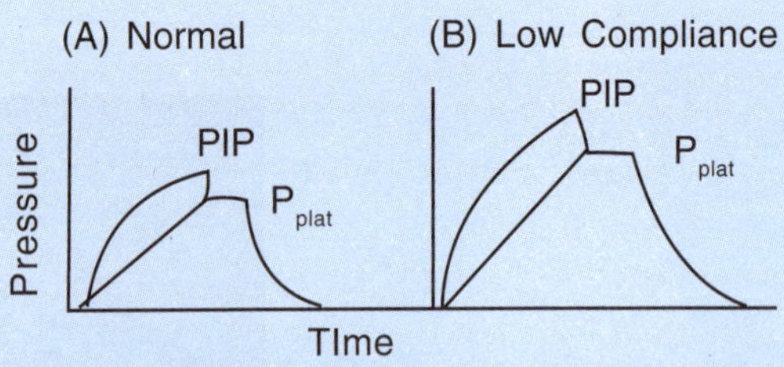

Fig. 22.5 Pressure time waveform showing normal (A) and decreased compliance (B).
Note that both the PIP and Pplat have increased with a normal gradient between the 2 pressures (B).

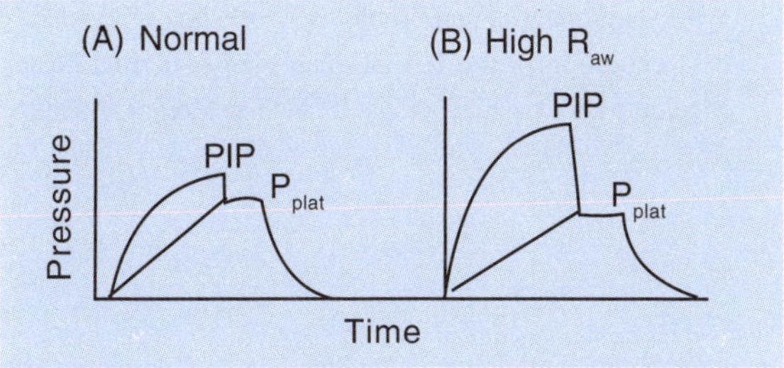

Fig. 22.6 Pressure-time scalar showing normal (A) and high resistance (B). Note that only the PIP has increased but Pplat remains the same resulting in a widened gradient between the two pressures.

7. **Circuit leaks**

- Air leaks are suspected on ventilator if low pressure, low volume and low flow alarms are activated and waveforms demonstrate the presence of a leak (Fig. 22.7).
- Minimal leaks around uncuffed tubes are expected and necessary to preserve tracheal mucosal integrity. If it is difficult to ventilate the patient on account of large leaks, it may be necessary to inflate the cuff further until leak is minimal, provided the cuff pressures do not exceed 20 mmHg. Other options include re-intubating with a larger tube or with a cuffed tube, if not done previously.
- Another common cause of leak is in the circuit where connections exist. These leaks can be determined by comparing the inspiratory and expiratory tidal volumes.

RESOLUTION OF PROBLEM MAY BE POSSIBLE

- Pneumothorax should be drained as quickly as possible if it is causing cardio-respiratory embarrassment.
- Bronchospasm should be treated with bronchodilators. Consider cardiogenic pulmonary edema and pulmonary emboli as a differential diagnosis for wheeze.
- Secretions need thorough toileting. It also suggests that humidification is not appropriate or that the patient might be developing ventilator associated pneumonia. Postural drainage and physiotherapy should be encouraged.
- If pulmonary edema is present, treat the underlying cause; consider ↑ PEEP, inotropes, vasodilators, diuretics.
- Change in body posture especially during early hours of morning when back care and sponging by the nurses is carried out is a prime time for accidental extubation and kinking of the tube.
- If lung disease has worsered, re-set ventilator and alarm settings as appropriate.

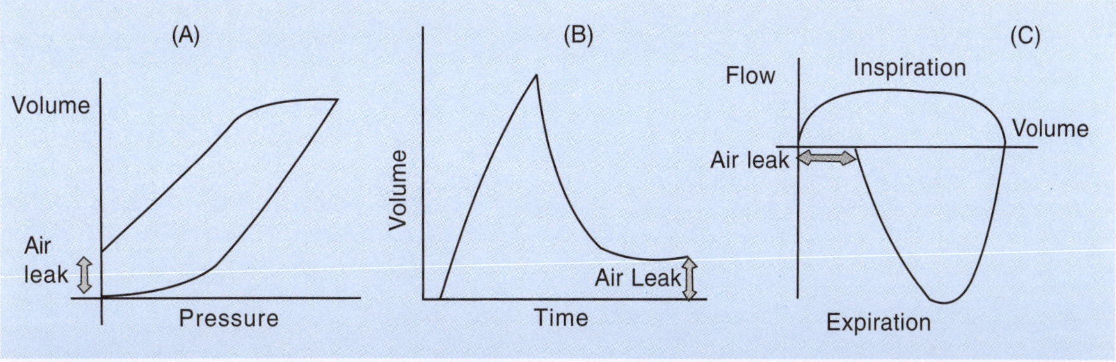

Fig. 22.7 Leak in the circuit as seen in pressure-volume (A), volume-time (B) and flow-volume (C) waveforms

REFERENCES

1. S. Pilbeam. Troubleshooting and problem solving. Chapter No.18 in Mechanical Ventilation: Physiological and Clinical Application. Fourth edition. Mosby Elsevier publication. p 391–413.
2. Restrepo RD, Deshpande VM. Essentials of Ventilator Graphics. RespiMedu 2000.
3. Workshop material and problems. Workshop of mechanical ventilation in the ICU. Department of Critical Care Medicine and Anesthesiology. Sundaram Medical Foundation.

23

Weaning and Extubation

- If a patient's spontaneous breathing capacity is capable of assuming his/her work of breathing, weaning (liberating) from mechanical ventilation may be considered.
- The time to initiate weaning is determined by improvement in the clinical status and sometimes by a clinical trial. The criteria for initiation of weaning and extubation in children rest on ill defined clinical factors and are not absolute.
- Once the need for mechanical ventilation is resolved, the ventilator can be discontinued. About 80% of children can be directly disconnected and do not need a slow programmed process. However, for some children, the process can be lengthy and complex.
- Weaning from the ventilator and extubation are usually considered together, although in some disease states such as Guillain Barre syndrome, airway support may be required for a longer period even after ventilatory support has ceased.

TRADITIONAL vs MODERN METHODS OF WEANING

- *Traditional methods depend on graded reduction in the level of support* over a period of days aiming to recondition the patient's respiratory muscles while concurrently avoiding fatigue.
- Numerous methods have been described. The method chosen depends largely on physician's experience and level of comfort. Some conventional methods include:

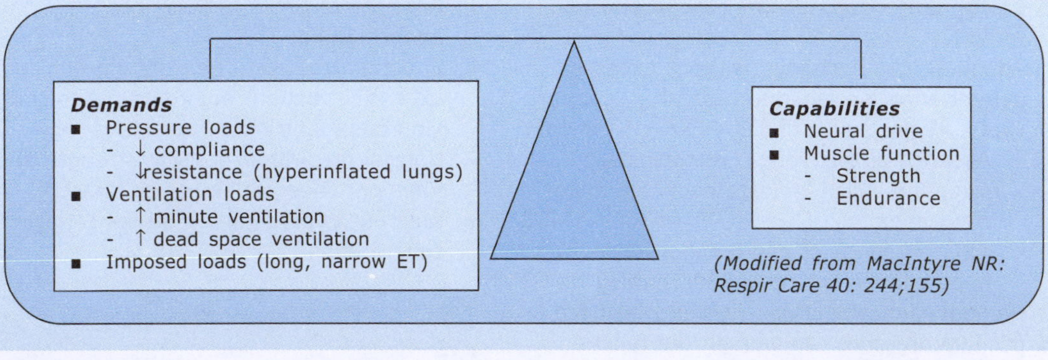

Fig. 23.1 The success of weaning is a balance between a patient's respiratory capabilities/reserve and demands on the respiratory system.

- IMV or SIMV
- IMV/SIMV with PSV

(With gradual reduction in IMV rate and pressure support levels)

- Adding PS to SIMV may be helpful since it can decrease the workload during spontaneous respirations, thus enhancing endurance conditioning of respiratory muscles without causing fatigue.
- Once the level of support is minimal, the patient's readiness to extubate may be assessed.
- Most clinicians do not place a patient on prolonged periods of CPAP prior to extubation as the resistance and WOB involved in breathing through a ETT can be substantial.
- In our PICU, the trend is to extubate patients from a low level of ventilatory support (e.g., SIMV rate of ~ 5/min, PS ~ 5 cmH_2O, PEEP ~ 5-7 cmH_2O).
- For infants and smaller infants who have been ventilated for > 48 hr, extubating to non-invasive CPAP of 5–8 cmH_2O is useful and is described in greater detail below.

MODERN METHODS OF WEANING: THE SPONTANEOUS BREATHING TRIAL (SBT)

- Reports even in children indicate that a prolonged gradual weaning process may be unnecessary: many may be "fast-tracked" when their disease process resolves, thus shortening time on ventilator and decreasing complications and costs.
- Daily assessment of the patient readiness to extubate will indicate if the patient meets the criteria in Table 23.1. An SBT may then be performed.
- Prior to any SBT trial, optimize the patient's breathing conditions by ensuring that the ET is patent and minimize dead space (Remove HME if present, is length of ETT too long?)

Table 23.1 Criteria for extubation

Major criteria	Minor criteria
1. The primary indication for intubation and ventilation must no longer exist. 2. The patient should be alert and responsive with an intact central respiratory drive and airway protective reflexes (cough and gag reflex). 3. Adequate gas exchange without excessive patient effort on minimal ventilatory support. (SpO_2 >94% in FiO_2 of 0.3, PEEP $\leq$ 5 cmH_2O). - Absence of tachypnea, retractions, sweating which indicate poor tolerance to weaning. - ABG: Absence of metabolic acidosis or hypercapnia, P/F ratio >300 mmHg 4. Hemodynamically stable (withdrawal from positive pressure can worsen the function of a failing heart).	1. No sedatives in last 4 hours 2. No gross metabolic derangements (low levels of PO_4, Mg, K can cause muscle weakness) 3. Absence of gross radiological abnormalities 4. Endotracheal secretions should not be excessive, patient must be able to cough vigorously and clear secretions 5. Normal respiratory muscle strength and function, chest wall must be intact 6. Rule out hypercatabolic states (e.g., severe sepsis)

- Careful bedside supervision of the initial 5-10 minutes of SBT is an important screening phase and will determine if the patient can tolerate a longer period of SBT.
- During the initial SBT screening, a clinical assessment of the patient's overall comfort level, mental status (alert vs agitated or drowsy), respiratory rate (progressively increasing rates are a bad sign) and pattern (regular vs periodic or jerky with accessory muscle use), hemodynamic stability (assess for new onset tachycardia/bradycardia, BP and extremity perfusion), gas exchange, presence of sweating (Table 23.2).
- If the initial trial is satisfactory, the SBT can be extended for 30 minutes.
- In children, SBT is carried out by any of the following methods:
  a. T-piece trials
  b. CPAP 5-8 cm ± minimal pressure support (PS) of 5-8 cm.

T-piece trials

- This is the oldest method of weaning.
- A T-piece may be applied by removing patient from ventilator and attaching a T-piece with O_2 flowing at 3 times the patient's minute ventilation.
- The T-piece trial may also be carried out through a ventilator where the mandatory rate is turned off and the machine is set on spontaneous/CPAP mode. On a ventilator, advantages are ability to monitor the exhaled tidal volumes, option for humidified O_2 and back up ventilation if the patient becomes apneic.
- *Patients with underlying heart disease or severe muscle weakness are less likely to tolerate weaning using the T-piece.*

SBT using low level CPAP/PS

- Although studies have shown that the extubation success rates are similar for SBT applied via T-piece or low level CPAP + PS, PICU physicians may be reluctant to subject infants and younger children to a trial of complete spontaneous breathing with either CPAP or T-piece circuit. The concern is about causing fatigue on account of the work of breathing imposed by the tracheal tube and the breathing circuit.
- Since smaller ETT have greater resistance on account of a smaller radius, the level of PS to overcome the WOB will depend on the ETT size. Accordingly, suggested PS levels depend on ET caliber.

Tracheal tube size		PSV level
3 mm ID	:	10 cmH_2O
4 mm ID	:	8 cmH_2O
5 mm ID	:	6 cmH_2O

Table 23.2 Clinical assessment during and on completion of the SBT

- Overall comfort level, presence of sweating
- Mental status (alert vs agitated or drowsy)
- Respiratory rate and pattern (regular vs periodic, jerky with accessory muscle use), WOB not excessive, tidal volumes (> 6.5 ml/kg= low risk of re-intubation)
- Hemodynamic stability (assess for new onset tachycardia/bradycardia, BP and extremity perfusion)
- Gas exchange satisfactory
- Effective cough

- *RSBI (Rapid Shallow Breathing Index)* score < 60-105 breath/min/L has a high likelihood of successful extubation. It is calculated using the formula *f*/VT where *f* = frequency and VT = tidal volume in liters (this index has been better validated in adults).

Criteria for terminating SBT

1. Inability to maintain gas exchange (SpO_2 less than 95% with 40% FiO_2 or needing more than 50% FiO_2 to maintain SpO_2 above 95%).

2. Inability to maintain effective ventilation (measured exhaled tidal volume less than 5 ml/kg or respiratory acidosis with pH less than 7.3 or increase in pCO_2 greater than 50 or increase of more than 10 from the baseline).
3. Increased work of breathing: increased respiratory rate and use of accessory respiratory muscle.
4. Other signs of distress include diaphoresis, heart rate greater than 90th centile for given age, change in mental status, systolic BP less than 3rd centile.

If the child fails an SBT, the next SBT should be done after assessing and rectifying both respiratory and non-respiratory reversible factors that are responsible for the failure. The next SBT should be tried only after 24 hours. Frequent SBT should not be tried over a single day. Even twice daily SBTs offer no advantage over testing once a day.

ADJUNCTS TO WEANING

1. Corticosteroids
   Routine administration of steroids has been shown to decrease the incidence of post extubation stridor, but not the need for re-intubation.
2. Use of non-invasive ventilation (NIV) as a bridge to extubation
   - NIV may act as a bridge to complete liberation from mechanical support. Careful patient selection and awareness of the limitations of NIV are important.
   - Use of CPAP via face mask or nasopharyngeal tubes provides positive pressure that can prevent small airways and alveoli collapse and consequent atelectasis post extubation.
   - Nasopharyngeal CPAP: In infants and smaller children, a tracheal tube may be inserted nasally up to the level of the tragus in order to deliver nasal CPAP.
   - Humidification should be provided. Tolerance is usually good. Ensure that the suction catheter is inserted only to the tip of the N-CPAP tube in order to prevent nasal mucosal trauma and bleeding.
   - Facial mask: CPAP can also be delivered through a snuggly fitting face mask.
   - The CPAP may be gradually discontinued in 24-48 hours.

FACTORS THAT CONTRIBUTE TO WEANING FAILURE

If a patient fails weaning attempts, a systematic approach is required to determine the likely causes.

1. **Respiratory factors**
   - Assess for abnormal imposed loads, e.g., are the lungs hyperinflated, is compliance reduced? Is there chest wall edema or abdominal distention that interferes with intercostal and diaphragmatic function?
   - Assess for diaphragmatic palsy/paresis especially in post cardiac surgical patients.
   - Consider tracheomalacia which may manifest as stridor that decreases with positive pressure. Air trapping on CXR and ventilator graphics provide additional clues.
2. **Cardiac factors**
   - Positive pressure provided by the ventilator decreases LV afterload, preload and also ↓WOB; all of these improve the function of a failing heart.
   - If, during weaning of PPV, hemodynamics worsen and/or pulmonary edema occurs, evaluate cardiac function. Diuretics, inotropes and afterload reduction may be useful prior to the next weaning attempt.
3. **Acid-base status**
   - Respiratory alkalosis depresses ventilatory drive whereas metabolic acidosis increases respiratory demand for compensation. This should be corrected before weaning.

4. **Metabolic status**
   - Hypophosphatemia, hypokalemia and hypomagnesemia can cause respiratory muscle weakness.
   - Hypothyroidism can cause decreased respiratory drive with possible respiratory muscle weakness.
5. **Drugs**
   - The child should be off all narcotics, sedatives and hypnotics. Aminoglycosides may rarely cause neuromuscular blockade and weaning failure.
6. **Nutrition**
   - Overfeeding can cause increased CO_2 production with excessive carbohydrate calories. Similarly, malnutrition with pre-existing nutritional deficiencies can cause respiratory muscle weakness and failure to wean.
7. **Psychological status**
   - Older children can have psychological ventilator dependence or can have lack of motivation to be weaned off the ventilator.

TECHNIQUE OF EXTUBATION

- Withhold feeds for at least 4 hours and empty stomach contents just prior to extubation.
- Perform thorough physiotherapy, postural drainage and endotracheal suctioning.
- Perform deep oral suctioning before deflation of the cuff to prevent oropharyngeal secretions trickling down into the trachea after extubation.
- Withdraw tube during positive-pressure inflation of 'Ambu' bag.
- Nurse child with head elevated; administer warm and humidified oxygen as required.

POST EXTUBATION COMPLICATIONS

1. Stridor: Usually self-limiting, rarely will require steroids and/or nebulized adrenaline. Dexamethasone (0.2 mg/kg x 3–4 doses Q6H, initiate 1st dose 12 hours prior to extubation. May be useful for patients with minimal peri-tubal leak, multiple intubations, prolonged intubation)
2. Upper lobe atelectasis: May be managed with postural physiotherapy, humidified O_2 and CPAP.

EXTUBATION FAILURE

- It is defined as re-intubation within 24 hours of extubation. The average pediatric failure rate is approximately 19%. The failure rate increases with increasing length of time on mechanical ventilation.
- Re-intubation can increase risk of ventilator-associated pneumonia.

ROLE OF TRACHEOSTOMY (See also chapter on tracheostomy)

- A tracheostomy is usually considered when it becomes apparent that the patient will require prolonged ventilator assistance.
- In children, there is no consensus as to when to perform a tracheostomy. In practice, whenever long-term ventilation is anticipated and usually after 7–14 days (if imminent extubation does not appear likely), a tracheostomy may be considered.
- The benefits of tracheostomy include greater ease of toileting (can be performed by parent), decreased dead space and consequent work of breathing. Improved patient comfort, better oral hygiene, ability to eat and drink orally is a great psychological boost and aids a sense of well being.
- Once the patient improves and decannulation is being considered, the tracheostomy can be initially uncuffed (observe for excessive coughing during swallowing liquids), then capped off. Some patients may require the tracheostomy to be downsized to a smaller tube prior to capping off. Close involvement with an ENT surgeon is important.
- If the patient can breathe and cough adequately around a closed tracheostomy, the chances of a successful decannulation are very high.

- Following removal of the tracheostomy cannula, the wound may be sealed with gauze over which a tight elastoplast is applied. This usually leads to satisfactory healing of the tracheostomy wound. Suturing the wound is generally not required.
- In the rare event that the patient requires reinsertion of the tracheostomy, a new tracheostomy tube may be inserted through the well-formed tracheostomy track. If re-cannulation is not possible, insert a lubricated endotracheal tube (can be maneuvred over a trimmed suction catheter if required). If this too is unsuccessful, the patient may need to be intubated orally.

REFERENCES

1. Pilbeam SP. Discontinuation of and Weaning from Mechanical Ventilation. In: Mechanical ventilation. Pilbeam and Cairo (eds). 4th ed. Philadelphia, PA 2006, Mosby Elsevier, 443-471.
2. Venkataraman ST: Mechanical ventilation and Respiratory Care. In: Pediatric Critical Care. Fuhrman and Zimmerman (eds). 3rd ed. Philadelphia, PA, 2006, Mosby Elsevier, 683-719.
3. MacIntyre NR, Cook DJ, Ely EW et al. ACCP/AARC/SCCM Task Force: Evidence Based Guidelines for Weaning and Discontinuing Mechanical Ventilator Support. *Chest* 120 (Suppl 6): 375S, 2001; Respir Care 47:69, 2002.
4. Heulitt MJ, Wolf GK, Arnold JH. Mechanical ventilation. Chapter 34 In: Rogers Textbook of Pediatric Intensive Care. 4th edition. David G Nichols. Lippincott Williams and Wilkins Publications. pp 508-531.

24

Disease Based Ventilation Strategy

- There are elements of both art and science involved in the application of mechanical ventilation. Just as a chef caters to his customer's palate, the clinician should customize ventilatory strategy based on the patient's disease and lung pathophysiology.
- A broad outline of the various strategies in certain specific lung diseases is outlined below.

1. Primary respiratory muscle failure

(E.g., neuromuscular disorders: Guillain Barre, muscle dystrophies)

- The principal difficulty in primary respiratory muscle failure is inadequate ventilation from weakness of the respiratory muscles (pump failure).
- Some patients also have ineffective cough and impaired ability to protect and clear their airway, placing them at risk for aspiration.
- The goals of respiratory support in patients with acute reversible neuromuscular diseases such as Guillain Barre syndrome are:
  1. Provision of respiratory assistance to maintain adequate minute ventilation.
  2. Avoidance of disuse muscle atrophy by encouraging spontaneous breathing as far as possible.
  3. Early tracheostomy to reduce dead space and WOB should be considered if no recovery of muscle strength is seen at 7-10 days.
- Non-invasive ventilation is much preferred in this group, provided adequate airway protective reflexes are present.
- Neuromuscular blockade must be avoided.
- Blood gases are a poor guide in decision making: the ABG may remain normal until late in the progress of illness and likewise, normalization of gases is not a good criterion to extubate a patient with neuromuscular disease.
- Controlled modes of ventilation may result in disuse muscle atrophy and delayed weaning from mechanical ventilation. Therefore, spontaneous breathing should be encouraged as much as possible.
- Useful strategies include modes that encourage "respiratory muscle conditioning" during the day and rest at night time to prevent fatigue.
- Modes such as SIMV with PS are useful as the spontaneous breathing efforts promote muscle conditioning and the level of assistance may be decreased from full to minimal in a gradual fashion.
- Furthermore, decreasing the trigger sensitivity (trigger more negative, –2 to –3 cmH_2O) to increase the work performed by the patient to trigger the ventilator is also sometimes used to improve respiratory muscle strength. However, a sufficient period of uninterrupted rest is essential in order to prevent muscle fatigue (typically overnight when

the SIMV rate may be increased and the trigger made more physiologic for the patient).

- Ventilatory settings and FiO_2 are usually kept to a minimum since the lung parenchyma is normal unless aspiration or VAP has occurred.
- Weaning in these patients involves a 2 step process:
  - *Wean from positive pressure ventilation* when respiratory muscle strength has improved, the lung mechanics and gas exchange are satisfactory.
  - *Wean from the artificial airway* when bulbar function improves as evidenced by ability to swallow oral secretions and adequate protective reflexes (gag and cough). Some patients can be weaned from the ventilator early but may need prolonged airway support.
- Following extubation, intermittent periods of mask NIV may be necessary in some patients.
- Tracheostomy may be considered as early as the end of the first week, unless the patient's muscle strength has begun to improve. Advantages of an early tracheostomy include ↓WOB by decreased dead space, improved tracheal toileting and oral hygiene and ability to feed by mouth which contributes greatly to patient well being and comfort.

2. Patients with chronic respiratory failure and hypoventilation

- Here, hypercarbia is the norm and the pH is normal due to high bicarbonate levels from renal compensation.
- Such a patient may acutely deteriorate from an intercurrent illness. They develop acute on chronic respiratory acidosis as the baseline high pCO_2 will be further elevated and the high pre-existing bicarbonate levels are insufficient to fully compensate for the higher pCO_2 levels. The arterial pH will be acidic with varying degrees of hypoxemia.
- The period of ventilation should typically be as short as possible during which time the precipitating infection is treated and aggressive postural physiotherapy is provided. Ventilator strategies should not aim to normalize the pCO_2, but rather maintain elevated pCO_2 levels provided the pH is normal.
- Oxygen must be administered cautiously as high inspired O_2 concentrations may abolish the backup hypoxic drive during weaning. Maintain the SaO_2 in the low 90s.
- PEEP is usually set at a relatively low level (3 to 5 cmH_2O).
- Minimize sedation, avoid aminoglycosides, check biochemical parameters (normalize PO_4, Mg^{++}, K^+, avoid alkalosis).

3. Disorders with airway obstruction

These may involve diseases of either the upper airway or lower airways.

Upper airway obstruction, e.g., epiglottitis, croup, post extubation stridor or burns *(See also Chapter on Upper Airway Obstruction)*

- The main aim in patients with upper airway obstruction is to provide an airway by bypassing the obstruction. This is done by intubating with an oro- or nasotracheal tube or by a tracheostomy. IPPV is generally not required as the lung mechanics are usually normal.
- The size of the ETT may be smaller than calculated for age.
- Specific measures where applicable such as antibiotics, steroids and humidification may be beneficial.
- Removal of the artificial airway may be considered when there is an adequate peri-tubal leak, usually after 48 hours.

Lower airway diseases

- Respiratory failure because of lower airway obstruction (e.g., bronchiolitis, asthma) poses specific problems during intubation and mechanical ventilation.

- Depression of cardiac output and hypotension after intubation may be multifactorial due to:
  - Application of positive airway pressure to an already hyperinflated lung with further impedance to venous return.
  - Tamponade effect because of dynamic hyperinflation and massive auto-PEEP (see below).
  - Pneumothorax.
  - Vasodilatation due to sedative drugs used for intubation.
  - Increased pulmonary vascular resistance.
- After intubation, massive "auto-PEEP" may also result from rapid manual ventilation.
- The above may be addressed by ensuring adequate filling prior/during intubation, avoiding overzealous manual ventilation and brief disconnection from the ventilator if hemodynamic instability occurs.

Lower airway diseases: Bronchiolitis

- No specific therapy is found to be useful in bronchiolitis apart from humidified oxygen.
- If child continues to be in respiratory distress with increased WOB, fatigue and hypoxemia, nasopharyngeal CPAP is a good option.
- CPAP of 6-10 cmH_2O will reverse the above complications. The level of CPAP may be titrated to decrease WOB and hypoxemia while avoiding further hyperinflation that may cause hemodynamic compromise. If > 9 posterior ribs on CXR are seen, reduce CPAP pressures.
- A pacifier may be used to encourage mouth closure and prevent loss of CPAP. Sedation with trichlorfos (25-30 mg/kg Q6hrly) and initiation of early continuous nasogastric feeds may help in better tolerance. Rule out hypoxia and hypercarbia prior to sedation.
- If the child progresses to respiratory failure despite CPAP, then intubation and ventilation are indicated.
- The ventilator strategies to be adopted will be similar to that of a patient with asthma.

Lower airway diseases: Asthma

- It is infrequent for asthmatics to require ventilation. *Considerations during asthma intubation are described above (see also Chapter 13).*
- Patients with asthma have predominantly ↑ time constants (TC) due to ↑ resistance, but may have heterogeneous lungs with some areas of collapse/pneumonia that have shorter TC.
- Goals of ventilation in asthma are:
  - Relieve respiratory muscle fatigue and reverse hypoxemia, if present.
  - Utilize lung-protective strategies that will avoid worsening dynamic hyperinflation and hemodynamic function.
- Strategies to implement these goals are:
  - Use low tidal volumes (5-7 ml/kg) to limit high plateau pressures.
  - PIP may be high but may be ignored as it reflects increased airways resistance.
  - Limit Pplat to ≤ 30-35 cmH_2O.
  - Accept high pCO_2 (permissive hypercapnia) if pH > 7.2.

☞ **REMEMBER** Plateau pressures (Pplat) are more significant than PIP as a marker of alveolar pressure and thus risk for barotraumas. Pplat may be high if compliance is decreased due to hyperinflation, excess PEEP, presence of pneumothorax, atelectasis, pneumonia.

- Mode of ventilation: Either volume targeted or pressure targeted modes may be used. Volume targeted modes guarantee volume delivery, but generated pressures may be high.
- PRVC mode may be useful since volume is guaranteed and decelerating flows result in lower MAPs and better distribution of gases to units with high resistance and long time constants. Set appropriate upper pressure limits.

- *Very long exhalation times* are essential in order to minimize air trapping: use low rates (10-14/min), long expiratory times, avoid reduction in inspiratory time below 0.5-0.6 sec.
- While setting low ventilator rates is easy, controlling the patient's spontaneous rapid respiratory rates on the ventilator may be difficult. Muscle relaxants may be occasionally used, but the mainstay of asthma ventilation is deep sedation and analgesia (ketamine 1 mg/kg/hr, midazolam, opioid) to decrease spontaneous respiratory efforts and increased airway reactivity (especially with suctioning).

> ☞ **REMEMBER** High $paCO_2$ in patients with extensive air-trapping is due to hyperinflation related dead space effect (V/Q mismatch) and responds better to lowering of ventilatory rates rather than higher rates.

- Frequent position change, head end elevation and gentle chest physiotherapy are important parts of ventilatory care of the asthmatic.
- Avoid the use of paralytic agents if possible (risk of critical illness myopathy that may be potentiated with concomitant use of steroids).
- Continue systemic steroids + bronchodilator therapy, preferably via in-line metered dose inhalers (MDI with spacer) in the inspiratory limb.
- Maintain hemodynamic stability with adequate filling and, if necessary, inotropy/vasopressor.
- Setting PEEP in the ventilated asthmatic is difficult and controversial.
  - Asthmatic patients already have excessive air-trapping and ↑ FRC and, logically, should not need more PEEP.
  - Soon after intubation, a low level of PEEP (2-4 cmH_2O) may suffice.
  - However, many patients require a higher level of PEEP to stent the airways open in order to overcome dynamic compression of the lower airways. This greatly helps in decreasing air-trapping.
  - External PEEP also aids the spontaneously breathing asthmatic to trigger the ventilator better.
- How to select the PEEP level?
  - Measure auto-PEEP with an expiratory hold.
  - Set the external PEEP to ~ $^2/_3$rd auto-PEEP, but not > 7-8 cmH_2O.
  - The plateau pressures (which reflect alveolar pressures) may help to fine tune external PEEP levels. Select the PEEP that results in the lowest Pplat.
  - Ventilator graphics, particularly flow-time scalars will help to titrate rates, E-times, PEEP.

> ☞ **REMEMBER** Catastrophic deterioration in a ventilated asthmatic is usually due to loss of airway (obstruction or displacement) or massive auto-PEEP or tension pneumothorax causing severe obstructive shock that may progress to cardiac arrest or pulseless electrical activity (PEA).
>
> - In the latter two conditions, both mechanical and manual ventilation will be difficult.
> - Rapidly rule out ET problems, then briefly disconnect the ET from the ventilator for ~ 30 sec. This will relieve massive auto-PEEP, if present. Proceed to needle thoracocentesis with a 16G cannula over the lung where air-entry is reduced. Get a stat CXR, consider a chest tube.

- Other complications are VAP, barotraumas, pulmonary edema, steroid induced myopathy.
- ***Fast track weaning:*** Once the patient is clinically better (lower plateau pressures, better flow-time graphics, less air-trapping on CXR), discontinuation from the ventilator should be rapid. Anticipate that the wheeze may persist or become more prominent during improvement; this should not deter weaning.

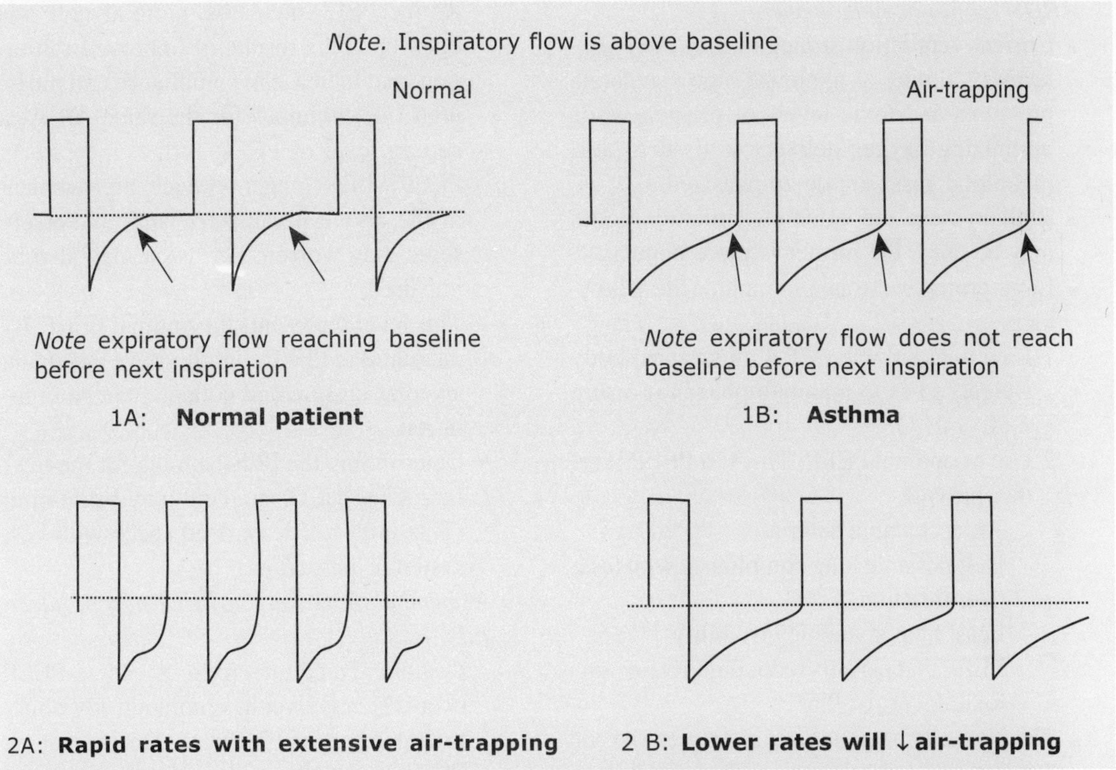

Fig. 24.1 Figures 1–2: Use of flow-time scalars on the ventilator graphics to minimize air-trapping (Figures modified from Ventilation ppt created by Dr Ram Rajagopalan, SMF, Chennai)

- The level of sedation should be rapidly reduced, and the patient extubated. Early extubation is important as the presence of the ET in the trachea may provoke more bronchospasm, particularly as sedatives are reduced.

4. Parenchymal lung disease: ARDS, pneumonia, aspiration

All the above diseases are associated with bilateral infiltrates, reduced compliance and hypoxemia. The prototype is ARDS (Acute respiratory distress syndrome): aka non cardiogenic pulmonary edema (*also see chapter on ARDS*)

- ARDS has multiple etiologies, both pulmonary (aspiration, inhalational burns, pneumonia) and non pulmonary (shock lung, sepsis, TRALI, post cardiopulmonary bypass).
- Although the lungs appear diffusely affected on CXR, the *pathology is heterogeneous*, with atelectatic segments interspersed with normal lung regions. This has important implications for ventilator induced lung injury (VILI): Normal lung segments get preferentially hyperinflated during PPV while the collapsed segments remain closed.
- Widespread atelectasis results in a reduced FRC with an increase in closing volume above FRC.
- Inadequate oxygenation occurs due to V/Q mismatching and intrapulmonary shunting.

ARDS ventilator management

- Current ventilation strategies are *"lung protective,"* aiming to minimize high ventilating pressures and toxic levels of oxygen while optimizing oxygen delivery to tissues. Normal blood gases are de-emphasized.
- Both pressure and volume ventilatory modes may be used; the former is more popular.
- Lung-protective strategies include the following:
  1. Low tidal volume (VT 6 ml/kg ideal body weight) so as to maintain plateau pressure < 30 cmH_2O
  2. Use of optimal PEEP: This is a PEEP level that provides
     - An acceptable saturation (86-90%)
     - Best possible lung compliance with least over-inflation
     - Least hemodynamic instability
     - PEEP that permits reducing FiO_2 to non-toxic levels (< 0.6)
- The above strategies have a greater risk of hypercapnia and hypoxemia than more conventional settings. "Permissive hypercapnia" is acceptable with no actual upper limit of pCO_2 as long as the pH is >7.15.
- A high level of PEEP is the mainstay of improving oxygenation in ARDS.
- PEEP improves compliance so that less ventilating pressures are required for the same change in volume. The high PEEP will prevent alveolar de-recruitment (closure) that can occur due to the low VT, particularly in dependent regions. PEEP also prevents cyclical opening and closure of alveoli, thus shear injury and release of inflammatory mediators is decreased (bio-trauma).
- *How to determine the optimal PEEP*
  - Increase PEEP gradually with a fixed level of ΔP (level of PIP above PEEP).
  - Monitor compliance (VTe), O_2 saturation and hemodynamics.
  - As the PEEP increases, more alveoli will open up. This results in improved saturation, and increase in compliance and measured tidal volumes for the same ΔP. At a certain level of PEEP, further increase in PEEP will no longer produce improvement in the above parameters, and conversely some may worsen. Perfusion may also be impaired.
  - This level represents the optimal PEEP. By maintaining PEEP slightly above this point, alveolar closure and collapse can be minimized.
  - Determining the PEEP aiming for the lowest $etCO_2$-$paCO_2$ gradient may be helpful. (This indicates least dead space with best systemic perfusion.)
- *Remember that excessive PEEP may be harmful!*
  - *Compliance can decrease* if excess PEEP over-distends alveoli: ventilation now shifts to upper part of PV curve (see chapter on Physiology)
  - Overinflated alveoli can decreased alveolar perfusion by compressing surrounding capillaries, worsen V/Q mismatch, thus increasing dead space and pCO_2.
  - Increased barotrauma risk
  - Hyperinflation can worsen hemodynamics by multiple mechanisms: decreased venous return, increased PVR, pulmonary hypertension resulting in right ventricular dysfunction; all culminating in decreased cardiac output (CO).
- In general, safe levels of PEEP are 7-10 cmH_2O in heterogeneous lung disease (e.g., pneumonia) and 10-15 cmH_2O in non-pulmonary ARDS where pathology is more diffuse.
- Since O_2 saturation may be low with the above strategies, attention to systemic oxygen delivery is important. It is essential to maintain a normal cardiac output (Optimize intravascular filling, use inotropes early, main-

tain high normal mean arterial pressures, monitor hemodynamics continuously with invasive arterial and central venous lines). Maintain hematocrit ≥ 30% to improve O_2 content.

- Sedate with benzodiazepine and opioid infusions to decrease metabolic demands.
- Modes with decelerating flow (PC/PRVC) are preferred for heterogeneous lung disease as they ensure higher mean airway pressure (MAP) for a lower PIP and cater to lung units with varying time constants. However, volume controlled ventilation is also widely used.
- *Decelerating flows* cater to the heterogeneous lung disease by permitting filling of lung units with both short and long time constants.
- Ensure long inspiratory time (at least one second) and normal for age rates. *Inverse ratio ventilation* can help in improving oxygenation.
- Prone ventilation has been shown to be beneficial in improving oxygenation for extrapulmonary ARDS if instituted early and for at least 20 hours a day. Not all patients improve. Discontinue if oxygenation worsens. Ensure that ETT is in lower $^{2}/_{3}{}^{rd}$ of trachea prior to proning (high incidence of tube dislodgement).
- *ETT suctioning protocol:* disconnecting the ETT from the vent can cause de-recruitment due to loss of PEEP. Options include minimizing suctioning unless strictly necessary; ventilator circuits with sealed ports for suctioning or using closed circuit suction catheters. Following suctioning, briefly ventilate at slightly higher tidal volumes in order to re-recruit alveoli.
- Summary: *Strategies to improve oxygenation (accept SaO_2 mid 80s to low 90s)*
  - Measures that increase MAP (↑ PEEP, PIP up to 30-35, longer Ti, decelerating flows with rapid rise time)
  - Decrease oxygen demands by sedation, consider muscle relaxants.
  - Select the "best PEEP."
  - Plateau pressure should not exceed 30 cmH_2O.
  - Ensure the hemodynamics and O_2 delivery to tissues are optimized (fluids, inotropes, hematocrit 30%)
  - Inverse I:E ratio ventilation, I:E ratio 1:1 to 1:2.
  - Prone ventilation.
  - Attempt to limit FiO_2 to < 0.6, however never withhold 100% O_2 to a hypoxic patient.
  - Rule out "DOPE" when the patient is condition worsens.
  - Nitric oxide (NO) at 20-40 ppm.
  - High frequency ventilation.
- Summary: *pCO_2 management*
  - Rule out "DOPE"
  - Low VT of 6 ml/kg will lead to elevated pCO_2 (accept high pCO_2 as long as pH > 7.15-7.2).
  - If pH < 7.2 secondary to ↑ pCO_2, increase ventilatory rate (up to 30-40/min)
  - If no improvement, sodium bicarbonate infusion may be given to raise pH.
  - Increase VT > 6 ml/kg provided plateau pressure are < 30-35 cmH_2O.

5. Ventilation of patient with heart failure, cardiogenic shock

Intubation and ventilation are usually initiated when circulatory shock is severe and/or associated with pulmonary edema.

How does positive pressure ventilation help?

- Decreases pulmonary congestion, decreases preload to failing heart
- Reduces afterload of the left ventricle, thereby improving cardiac output.
- Opens the alveoli in pulmonary edema, ↓WOB, improves compliance and oxygenation.

- Improves systemic oxygen delivery by taking over work of breathing and diverting cardiac output from respiratory muscles to the peripheral tissues.
- Ventilation in conjunction with judicious sedation will reduce metabolic demands.

Cardiogenic shock: Strategies in ventilatory management

- Intubate and initiate controlled ventilation with sedation early for a patient in cardiogenic shock who fails to improve with other supportive measures.
- PEEP should be sufficient to recruit lung and improve pulmonary edema (5-8 cmH_2O): excessive PEEP will ↑ PVR and worsen right ventricular function.
- Ventilation may be weaned only when inotropic requirement is minimal (5 mcg/kg/min of dopamine or dobutamine).

6. Postoperative ventilatory management after repair of congenital heart disease

Strategies:

- Many infants and children require mechanical ventilation after open heart surgery. This ventilation is usually for a short period till the child is hemodynamically stable. Prolonged intubation and mechanical ventilation are more likely in infants, complex heart lesions, prolonged bypass and circulatory arrest times, post-operative respiratory failure and hemodynamic instability.
- In the immediate post-operative period, tidal volume should be at least 6-8 ml/kg. Adequate PEEP (3-5 cmH_2O) should be applied to prevent atelectasis. The ventilator rate should be appropriate for the age and can be weaned as haemodynamic function improves.
- Strategies to reduce pulmonary vascular resistance (PVR) include maintaining low normal pCO_2 (30-35), low PEEP, high FiO_2.
- In patients with a marginal cardiac output, high airway pressures are to be avoided. PEEP helps in reducing afterload and thereby the cardiac output.
- In patients who have undergone a Fontan procedure, early extubation is desirable, and if that is not possible, then spontaneous ventilation should be encouraged using PS/CPAP or NIPPV. Since the right ventricle is bypassed, these patients depend totally on venous return for forward flow to the pulmonary circulation. High pulmonary or airway pressures will therefore impede systemic venous return and also reduce pulmonary blood flow (PBF) from ↑ PVR. Hence airway pressures must be kept at a minimum.
- Following the Glenn procedure, the pCO_2 should be maintained at around 40 mmHg to avoid reduction in cerebral blood flow and cerebral ischemia.

Failure to wean children following cardiac surgery may be due to:

a. Heart failure or residual defects
b. Airway abnormalities like tracheobronchomalacia.
c. Diaphragmatic palsy/paresis.

REFERENCES

1. Venkataraman ST. Mechanical ventilation and Respiratory Care. In: Pediatric Critical Care. Fuhrman and Zimmerman (eds). 3rd ed. Philadelphia, PA, 2006, Mosby Elsevier, 683-719.
2. Heulitt MJ, Wolf GK, Arnold JH. Mechanical ventilation. In: Rogers Textbook of Pediatric Intensive Care. David G Nichols (Ed). 4th ed. Philadelphia, PA, 2008. Lippincott, Williams and Wilkins, 508-531.

25

Getting Started: Setting up the Ventilator and Care of a Ventilated Patient

- Artificial ventilation is a demanding procedure, which requires all the technical resources of the Intensive Care Unit.
- Wall outlets for oxygen, purified air and suction, monitors with abilities to track continuous HR, RR, Sao_2, invasive monitoring, facilities for immediate blood gas analysis and bedside X-ray are essential.
- Trained medical and adequate nursing staff should be available around the clock.

ANATOMY OF THE VENTILATOR

Ventilator hardware: The gases and control system

- Most modern ventilators are powered by compressed gases and electricity.
- Compressed air may be provided either centrally from a wall outlet or via stand alone compressors that are attached to the ventilator.
- Oxygen is supplied either centrally from a wall outlet or from bulk O_2 cylinders.
- The O_2 and air are delivered at prescribed pressures (60 psi: pounds per square inch) that, apart from supplying gas for exchange, also are a source of the ventilator power to propel gases into the patient's lungs.
- Both air and O_2 are cold and dry and must be warmed and humidified prior to delivery to the patient's lungs.
- A control system consists of sophisticated software that ensures that the pattern of breath output by the ventilator is the same as that which is set by the caregiver.

Ventilator hardware: Monitors

- All ventilators will have pressure gauges and volume and flow sensors to monitor the function of the ventilator and assess the patient's breathing efforts.
- Signals interpret patient-ventilator interaction and control the ventilator output.
- Alarms that indicate high and low pressure, volume and oxygen concentrations are universal.
- Many modern ventilators also have a graphical package that can accurately assess patient-ventilator interaction and function and indicate problems much before clinical signs are manifest.

Ventilator hardware: The ventilator circuit

- Reusable vs disposable circuits. Either may be used provided sterility is ensured. There is no role for routine changes of the ventilator circuit unless visibly soiled. Frequent changes predispose to a higher incidence of VAP.
- Connect a ventilator circuit that has a heated wire in the inspiratory limb, preferably in the expiratory limb as well: this prevents condensation of the heated humidified gases in the tubing (rain-out) which can lead to potential problems with triggering and a higher VAP rates.

- Ensure functioning humidifier or a HME device in older children.
- Ensure that water traps are present in both limbs and that these are placed in a dependent position so that excess water in the circuit is drained and does not inadvertently flow into the patient's lungs.
- Remember the "compressible volume" of ventilator circuit.
  - The pre-set tidal volume that leaves the inspiratory port of the ventilator is divided between the circuit and the patient's lungs. In infants, the volume that remains in the circuit represents a much larger proportion of the smaller pre-set tidal volume.
  - The compressible volume never reaches the patient but is compressed and then distends the circuit during positive pressure ventilation.
  - Circuits that are soft will have a greater compressible volume and distend more with less volume reaching the patient. Stiffer circuits distend less, more of the pre-set volumes reach the patient and are preferred especially in infants.
  - The manufacturer may specify the compressible volume (varies from 0.8 to 2 ml/cmH_2O).
  - Prior to connecting the patient to the ventilator, ensure that a *system self-check* has been performed with the circuit and the test lung in place. This calculates the compressible volume of the circuit and will factor this calculation while displaying the VTe.
  - Overall, it may be prudent to ventilate infants < 8 kg in the pressure control mode if circuit compressible volume is thought to be leading to hypoventilation, particularly when hypercapnia is an issue.

Ventilator hardware: Humidification

- With nose breathing at rest, inspired gases become heated to 36°C and are about 80% to 90% saturated with water vapour by the time they reach the carina, largely due to heat transfer in the nose.
- If totally dry gases were inspired and fully saturated gases exhaled, the total water loss from ventilation at rest would be about 300 ml/day in the average adult.
- Bypassing the nose with an endotracheal tube and not humidifying gases causes water loss, hypothermia, inspissation of airway secretions, destruction of airway epithelium and atelectasis.
- All patients with an artificial airway (endotracheal or tracheostomy tube) should receive continuous humidification of inspired gases.
- This may be accomplished using either a heated humidifier or a heat and moisture exchanger (HME). The chosen device should provide a minimum of 30 mg H_2O/L of delivered gas at 30°C.
- Heated humidifiers operate actively to increase the heat and water vapour content of inspired gas.
- HMEs are also known as hygroscopic condenser humidifiers, or artificial noses. HMEs operate passively by storing heat and moisture from the patient's exhaled gas and releasing it to the inhaled gas.
- Heated humidifiers are preferred in most instances to an HME device in children as the resistance and consequent WOB may be higher with an HME. There is some evidence, however, that HME may lead to a lower incidence of VAP as the dry tubings are less prone to bacterial overgrowth.
- Because condensate in the circuit is infectious waste, it should never be drained back into the humidifier reservoir.
- Contraindications for HME:
  - Tracheal secretions that are copious, tenacious or thick.
  - Patients with an expired tidal volume less than 70% of the delivered tidal volume (e.g., uncuffed ETT or large bronchopleurocutaneous fistulas)

- Body temperatures less than 32°C.
- High spontaneous minute volumes.
- An HME must be removed from the patient circuit during aerosol treatments when the nebulizer is placed in the patient circuit.

- Hazards and complications of humidification devices
  - Temperature disturbances: Hyperthermia with thermal injury to airway with heated humidifiers. Select appropriate temperature settings.
  - Under-hydration and impaction of mucus secretions. Ensure adequate water level.
  - Hypoventilation and/or alveolar gas trapping due to mucus plugging of airways.
  - Possible hypoventilation due to increased dead space via HME. The HME selected should be appropriate to the patient's size and tidal volume.
  - Inadvertent tracheal lavage from pooled condensate in patient circuit. Keep water traps in a dependent position.
  - Patient ventilator dysynchrony and improper ventilator performance due to pooled condensation in the circuit with heated humidifiers.
- HME vs heated humidifier
  - HMEs are better suited for short term use (= 96 hours) and during transport.
  - Heated humidifiers should be used for patients requiring long term mechanical ventilation (> 96 hours) or for patients who exhibit contraindications for HME use (see above).
  - Heated humidifiers preferred in young children and infants.

INITIAL VENTILATOR SETTINGS

1. **Before connecting the patient to the ventilator**
   - Have the ventilator perform a "System Self Check" with the circuit and a test lung in place prior to connecting the patient. This will measure the "compressible volume" (see above: ventilator circuit) of the circuit and factor this value during tidal volume measurements.
   - Pressure controlled ventilators are preferred in infants < 8 kg as the tidal volumes in small infants (30-100 ml) may be much less than the relatively large volume of the ventilator circuit. Volume may also be lost because of a leak around an uncuffed tube.
   - There is no precise method to predict the initial requirements of PIP until the extent of the patient's pulmonary dysfunction is established. An adequate chest rise, good oxygenation and hemodynamic stability will determine the setting.
   - Once the preliminary settings are made, the patient is connected to the ventilator. The optimum PIP and tidal volume are then assessed by listening to the air entry and exit, observing chest excursion and performing an arterial blood gas analysis.
   - Ensure functioning humidifier or an HME device. An HME may be appropriate in older children, unless tracheal secretions are excessive.
2. **Provision of adequate alveolar ventilation (CO_2 removal)**
   - Select ventilator rate: As per disease and physiologic norm for age.
   - Volume controlled ventilation: Select tidal volume: 6-8 ml/kg. This may be further adjusted based on chest rise, air entry and blood gases.
   - Pressure controlled ventilation: Select PIP: 10-20 cmH_2O above PEEP. The selected PIP should be sufficient to produce a satisfactory chest rise. The tidal volumes generated will depend on the ΔP (difference between PIP and PEEP) and also the lung mechanics.
   - Select Inspiratory time (I:E ratio): Age specific norm resulting in I:E ratio ≈ 1:2 (in obstructive lung disease, prolonged expiratory time and slow rates may be required).
3. **Maintenance of adequate oxygenation**
   - In a hypoxemic patient, set the initial FiO_2 high at 0.6-1.0. Once oxygenation improves,

one should bring the FiO_2 to non-toxic levels ($FiO_2 < 0.5$).

- PEEP: 5 cmH_2O or higher as needed. Optimal PEEP should recruit collapsed lung units and improve compliance and oxygenation while avoiding hemodynamic impairment and over-inflation.
  - In general, in diseases with ↓compliance, PEEP levels are titrated to above end points.
  - In heterogeneous lung disease, limit PEEP to 7-10 cmH_2O; in more diffuse lung disease, PEEP of 10-15 cmH_2O can safely be used. Target SaO_2 90% with FiO_2 0.5-0.6.
  - In lower airways disease, PEEP is initially set low and then titrated to levels of auto-PEEP (see chapter on Disease Based Ventilation).
  - Assess adequacy of oxygenation (color, pulse oximetry), compliance (change of volume for the given ΔP) and signs of perfusion.
  - The final selected PEEP should result in adequate lung volumes: counting eight to nine posterior rib spaces on CXR is a useful guide.

4. **Setting appropriate alarm settings**
   - As soon as the final adjustments of the ventilatory settings have been made, it is essential to set the high and low pressure and volume alarms on the ventilator. This is often forgotten as it is considered unimportant by caregivers.
   - Common sense will dictate the alarm settings. If the alarms are set in a very narrow range, early events will be picked up, but many false alarms may occur: real events may thus be ignored by caregivers.
   - Likewise, if the alarm limits are too wide and extreme, life threatening events may not result in any alarms until too late.
   - High pressure alarm:
     - This should be based on the patient lung mechanics. The high pressure limits are usually set 8-10 cmH_2O above the set PIP. When the high pressure alarm is activated, inspiratory flow to patient ends and excess gases are vented out. The high pressure alarm is also activated when the patient coughs.
     - A new onset persistent high pressure alarm signifies worsening of lung mechanics (increase in the resistance or decrease in compliance) or ET related issues (secretions, patient biting the tube).
   - *Low pressure alarm*
     - This is usually set 5 to 10 cmH_2O below the PIP. This alarm indicates that the circuit pressure has fallen significantly usually because of leaks in the system.
     - The common causes of leak are disconnections at any point along the ventilator circuit. Check all connections for leaks, disconnections.
     - Leaks most often occur around the humidifier, at water traps or at any point where joints are present. Leaks can also develop around the ET cuff if it is not adequately inflated or when lung compliance worsens.
     - Large leaks may result in inadequate ventilation and also interfere with flow cycling, especially if the child is on pressure support.

ASSESSMENT AND MONITORING OF A VENTILATED PATIENT

1. **Clinical assessment**
   - Assess frequency and strength of both mechanical and spontaneous breathing.
   - Synchronization with the ventilator.
   - Chest wall excursion and adequacy of air entry/exit.
   - Observing and documenting vitals of the patient (BP, HR, temperature, respiratory rate, distal and central pulses should be done at least every hour and more often if required).

- Abdominal distension, bowel sounds and gastric aspirates.
- Neurobehavioral activity.
- Readiness for weaning.

2. **Interpretation of the central venous pressure (CVP) measurement during positive pressure ventilation (PPV)**
   - Remember that the measured CVP value on the monitor will increase proportional to the intrathoracic positive pressure: this occurs even though the venous return actually decreases during PPV. The CVP should be measured at end expiration.
   - A high CVP does not rule out hypovolemia; however, a low CVP on PPV in a patient with hemodynamic instability indicates significant hypovolemia and mandates immediate fluid resuscitation.

3. **Ventilator assessment**
   - Mode of ventilation and the breath type must to be documented.
   - Assess whether the set trigger/sensitivity is comfortable for the patient and all breathing efforts are assisted without over-triggering.
   - Assess the mechanical and spontaneous VTe, rates and minute ventilation.

4. **Radiological assessment**
   - X-rays should be done at least once daily in the acute stage and whenever acute deterioration occurs. In a stable ventilated patient, less frequent X-rays are acceptable.
   - The following should be looked for in the CXR of a ventilated patient.
     - Position of ET tube tip (lower $^{2}/_{3}$rd of trachea, ≈ at the level of the 2nd rib), position of nasogastric tube.
     - Overall lung volume, evidence of hyperinflation.
     - Air leak syndromes: Interstitial emphysema, pneumothorax etc.
     - Presence of new infiltrates, atelectasis, pulmonary edema.
     - Heart size, presence of chest wall edema.

5. **Laboratory Investigations**
   - Arterial blood gas (ABG)
     - Perform an ABG within 20-30 minutes of initiating ventilation and ideally after major setting changes.
     - Repeat ABG every 4-6 hours thereafter, or earlier if there is a marked change in condition.
     - Stable ventilated patients may need less frequent ABG, depending on the clinical status.
     - Maintain disease specific goals: Decreasing ventilator induced lung injury (VILI) has a higher priority than attempting to achieve normal blood gases.
   - Others laboratory tests: Hemogram, biochemical parameters as clinically indicated
   - Microbiological testing for suspected ventilator associated pneumonia (VAP) or tracheobronchitis:

> ☞ **REMEMBER** It is important to differentiate between bacterial colonization vs invasive nosocomial pneumonia (see chapter on Hospital Acquired Infections).

     - ET tubes get rapidly colonized by the patient's throat flora (usually GNB in the ICU patient).
     - While colonization is frequent, invasive pneumonias are less common.
     - A positive growth of micro-organisms from ETT secretions may be confusing and should not automatically be labeled as VAP or lead to unnecessary antibiotic prescribing unless the patient has other evidence of VAP.
     - Whenever a VAP is suspected, a protected bronchoscopic sample of the involved area is cultured.
     - An alternative is obtaining a protected sample of the lower respiratory tract secretions by a 'tube in tube method" or mini BAL.

FEEDING AND NUTRITION

- Oral feeds of a ventilated child with an ETT is not possible since the tube interferes with normal swallowing.
- However, the majority of ventilated children may be fed enterally via a nasogastric tube.
- The few patients in whom enteral feeds are not possible (ileus, abdominal pathology) should receive parenteral nutrition.
- Whichever the route chosen, an attempt to meet the required calorie and protein requirements must be made. High carbohydrate containing diets should be avoided as it may result in increased CO_2 production.

GENERAL CARE OF A CHILD ON VENTILATOR

- The head-end of the child should be elevated by 30-45°. This is one of the most efficient and cost effective methods of preventing micro-aspiration and VAP.
- Frequent position change. The patient must be turned on to the left and right lateral positions every 2 hours. This may require two personnel, one to ensure airway stability and the other person to turn. After turning, prevent the patient rolling back to supine position by propping with pillows or rolls. Ensure that the patient is in a comfortable position.
- Keep the ventilator circuit free from condensate by ensuring that the water traps and in a dependent position to facilitate optimal drainage of collected moisture/"rain out." Ensure that the condensate does not drain into the patient's ETT.

Care of tubes

- Ensure that the tapes are secure and check marking at lip/nose. Verify position on CXR.
- The tracheal tube or the tracheostomy cuff pressure should be checked every 8-12 hours (every shift) to ensure that the cuff pressure does not exceed 20-25 mmHg.
- If cuff pressure measurement is unavailable, ensure that a palpable leak is felt when the PIP is 20 cmH_2O.
- Keeping the cuff pressure below this level helps in reducing the risk of tracheal mucosal ischemia and consequent necrosis associated with over-inflated tube cuffs or large ETT with the risk of post-extubation stridor. This is particularly important in hypotensive patients where cuff pressure may be higher than the capillary pressure of the trachea resulting in significant tracheal mucosal damage.

Suctioning the ETT and oral cavity

- The ET may be suctioned when secretions are thought to be excessive.
- A clean technique (clean, non-sterile gloves with "hand-rub" disinfection) is adequate and does not increase the risk of VAP compared to a sterile technique.
- Frequent suctioning of oral and deep pharyngeal secretions by a Yankauer suction apparatus has an important role (often overlooked) in minimizing trickling down of pharyngeal secretions, thus preventing micro-aspiration and VAP.
- Thrice daily oral hygiene with 2% chlorhexidine is important to decrease the incidence of VAP.

Keeping the patient comfortable

- Intubation, ventilation along with all of the monitoring paraphernalia, unfamiliar environment, loud alarms etc., are highly anxiety provoking, frightening and can have adverse long term psychological impacts on children.
- It is humane to alleviate pain and anxiety and the majority of patients can be adequately analgesed and sedated by a combination of benzodiazepine and opioid infusion. In our PICU, a combination of midazolam 1-2 mcg/kg/min and morphine 30-60 mcg/kg/min is the standard regimen in ventilated children.
- However, ensure that agitation or "fighting" is not due to correctable systemic causes such

as hypoxemia or cerebral hypoperfusion. Ensure that the ET tube is patent, in good position and well secured, the ventilator settings are appropriate and no complications have occurred.

- The need for muscle relaxants is exceedingly uncommon because of the risk of critical illness polyneuro/myopathy and the availability of safe and effective sedative agents.
- Good sedation analgesia protocols should be followed and "drug holidays" and appropriate weaning planned.
- Both sleep deprivation and sedation withdrawal are common reasons for agitation and this should be taken care of.
- Pressure areas and bony prominences should be well protected to prevent sores from developing.
- Oral and eye care along with general hygiene should be maintained.
- The caregivers should try and maintain a pleasant ICU ambience. Care should be taken to maintain asepsis for all procedures.
- Frequent visit by parents and touch and play therapy should be encouraged if the child is awake.

DETERIORATION IN VENTILATED PATIENTS

(See chapter on Trouble-shooting a ventilated patient)

Acute deterioration

- D – Displaced tube: esophagus, right main bronchus
- O – Obstructed tube
- P – Pneumothorax, pneumopericardium
- E – Equipment failure, disconnection

Gradual deterioration

- Partial tube occlusion
- Sepsis, pneumonia
- Myocardial dysfunction, pulmonary edema
- Biochemical: Disturbances in glucose or electrolytes, metabolic alkalosis

COMPLICATIONS OF ASSISTED VENTILATION

Numerous complications may contribute to patient morbidity and mortality.

1. **Related to increased airway pressures and lung volume**
   - Barotrama/volutrama
   - Pulmonary interstitial emphysema, pneumothorax
   - Pneumopericardium, pneumoperitoneum, subcutaneous emphysema
   - Decreased cardiac filling and poor perfusion
   - Other organ dysfunction: Renal, hepatic, CNS
   - Pulmonary parenchymal damage.
2. **Related to endotracheal/tracheostomy tube**
   - Tracheal mucosal damage
   - Sinusitis/middle ear infection (nasal ET tubes)
   - Laryngeal edema, subglottic stenosis
3. **Nosocomial infections**
   - Ventilator associated pneumonia
   - Ventilator associated tracheobronchitis
   - Sepsis
4. **Mechanical operational problems**
   - Mechanical ventilator/compressor failure
   - Alarm failure or inappropriate limits
   - Inadequate humidification

Prevention of ventilator associated pneumonia: The VAP bundles

- Elevation of the head of the bed 30-45°.
- Daily assessment of sedation and "sedation holidays" where the doses of sedative drugs are decreased or ceased.
- Daily assessment of readiness to extubate.
- Peptic ulcer disease (PUD) prophylaxis.
- Oral care protocol with chlorhexidine-based mouth wash at least thrice daily and frequent pharyngeal secretion clearance.

REFERENCES

1. Venkataraman ST: Mechanical ventilation and respiratory care. In: Pediatric Critical Care. Fuhrman and Zimmerman (Eds). 3rd ed. Philadelphia, PA, 2006, Mosby Elsevier, 683-719.

2. Martin LD, Bratton SL, Walker LK. Principles and Practice of Respiratory Support & Mechanical Ventilation. In: Rogers Textbook of Pediatric Intensive Care. 3rd ed. William & Wilkins, 1996

3. AARC Clinical Practice Guidelines. Humidification during Mechanical Ventilation. *Respir Care* 1992(8); 37:887-890

26

Non-Invasive Positive Pressure Ventilation

- Non-invasive ventilation (NIV) is the delivery of mechanical ventilation to the lungs using techniques that do not require an endotracheal airway.
- NIV is attractive because it has the potential to avoid complications of conventional ventilators such as intubation complications, ventilator associated pneumonia (VAP), post extubation stridor etc (Table 26.1).
- The three basic methods by which NIV can be delivered are:
  - Negative pressure ventilation
  - Abdominal displacement ventilation and
  - Positive pressure ventilation.

The chapter will only cover ***non-invasive positive pressure ventilation (NIPPV)*** which is widely used in both adult and pediatric intensive care units (PICU).

The two methods by which NIPPV can be delivered are:

1. Continuous positive airway pressure (CPAP).
2. NIPPV using stand alone NIV machine or using the conventional ventilator

Table 26.1 Advantages of NIPPV

Acute care settings	Chronic care settings
▪ Reduces need for intubation	▪ Alleviates symptoms of chronic hypoventilation
▪ Reduces incidence of nosocomial pneumonia	▪ Improves duration and quality of sleep
▪ Shortens ICU stay	▪ Improves functional capacity of the lungs
▪ Preserves airway defences	▪ Prevents disuse atrophy of respiratory muscles
▪ Improves patient comfort	▪ Prolongs survival
▪ Allows direct oral feeds, permits communication and improves sense of well being	
▪ Reduces costs	
▪ Reduces need for sedation	

INDICATIONS FOR NIPPV

a) *Acute hypoxemic respiratory failure (AHRF)*

- This is the commonest use of NIPPV in pediatric patients. Examples of AHRF include pneumonia, atelectasis, asthma and episodes of acute hypoxemia in chronic conditions like cystic fibrosis.
- Careful selection of these patients when they have moderate degrees of hypoxemia is important.
- Children with severe hypoxemia (such as ARDS) should never be given NIPPV.

b) *To facilitate early extubation*

- Children on invasive ventilation whose disease process has improved but not resolved and continue to require moderate levels of positive pressure can be extubated to NIPPV.

c) *Obstructive airway disease*

- Patients with dynamic upper airways obstruction such as laryngomalacia and tracheomalacia may benefit from positive pressure applied via NIPPV that acts to splint open the airways. NIPPV should not be used in those with fixed airway obstruction, e.g., subglottic stenosis, webs.

d) *Neuromuscular disorders*

- NIPPV has been extensively studied in the children with Duchenne muscular dystrophy and Guillain Barre syndrome provided their bulbar functions and airway protective reflexes are preserved. In these disorders, NIPPV prevents ventilator dependency and atelectasis by improving functional residual capacity.

e) *Cardiogenic pulmonary edema*

- CPAP applied via mask decreases the afterload of the failing heart, improves WOB by recruiting fluid filled alveoli, thus improving lung compliance and oxygenation.

f) NIPPV has an important role in immunocompromised patients with decompensated respiratory disease as VAP rates are much lower.

MECHANISM OF NIPPV MODES

- *In CPAP, a continuous positive pressure* is delivered during the spontaneous respiratory cycle.
- In NIPPV, *two levels of positive pressure* are delivered, viz: IPAP and EPAP
  - IPAP: Inspiratory positive airway pressure.
  - EPAP: Expiratory positive airway pressure (which functions like PEEP).
  - The difference between the two levels of pressure generates the pressure support and tidal volume.

TYPES OF VENTILATORS THAT DELIVER NIPPV

- NIPPV can be delivered by a conventional ICU ventilator (where the operator can set the IPAP and EPAP) or through portable stand alone NIV ventilators.
- These portable ventilators are pressure targeted or volume targeted; the former is more common. The pressure targeted ventilators are also known as BiLevel CPAP ventilators or BiPAP.

BiLevel CPAP or pressure targeted ventilators (PTV)

- They have a single tubing gas delivery system that uses an intentional leak port for patient exhalation instead of a true exhalation valve; this allows continuous flow of gas through the small leak port to help maintain pressure levels and flush the exhaled gases from the circuit.
- PTVs may be flow or time triggered, pressure limited, flow or time cycled ventilators.
- They are designed to increase minute ventilation and improve gas exchange with delivery of an IPAP (range: 2-30 cmH_2O) and EPAP (range: 2-30 cmH_2O).
- Most PTV can be operated with following modes:

  a) *CPAP mode*
  - The patient breathes spontaneously at a preset baseline pressure.
  - The patient controls both the rate and depth of breathing.
  - When the patient's respiratory effort is sensed by flow sensors, flow through the circuit is increased to maintain a stable preset pressure.

  b) *Assist/Spontaneous mode (S)*
  - Here, apart from the set EPAP, a change to the set IPAP is delivered whenever the patient makes an inspiratory effort.
  - However, if the patient were to become apneic, there is no back up rate which the ventilator can deliver.

- Therefore this mode can be used only in patients with a stable respiratory drive.

c) *Assist Control/Spontaneous-timed mode (S/T)*
- This is similar to assist mode but also has a back up rate that needs to be set.
- If a patient fails to make an inspiratory effort within a set interval, the machine triggers inspiration to the set IPAP.

d) *Control mode*
- The control mode delivers pre-set pressure targeted breaths based on the control settings and not on the patient efforts.
- The clinician sets the IPAP and EPAP, the number of breaths per minute, and the inspiratory time percent (IPAP %).
- The breaths are time triggered to the IPAP based on the set rate. IPAP then cycles to EPAP based on the IPAP % period.
- In all the modes the tidal volume delivered will depend on the gradient between IPAP and EPAP, the inspiratory time, the patient's inspiratory effort and lung mechanics.

OXYGEN DELIVERY AND CO_2 ELIMINATION DURING NIPPV

NIPPV has several **limitations** compared to conventional ventilation and cannot be used in severe respiratory failure.

1. *The oxygen delivery is variable*
   - The FiO_2 is not measured in most NIV machines.
   - When supplemental oxygen is required, it must blend into the system through the mask or through the additional port near the outlet.
   - Therefore the FiO_2 may vary and is affected by four factors:
     - Oxygen flow rate.
     - Type of leak port in the system.
     - Site where the supplemental oxygen is introduced into the circuit.
     - IPAP and EPAP.
   - Higher oxygen flow rates result in higher oxygen concentrations.
2. *Rebreathing of CO_2 is a concern with any NIPPV that uses a single circuit gas delivery system* because exhalation occurs through a single leak port and depends on the adequate continuous flow of gas in the circuit.
   - If gas flow is inadequate, flushing of exhaled gas may be incomplete and patient may rebreathe the exhaled gas.
   - The flow of gas depends on the EPAP settings and the patient's I:E ratio.
   - At low EPAP settings (< 4 cmH_2O) and faster respiratory rates, flow may not be adequate to flush the CO_2.

NIPPV INTERFACES

- An interface is a device that permits the tubing of the machine to be connected to the patient.
- Examples of NIPPV interfaces
  - Nasopharyngeal tubes (endotracheal tubes inserted with depth of insertion from nose to tragus) or nasal prongs to deliver CPAP.
  - Oronasal/nasal mask to deliver NIPPV.
  - Newer interfaces like helmets and full face masks are also available.
- In addition to the interfaces, mouth seals and lip seals are provided to prevent mouth leakages during nasal ventilation.

INITIATION AND TITRATION OF NIPPV

- The intitiation of NIPPV has to be done in a controlled manner as many children do not tolerate the tightly applied interfaces with high gas flow blasting on the face.
- It is helpful for caregivers to enlist parental support and spend some time in familiarizing the child with the interface and the device.
- They should gain the trust and gauge the compliance of patient. The interface is initially gently applied against face without fastening the head straps.

- During this period, constant reassurance and encouragement is necessary. The interface may be changed if the patient is uncomfortable with the one used.
- Following this, the parents/caregivers should slowly initiate the NIPPV at a lower settings and gradually increase it rather than beginning at the higher target pressures. It is best to start with low levels of EPAP alone and then gradually increase EPAP and finally dial in the IPAP. This helps in establishing a good seal between the child's face and the interface without any leak.
- The headgear straps are only adjusted and tightened once the patient is comfortable. This may take some time and needs continuous monitoring.
- A nasogastric tube may be inserted to initiate feeds and it can be used to decompress stomach in between feeds.
- A mild sedative agent (trichlorofos) can be given if the child is not tolerating the interface provided hypoxia is not the cause for agitation.
- Over the initial 2 hours, the set pressures may be titrated by continuous monitoring of clinical parameters such as heart rate, respiratory rate, breathing pattern, breathing sounds and chest excursion along with O_2 saturation and blood gases.
- A decrease in heart rate by approximately 20% from the baseline, 10% reduction in respiratory rate with improvement in work of breathing, saturation and blood gases within 1–2 hours of initiation of NIPPV indicate that the patient is benefiting from and tolerating the device satisfactorily.

CONTRAINDICATIONS FOR NIPPV

- Hemodynamic instability
- Impaired mental status with poor respiratory drive
- Moderate to severe bulbar weakness
- Inability to handle oral secretions
- Inability to tolerate the mask
- Refractory hypoxemia
- Upper gastrointestinal bleed

NIPPV is best for patients who are sick but not too sick.

MONITORING DURING NIPPV

- Close monitoring is the rule. It is important that patients who fail NIPPV (not improving or worsening) should be immediately shifted to invasive ventilation. Deaths have been reported from failure to recognize that the patient is deteriorating on NIPPV.
- Monitor HR, RR, BP, pulse oximetry, alertness and comfort level.
- Other variables to be monitored:
  - Adequacy of seal
  - Patient agitation and discomfort
  - Skin irritation, pressure points
  - Gastric distension
- Ensure that humidification is adequate.
- Nurses and duty doctors must be fully aware of signs of deterioration.

WEANING OF NIPPV

Two methods may be employed:

- Once steady improvement of clinical condition has begun, NIPPV settings are lowered. The IPAP levels are weaned first followed by EPAP.
- The second option is intermittent discontinuation of NIPPV for brief periods (30-60 min).
- If tolerated, the duration of discontinuation may gradually be increased until patient is off for 3-4 hr.
- Eventually, NIPPV may be provided only at night-times when the patient is asleep.
- Intermittent NIPPV allows re-conditioning of the respiratory muscles while simultaneously preventing fatigue by permitting a sufficient period of rest.

COMPLICATIONS

- Epistaxis due to absence of humidification
- Eye irritation
- Intolerance due to high gas flows
- Gastric distension
- Sinusitis

Remember, NIPPV may have life threatening consequences if:

- *The expiratory ports are closed.*
- *Over reliance on NIPPV when disease is worsening.*
- A patient who demonstrates continued respiratory distress despite maximum support, poor tolerance of mask, onset of hemodynamic instability or excessive airway secretions requires immediate intubation or else can progress to cardiorespiratory failure and death.
- NIPPV is a good option to conventional ventilation in carefully selected patients in select conditions.

REFERENCES

1. Liesching T, Kwok H, Hill SN. Acute applications of Non invasive positive pressure ventilation. Review article: Chest ,124;2:Aug 2003: 609-712.
2. Sangeeta Mehta and Nicholas S Hill. Non-invasive Ventilation. J Respir. Crit Care Med Volume 163, Number 2, February 2001; 540:577.
3. Non invasive ventilation in acute respiratory failure. British Thoracic Society Standards of Care Committee. Thorax 2002; 57:192-211.

27

High Frequency Oscillation Ventilation (HFOV)

INTRODUCTION

- *What is HFOV?*
  Mechanical ventilation that uses supra-physiological breathing rates and very low tidal volumes (0.5-2 ml/kg) is called HFOV. The tidal volume is barely greater than the dead space, hence alternative mechanisms of gas transport are required to explain the effect of HFOV.
- In conventional ventilation, the inspiration is active and expiration is passive, very similar to normal breathing. In HFOV, both inspiration as well as expiration is active. This facilitates independent oxygenation and ventilation.
- Oxygenation is achieved by sustained inflation and recruitment of the lungs by the application of continuous distending pressure.
- Ventilation is achieved by the imposition of an oscillating waveform with variable frequency and amplitude.
- HFOV is not as yet proven to be of benefit in the *elective treatment* of respiratory failure. Furthermore, the main concern when HFOV is used relates to worsening cardiac output due to constant high airway pressures.
- Also some infants do not tolerate the extra handling involved in switching ventilators or simply may not respond to HFOV. If no improvement is seen with HFOV, do not persist for too long, consider reverting back to conventional ventilation.

BENEFITS OF HFOV OVER CONVENTIONAL VENTILATOR

- Conventional ventilation works on the principle of producing pressure changes to cause bulk flow of gas in and out of the lungs. The large volumes and pressures may cause ventilator induced lung injury (VILI).
- The various types of VILI include:
  a. Barotrauma: trauma caused to lungs due to high airway pressures.
  b. Volutrauma: trauma caused to lungs due to high volumes, particularly at end-expiration.
  c. Atelectrauma: trauma caused due to shearing forces due to cyclic closing and opening of alveoli.
  d. Biotrauma: The cumulation of all the insults result in extensive release of inflammatory mediators which can then trigger multiorgan failure.
- HFOV can decrease VILI in the following manner:
  a. Smaller tidal volumes prevent volutrauma.
  b. Barotrauma is less as pressure gets damped by the time it reaches the terminal airways and alveoli. This is in contrast to conventional ventilator where there is no dampening.
  c. Atelectrauma and shearing injury is minimal during HFOV as the cyclic opening and closing of alveoli which occurs in conventional ventilator is reduced. The sustained pressures

during HFOV opens even more previously inaccessible alveoli with more surface area for oxygenation and ventilation. This improves V/Q matching. The lower distending pressures do not traverse either the lower or upper inflection points, thus preventing both atelectasis as well as over-distension.

d. Biotrauma and multiorgan failure is also reduced.

CLASSIFICATION OF DEVICES

- High frequency oscillation ventilation
- High frequency jet ventilation
- High frequency flow interrupters

- Of all these devices, the most widely used is the SensorMedics A and B HFOV machine. Also in the market are ventilators which combine conventional and high frequency but they do not possess all the features of a complete HFOV.
- The SensorMedics A machine is useful for children up to 30 kg. The SensorMedics B machine is used for older children and adults; it is not recommended for use in children < 10 kg.

MECHANISM OF GAS EXCHANGE

Gas transport under non-physiologic conditions

- Bulk flow can provide some conventional gas delivery to proximal alveoli with low regional dead space volumes.
- Gas exchange also occurs in areas of coaxial flow: this describes regions where gas flows in two directions (gas in the centre which flows inward and gas on the periphery flows outward).
- Taylor dispersion produces mixing of fresh and residual gas.
- Pendelluft results in mixing of gases between lung regions with different impedances.

Principle of HFOV (Fig. 27.1)

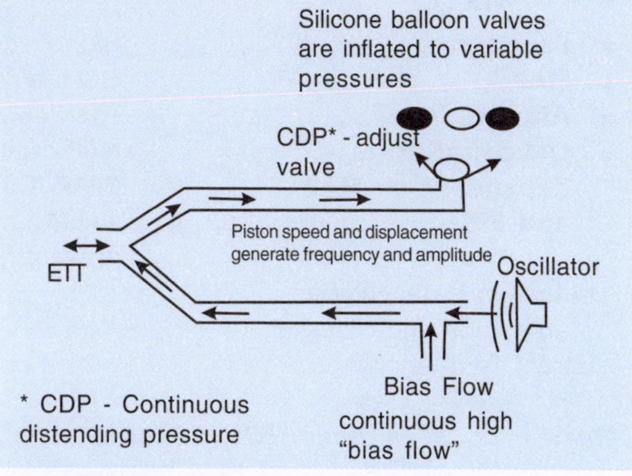

Fig. 27.1 Principle of HFOV

- Silicone balloon valves are inflated to variable pressures to generate continuous distending pressure (CDP) in the expiratory circuit.
- There is continuous high "bias flow" in the circuit: This is very important for maintaining the continuous distending pressure and interruption of this flow even for 0.4 sec results in lung derecruitment.
- Piston speed and displacement generate frequency and amplitude and vary ventilation.
- Inspiration and expiration are both active phases.

CLINICAL INDICATIONS FOR STARTING HFOV

Requirements for high FiO_2 (> 0.6) and pressures (MAP >16 cmH_2O) to maintain adequate oxygenation and ventilation in a patient who is not clinically improving.

STARTING A PATIENT ON HFOV

The continuous high intrathoracic pressures on HFOV can cause significant low cardiac output (CO) and it is essential to optimize CO with volume ± inotropes prior to HFOV initiation.

- Start with FiO_2 of 1.0.

Table 27.1 HFOV terminology

▪ **Frequency**	- High frequency ventilation rate (Hz, cycles per second)
▪ **MAP**	- Mean airway pressure (cmH_2O)
▪ **Amplitude**	- The Power or delta P is the variation around the MAP
▪ **Oxygenation is dependent on MAP and FiO_2**	- MAP provides a constant distending pressure equivalent to CPAP. This inflates the lung to a constant and optimal lung volume maximising the area for gas exchange and preventing alveolar collapse in the expiratory phase.
Ventilation is dependent on amplitude and to lesser degree, frequency.	

Remember, when using HFOV, CO_2 elimination and oxygenation are independent

- MAP should be 2-3 cmH_2O greater than MAP on the conventional ventilation.
- Amplitude is set at 20-40, titrated to presence of vibration or "*wobble*" in lower abdomen.
- Frequency is set according to the patient's age and weight (see Table 27.2)

Table 27.2 Choosing the frequency setting

Patient weight	Hertz
Preterm neonates	10-15
Term neonates	8-10
Children	6-8
Adults	5-6

- Increase MAP by 1-2 cmH_2O to achieve optimal lung volume. Optimal lung volume is determined by:
  - Increase in O_2 saturations allowing the FiO_2 to be weaned
  - Diaphragm is at T9 on chest radiograph

AFTER PLACING A PATIENT ON HFOV (TABLE 27.3)

- Once on the oscillator, monitor oxygen saturations, perfusion and get a blood gas within 20 minutes.
- You should be able to wean the FiO_2 to < 0.6 within the first 12 hours of HFOV.
- Follow CXR to assess the lung expansion
  - If the diaphragm is between 8 and 8½ ribs and sats > 90%, maintain MAP and FiO_2.
  - If the diaphragm is between 9 and 9½ ribs, wean the MAP by 1 cmH_2O.
- If unable to wean FiO_2, consider a recruitment maneuver (sustained inflation) or increasing the MAP.

Table 27.3 Making adjustments once established on HFV

Poor oxygenation	Over-oxygenation	Poor ventilation (high CO_2)	Over-ventilation (low CO_2)
Increase FiO_2 Increase MAP (1-2 cmH_2O)	Decrease FiO_2 Decrease MAP (1-2 cmH_2O)	Increase amplitude Decrease frequency (1-2 Hz) if amplitude maximal	Decrease amplitude Increase frequency (1-2 Hz) if amplitude minimal

VARIABLES THAT CONTROL VENTILATION

a) Tidal Volume (ΔP or amplitude)
   - The power controls and regulates the force and distance with which the piston moves from baseline.
   - The degree of deflection of the piston (amplitude) determines the tidal volume.
   - This deflection is clinically demonstrated as the "wobble" seen in the patient.
   - The wobble factor can be utilized in assessing the adequacy of set amplitude.

b) Frequency (λ) (Table 27.2)
   - Referenced in Hertz (1 Hz = 60 breaths/second)
   - Range: 3-15 Hz.
   - Adjustments in frequency are made in steps of ½ to 1 Hz.

c) For improving ventilation, initially increase the amplitude. Amplitude can be increased to more than 3 times the MAP. If CO_2 removal is still problematic, then the frequency can be reduced. Reduce frequency in steps of 0.5 to 1 Hz.

d) If high pCO_2 still a concern, deflate the ETT cuff in order to produce a moderate leak.

INDICATIONS FOR HFOV

1. ARDS/ALI
   HFOV in ARDS helps to utilize aggressive alveolar recruitment and utilizes the open lung strategy *("Open the collapsed alveoli and keep them open")*
2. Other conditions where HFOV may be useful
   - Meconium aspiration
   - Hyaline membrane disease, BPD
   - Extensive atelectasis, lung hypoplasia
   - Air leak syndromes: This is never a primary diagnosis but a result of diffuse alveolar disease. Open lung strategy helps in resolution of the air leaks.
     - There are occasional patients in whom air leak can be refractory.
     - In such patients, the patient is removed form HFOV and by manual inflation a *"leak pressure"* is identified above which air bubbles appear in the thoracotomy drainage tube. If the leak pressure is > 15 cmH_2O, a period of permissive hyperoxia is undertaken.
     - Here the pressure is set below the leak pressure and FiO_2 is set high so as to achieve saturations between 85-90% despite the lower MAPs. The air leak will usually decrease within next 24 hr.
   - Persistent pulmonary hypertension and congenital diaphragmatic hernia.

SEDATION AND NEUROMUSCULAR BLOCKADE

- Transitioning a patient from CMV to HFOV usually indicates that the respiratory distress has worsened.

- The greater the amplitude, the greater the CO_2 clearance.
- The lower the frequency, the greater the CO_2 clearance.
- The lower the frequency setting, the larger the volume displacement.
- The higher the frequency setting, the smaller the volume displacement.

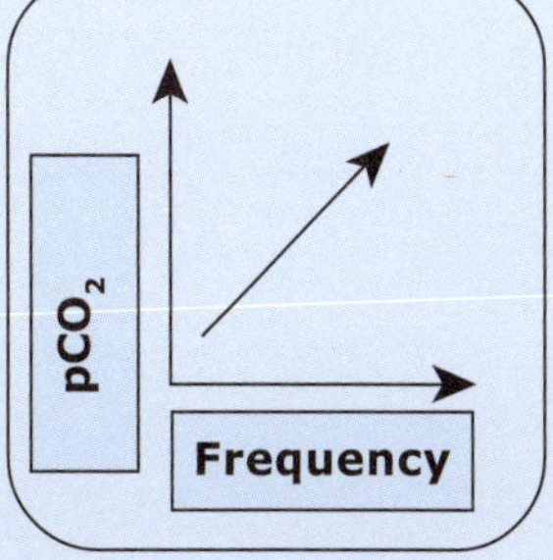

Fig. 27.2 Determinants of CO_2 clearance

- To facilitate 'capturing' the patient, additional sedation may be required; in older children, brief periods of neuromuscular blockade may be required.

POTENTIAL COMPLICATIONS AND DISADVANTAGES OF HFOV

- Potential to cause decreased cardiac output is a major concern.
- Necrotizing tracheobronchitis: This may be avoided by adequate humidification of the high flow inspiratory gases.
- Pneumothorax, air leaks
- Migration/displacement of tracheal tube
- Bronchospasm
- Acute airway obstruction from mucus plugging, secretions, blood clots
- Complications of the high-dose sedation +/- muscle relaxants

REFERENCES

1. John H Arnond. High-frequency ventilation in the pediatric intensive care unit. Pediatr Crit Care Med 2000; Vol 1:93–99.

28

Approach to a Child in Shock

DEFINITION

- Shock is defined as a syndrome of cardiovascular dysfunction characterized by the inability of the circulatory system to provide adequate oxygen and nutrients to meet the metabolic demands of vital organs, clinically recognized by inadequate perfusion.
- It is important to note that the definition of shock does not depend on the blood pressure. A child in shock can have normal, high or low blood pressure.
- Shock, if not recognized and treated appropriately, can progress to death from cardiovascular and multiorgan failure.

PHYSIOLOGY OF SHOCK

- Inadequate tissue oxygenation due to inadequate perfusion leads to tissue hypoxia, anerobic metabolism, tissue acidosis and organ damage.
- Hypoxic-ischemic injury to tissues is the final common determinant in all forms of shock.
- While oxygen delivery (DO_2) depends on cardiac output (CO) and oxygen content (CaO_2), tissue oxygenation also depends on oxygen extraction (OE). OE may be impaired in certain forms of shock despite adequate or increased CO and DO_2.

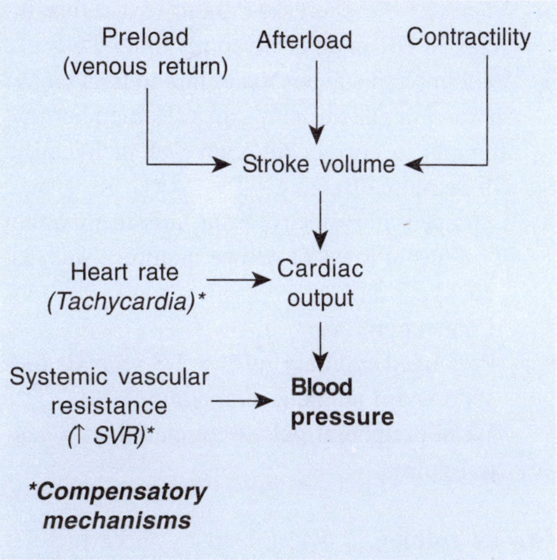

Fig. 28.1 Determinants of blood pressure

The determinants of oxygen delivery to tissue can be summarized by the following relationships:

Oxygen delivery (DO_2) = Cardiac output (CO) × Oxygen content (CaO_2)

↓ CO = Stroke volume (SV) × Heart rate (HR)

↓ $CaO_2 = 1.34 \times Hb \times SaO_2 + (0.003 \times paO_2)$

Oxygen content of the blood can be improved by optimizing the Hb content and also to some extent by administering supplemental oxygen.

- Oxygen administration may be required even if the patient is not hypoxemic: CaO_2 will increase by increasing dissolved oxygen in the blood.

Cardiac output (CO) is the product of stroke volume (SV) which is the volume of blood ejected with each cardiac contraction, and heart rate (HR).

- In children, low CO is generally due to low SV rather than low HR.
- When the SV decreases, there is a reflex increase in HR in an effort to maintain CO.
- A common mistake is to attempt to treat tachycardia in a patient with shock. Remember that attempts to correct the cause of tachycardia will be more effective.
- If compensatory tachycardia fails to maintain CO, signs of low CO will be manifest, such as:
  - Tachycardia.
  - Cool extremities.
  - Prolonged capillary refill > 2-3 seconds (despite warm ambient temperature).
  - Weak peripheral pulses compared with central pulses.

Stroke volume is determined by three factors: Preload (end-diastolic volume), contractility and the afterload.

Inadequate preload is the most common cause of low SV and therefore low CO.

- It is important to understand that preload basically means the effective circulating volume and not the total blood volume.
- Inadequate preload can result from obvious losses in circulating volume as in hemorrhagic shock, diarrhea and vomiting.
- Inadequate preload may also result from occult losses as in septic shock where capillary leak, venodilation and maldistribution of blood flow (resulting in relative hypovolemia) may occur.
- Maldistribution and abnormal blood flow is also called *distributive shock* (see types of shock below), which can occur with normal, low or increased total blood volume.
- This may be encountered in neurogenic and anaphylactic shock apart from septic shock.

Decreased myocardial contractility (myocardial dysfunction) may be due to a congenital intrinsic problem with the cardiac pump (some forms of congenital heart diseases) or due to acquired causes such as inflammation of the heart muscle (myocarditis), circulating myocardial depressants (as in septic shock) or secondary to myocardial hypoxemia causing dysfunction (hypoxic-ischemic injury following cardiac arrest, prolonged hypoxemia due to any cause).

Increased afterload is an uncommon primary cause for low cardiac output. This component most often occurs in response to decreased CO and is a compensatory mechanism that serves to maintain perfusion pressures to vital tissues such as brain and heart.

CATEGORIES OF SHOCK

Shock can be categorized by its effect on the systolic blood pressures (SBP) into two broad forms:

- **Compensated shock**
  - Compensated shock is a clinical state where the SBP is maintained within normal range with signs of inadequate tissue perfusion being present.
  - BP is maintained secondary to compensatory mechanisms (increased HR and increased SVR) that attempt to maintain adequate perfusion to brain and heart at the cost of inadequate perfusion to skin, skeletal muscle, gut and kidneys (Table 28.1).
  - It is important to note that children with compensated shock may be critically ill with severe shock despite the SBP being normal.
  - Although the SBP is normal in compensated

Table 28.1 Compensatory mechanisms in shock

Compensatory mechanisms	Tissue/ organ	Signs
Increased heart rate	Heart	Tachycardia
Increased SVR	Skin	Cold, pale, diaphoretic
	Circulation	Delayed capillary refill
	Pulses	Weak peripheral pulse, narrow pulse pressure, elevated DBP
↓ splanchnic blood flow	Kidney, intestine	Oliguria, vomiting, ileus

shock, the diastolic blood pressures (DBP) may be normal or high.

- **Hypotensive shock** (previously called decompensated shock)
  - Hypotensive shock develops when the physiological compensatory mechanisms fail and is a late finding in most types of shock.
  - This may signal irreversible organ injury and impending cardiac arrest.
  - Clinically it is characterized by impalpable radial or brachial pulses, impalpable or weak central pulses and low SBP (< 5th centile for age, Table 28.2).
  - Warning clinical signs that predict progression of shock from compensated to hypotensive shock to impending cardiac arrest are deterioration in the mental status, loss of peripheral pulses, inappropriate bradycardia and absent central pulses.

Shock should be clinically diagnosed before hypotension occurs by carefully assessing patients at risk of shock (fluid losses, fever etc) by evaluating clinical signs which include hypothermia or hyperthermia, altered mental status, with peripheral vasodilatation (warm shock), or cool extremities with capillary refill > 2 seconds (cold shock).

TYPES OF SHOCK

There are four types categorized clinically:

- Hypovolemic
- Distributive
- Cardiogenic
- Obstructive

Table 28.2 Lower limit of SBP for age

Age	SBP (mm Hg)
Term neonates	< 60
1-12 months	< 70
1-10 yr	< 70 + (2 × age in yr)
>10 yr	< 90

Table 28.3 Normal heart rates by age (beats per minute, BPM)

Age	Awake rate	Sleeping rate
Newborn to 3 months	85-205	80-160
3 months-2 yr	100-190	75-160
2-10 yr	60-140	60-90
>10 yr	60-100	50-90

ASSESSMENT OF A PATIENT WITH SUSPECTED SHOCK

Airway

- Categorize airway as: Clear/maintainable by simple measures/compromised (needs advanced intervention such as intubation).

Table 28.4 Physiology of each category of shock

Category of shock	Preload	Contractility	Afterload
Hypovolemic	Decreased	Normal or increased	Increased
Distributive	Normal or decreased	Normal or decreased	Variable
Septic shock	Decreased	Normal or decreased	Variable
Cardiogenic	Variable	Decreased	Increased

- If the airway is significantly compromised in a patient with shock, remember that
  - The shock state is at an advanced stage, and
  - The patient is at risk of severe brain hypoxia and may need urgent interventions, both to stabilize airway and circulatory status

Breathing

- Patterns of breathing may provide useful information, both at initial presentation and during correction with fluids.
- Some patients may have "quiet" tachypnea (rapid respiratory rates with normal mechanics of breathing) due to associated metabolic acidosis.
- Other patients in shock may have increased "work of breathing" (WOB) when there is lung parenchymal involvement (pneumonia as the focus, or pulmonary edema which may be cardiogenic/non-cardiogenic).

Circulation

- Assess heart rate (HR) and assess if appropriate for age (see normal ranges as in Table 28.3).
- Patients in shock are usually tachycardic both during the compensated and hypotensive stage. Bradycardia is usually a preterminal event.
- Relative bradycardia for the degree of shock can be seen in children with specific shock states (dengue shock syndrome and spinal shock) and also in children who are on drugs which decrease heart rates (beta blockers).
- Assess rhythm: Usually regular unless associated with arrhythmias
- Assess blood pressure: Systolic, diastolic and mean blood pressure.
- Systolic blood pressure (SBP) for age: This may be normal/high/low.
- Assess pulse pressure (PP = SBP – DBP): Usually about 40 mmHg in adults.
- The pulse pressure depends on the DBP and may be assessed in relation to the SBP
  - A narrow PP due to a rise in DBP is associated clinically with cold peripheries and narrow pulse pressure.
  - A narrow PP may be seen in cold septic shock, dengue shock, hypovolemic shock and cardiogenic shock (DBP > 2/3 SBP).
  - A wide PP is usually clinically associated with warm extremities and bounding pulses.
  - A wide PP may be seen in warm septic shock, anaphylactic shock, neurogenic shock (DBP < ½ SBP or PP > ½ SBP).
- Assess the pulse volume, i.e., strength of central pulse (carotid, brachial, femoral) versus peripheral pulse (radial, dorsalis pedis, posterior tibial).
  - All pulses may be bounding in distributive shock.
  - Central pulses may be better felt compared to weak peripheral pulses in compensated shock.

- Central pulses may also become weak or impalpable as shock progresses.
- Assess capillary refill time (CFT). Normal CFT < 2 seconds. May be delayed to > 3 sec in cold shock, a rapid or "flash" CFT is seen in warm shock.
- Assess skin colour and temperature: Cold, mottled, cyanosed extremities in cold shock, warm, flushed extremities in warm shock.
- Assess for presence of cyanosis which may be peripheral cyanosis (indicating poor peripheral perfusion), or central cyanosis (respiratory failure with shock, abnormal hemoglobins).
- Assess end-organ function
  - Brain perfusion: Assess for altered mental status, irritability, lethargy, agitation, seizures, coma, hypotonia.
  - Renal hypoperfusion: Easily assessed by catheterizing and measuring hourly urine output. Because the kidneys receive the second highest blood flow in the body, measurement of urine output is a simple, inexpensive method of assessing adequate perfusion status.
  - Urine output may be unreliable in the presence of osmotic diuresis (hyperglycemia, mannitol), or recent diuretic use. Oliguria is defined as urine output < 1 ml/kg/hr.

SIGNS OF SPECIFIC TYPES OF SHOCK

1. **Hypovolemic shock** (GI losses, hemorrhage, diuresis as in diabetic ketoacidosis or diabetes insipidus, burns, capillary leak)
   - History suggestive of obvious losses (diarrhea, vomiting, bleeds, inadequate intake, diuresis) or in the setting for occult losses (burns, capillary leak, sepsis)
   - Quiet tachypnea
   - Tachycardia
   - Hypotension or normotension with narrow pulse pressure
   - Variable pulse volume (normal/low) depending on stage/severity of shock
   - Delayed capillary refill
   - End organ perfusion abnormalities: Cold extremities, altered mental status, oliguria
   - Favorable response to fluids, hypovolaemic arterial trace, improvement on leg raising and pressure over liver (equivalents of fluid bolus).
2. **Distributive shock** (anaphylactic, septic, neurogenic shock)
   - Tachycardia
   - Usually quiet tachypnea
   - Normotensive or hypotension with wide pulse pressure
   - Bounding peripheral pulses
   - Brisk or delayed capillary refill
   - Warm, flushed extremities
   - Altered mental status
   - Oliguria
   - Presence of associated symptomatology

Septic shock

Most patients are warm and vasodilated; however, some patients may be cold and vasoconstricted. The clinical diagnosis of septic shock is made in children who have:

- Suspected infection manifested by hypothermia or hyperthermia, and
- Clinical signs of decreased perfusion including any of the following:
  - Decreased mental status
  - Prolonged capillary refill > 2 seconds (cold shock) or flash capillary refill (warm shock)
  - Diminished peripheral pulses (cold shock) or bounding peripheral pulses (warm shock)
  - Mottled cool extremities (cold shock)
  - Decreased urine output < 1 ml/kg/hr

Anaphylactic shock: Rash, urticaria, angioedema, nausea/vomiting, bronchospasm.

Neurogenic shock: Setting of head injury or spine injury, hypotension with bounding pulses, relative bradycardia or absence of tachycardia, respiratory muscle weakness.

3. **Cardiogenic shock**: Suspect in the presence of congenital heart disease, myocarditis, cardiomyopathy, arrhythmias, sepsis, poisoning, drug toxicity, myocardial contusion, any prolonged shock with poor perfusion to the myocardium will eventually lead to cardiogenic shock.
   - Tachypnea with increased work of breathing.
   - Tachycardia with or without a gallop rhythm.
   - Normal or low blood pressure with narrow pulse pressure (unless in warm septic shock and associated myocardial dysfunction).
   - Weak or absent peripheral pulses.
   - Delayed CFT.
   - Cold extremities, altered mental status, oliguria.
   - Hepatomegaly, jugular venous distension, basal lung crackles and cyanosis may be present.
   - Adverse response to rapid fluid challenge.

☞ **REMEMBER** The combination of tachycardia and poor perfusion with abnormal mechanics of breathing is highly suggestive of cardiogenic shock.

4. **Obstructive shock** secondary to conditions such as cardiac tamponade, tension pneumothorax, duct dependant lesions, massive pulmonary embolism.
   - *Cardiac tamponade*: Muffled or diminished heart sounds, pulsus paradoxus, distended neck veins. Small QRS complexes on ECG.
   - *Tension pneumothorax*: Respiratory distress, hyper-resonance on the affected hemithorax, diminished breath sounds, tracheal deviation to the opposite side and rapid evolution from tachycardia to bradycardia as cardiac output falls.
   - *Duct dependant lesion* (coarctation, interrupted aortic arch): Presents usually during the first 2 weeks of life with poor systemic perfusion, congestive heart failure, absent femoral pulses, respiratory failure with pulmonary edema or apnea.

SOME COMMON TERMINOLOGIES UNIVERSALLY USED TO DESCRIBE THE STATE OF SHOCK

- **Fluid refractory shock**: Signs of shock persisting despite 60 ml/kg of appropriate fluid resuscitation in the first hour of presentation OR shock that persists despite restoring normovolemia as evidenced by a CVP > 12 mmHg or adequate chamber filling on ECHO.
- **Cold septic shock**: Decreased perfusion manifested by altered mental status, capillary refill > 2 seconds, diminished peripheral and/or central pulse volume, mottled cool extremities and decreased urine output < 1 ml/kg/hr.
- **Warm septic shock**: Decreased perfusion manifested by altered mental status, flash capillary refill, bounding peripheral pulses, warm extremities, decreased urine output < 1 ml/kg/hr and metabolic acidosis or elevated lactate.
- **Fluid refractory/dopamine-resistant shock**: Shock persists despite > 60 ml/kg fluid resuscitation and dopamine infusion of 10 μg/kg/min.
- **Catecholamine resistant shock**: Shock persists despite use of the direct acting catecholamines, epinephrine or norepinephrine.
- **Refractory shock**: Shock persists despite goal directed use of inotropic agents, vasopressors, vasodilators, and maintenance of metabolic (glucose and calcium) and hormonal (thyroid, hydrocortisone, insulin) homeostasis.

MANAGEMENT OF SHOCK

(Also refer to specific chapters on septic shock, dengue shock, cardiogenic shock and inotropes). Management consists of supportive interventions which are geared to the underlying cause of the shock.

1. Stabilize the airway and breathing.
   - Administer oxygen by non-rebreathing mask.

- Consider intubation for low GCS < 8, unstable airway, hypoxemia or hypercarbia and refractory shock.

2. Establish early intravenous access. Two IV lines preferred. Intraosseous cannula if rapid peripheral access not obtained.
3. Resuscitate with rapid boluses of 20 ml/kg isotonic crystalloid such as saline or Ringer's lactate, unless in cardiogenic shock. Consider colloid.
4. Early antibiotics must be given in suspected septic shock after drawing cultures.
5. Establish central and invasive arterial lines. Monitor CVP, arterial lactate and mixed venous saturations.
6. Consider inotropes/vasopressor if shock persists despite adequate fluid resuscitation.
7. Consider early inodilators in cardiogenic shock.

Key Messages

- Early recognition of shock and intervention is critical in halting progression from compensated to hypotensive shock to cardiorespiratory failure.
- Treatment goal for shock is to prevent end-organ injury and halt the progression of cardiopulmonary failure and cardiac arrest.
- Blood pressure in shock can be normal, high or low. Hypotensive shock is a late finding and may signal irreversible organ injury or impending cardiac arrest.
- Increased work of breathing differentiates cardiogenic shock from hypovolemic shock which is characterized by quiet tachypnea. Other features include hepatomegaly, jugular venous distension, basal crepitations and gallop rhythm.
- Consider duct dependant lesions in a neonate with shock and intervene early with prostaglandins.

REFERENCES

1. Ralston M, Hazinsky MF, Zaritsky AL, et al (Eds): Pediatric Advanced Life Support Provider Manual. Dallas, TX, American Heart Association, 2006–2007
2. PR Dellinger, MM Levy, J Carlet, et al. Surviving Sepsis Campaign: International guidelines for management of severe sepsis and septic shock: 2008. *CCM* 2008; 36 (1):296-327
3. Circulatory blood flow: The ICU book. 3rd edition. Lippincott Williams & Wilkins, Baltimore 2007, pp 3-16.

29

Pediatric Septic Shock

- Septic shock is a form of *distributive shock.*
- It is caused by invasion of micro-organisms and is exaggerated by the body's immune response to the infection resulting in the release and activation of inflammatory mediators (cytokines).
- The cytokines mediate some of the typical changes of septic shock such as vasodilatation and capillary permeability.

1. **Definitions**
   - In the early stages, the patient may exhibit features of SIRS *(systemic inflammatory response syndrome)* which is a non-specific response to infection, trauma, surgery, burn etc.
   - *SIRS* comprises 4 components *(4 Ts)*:
     - Temperature changes: Fever or hypothermia
     - Tachycardia
     - Tachypnea
     - Total WBC changes: leucocytosis or leukopenia
   - *Sepsis:* SIRS with a suspected or proven infection.
   - *Severe sepsis*
     - Sepsis plus cardiovascular dysfunction or ARDS (Acute respiratory distress syndrome) OR
     - Sepsis with 2 or more organ failures.
   - *Septic shock*
     - Sepsis + Cardiovascular dysfunction* despite administration of ≥ 40 ml/kg isotonic fluid in 1 hour.
   - *Cardiovascular dysfunction** may be defined as:
     - Hypotension (SBP < 5th centile for age or need for vasoactive medication to maintain BP)

     OR any 2 of the following:
     - Unexplained metabolic acidosis (BE > -5 or lactate > twice upper limit of normal)
     - Oliguria: urine output < 0.5 ml/kg/hr
     - Capillary refill > 5 sec
     - Core to peripheral temperature gradient > 3°C.
2. **The pathophysiology** and response to therapy in septic shock are highly age dependent.
   Septic shock results in organ hypoperfusion due to multiple mechanisms:
   - *Hypovolemia:*
     - Abnormal vascular permeability (capillary leak) with loss of plasma into the interstitial compartment.
     - Decreased intake/excess losses from vomiting/diarrhea
   - *Altered systemic vascular resistance (SVR).*
     - Many patients have abnormally low SVR with arterial and venodilation resulting in increased capacitance and excess pooling of blood, further worsening of hypovolemia, wide pulse pressures, warm extremities with bounding pulses and early onset hypotension.
     - Some children are cold with elevated SVR.

- *Cardiac output (CO)* may be increased (hyperdynamic), normal or decreased. Although myocardial dysfunction is common, stroke volume can be normalized by aggressive volume resuscitation.
- *Maldistribution of blood flow* with some areas of excess flow (typically skin and skeletal muscle) co-existing with other organs/tissues that are inadequately perfused (especially the gut and splanchnic vasculature).

3. **Risk factors for sepsis**
   - Extremes of age, compromised immune system, malnutrition, asplenia, chronic antibiotic or steroid use.
   - Any insult (shock, trauma, burn, pancreatitis) that makes the gastrointestinal tract permeable to gram negative bacteria puts individuals at risk for sepsis.
4. **Causative organisms**
   - Gram negative and positive bacteria
   - Fungi, anaerobes
   - Viral septic shock
5. **Priorities of initial management are 3-fold** and include:
   - Early recognition of septic shock.
   - Early aggressive fluid and vasoactive medications aiming to normalize disordered hemodynamics within the first 6 hours.
   - Early appropriate antibiotics (within the 1st hour of diagnosis), identification of focus and source control (e.g., drainage of abscess/debridement of necrotic tissue where appropriate).
6. **Recognition of septic shock (Box 29.1)**
   - Rapid recognition of septic shock is essential to improve outcomes.
   - *Septic shock is a clinical diagnosis* and laboratory data are of limited utility in establishing the diagnosis.
   - Signs of early septic shock may be subtle and the progression rapid and there is a danger of overlooking the diagnosis in a busy outpatient or emergency department.
   - Any change in mental status (*altered alertness,* poor eye contact, inconsolable cry, excessive sleepiness or lethargy, unarousable) of a febrile child should prompt immediate consideration of septic shock.
   - For children, changes that occur *before* the onset of hypotension are the recognized clinical triad of hyper- or hypothermia, altered mental status and peripheral vasodilation ("warm" shock) or vasoconstriction ("cold" shock).
   - In 'warm shock,' bounding peripheral pulses and flash capillary refill may occur in conjunction with evidence of decreased perfusion, including decreased urine output, altered mental status and metabolic acidosis.
   - Patients with 'cold shock' have diminished peripheral pulses and prolonged capillary refill in conjunction with decreased perfusion.
   - Cultures of blood or any other body fluid suspicious of being infected should be taken prior to antibiotics being given. Identification of the organism causing the shock is useful in narrowing antibiotic medication later in treatment.
7. **Initial management (Box 29.2)**
   - The initial ABC's should be addressed as per Pediatric Advanced Life Support (PALS) guidelines and the Guidelines for the hemodynamic support of pediatric and neonatal septic shock outlines by the American College of Critical Care Medicine in 2009.
   - 100% Oxygen should be delivered to all patients by a non-rebreathing mask (NRM) and the need for a definitive airway should be assessed.
8. **Antibiotic therapy**
   - Due to the rapid progression of sepsis and multiorgan dysfunction, initiating appropriate antibiotics promptly will save lives.

Box 29.1 Recognize septic shock

A. Recognize septic shock:
- **Core temp** (oral/rectal/esophageal): < 98°F or > 101.5°F
- **CNS**: Change in mental status: Altered alertness, inconsolable, inability to recognize parents, unarousable
- **Breathing**: "Quiet" tachypnea or ↑ WOB
- **Threshold HR***: < 1 yr: < 100/min OR > 180/min; > 1 yr: < 80/min OR > 160/min

  *Correct HR for fever: HR increases by 10% of baseline for each degree rise of temp over 100°F
- **BP**: Low systolic BP or mean BP (MAP preferred) (See Box 29.5)
- **Peripheral perfusion**: Cold peripheries, central ± peripheral pulses feeble/absent with CFT > 3 sec *(cold shock)* OR warm extremities, bounding pulses with flash CFT < 1 sec *(warm shock)*
- **Urine output**: ask parent if urine output is normal or decreased in last 6 hr?
- **Metabolic acidosis**: Base deficit > - 5 or lactate > twice upper limit normal

B. Any of the following indicate a moribund state:
- Core temp low, low SBP/MAP, central pulse feeble, poor response to pain, bradycardic: Intubate STAT, initiate adrenaline 0.3-0.5 ml/kg/min early

- At least 2 sets of blood samples must be drawn for culture, one set from existing central lines (if present) and the second from a peripheral site. Ensure that aseptic precautions (sterile gloves, skin prep) are used in order to prevent contamination by skin flora.
- Initially the selection of antibiotics is empiric and should be broad spectrum (see Ch. 71).
- Choice of empiric antibiotic should be based on a consideration of:
  - The suspected site/focus of infection.
  - The suspected organism.
  - Whether the infection was acquired in the community or a hospital setting.
  - Host factors: Immune status, co-morbid conditions.
  - The local antibiotic resistance patterns.
- De-escalation based on sensitivities is an essential component of therapy.

9. **Fluid resuscitation (Box 29.4)**
   - Early fluid resuscitation is the cornerstone of septic shock treatment.
   - Venous access must be established as quickly as possible; if unsuccessful, proceed rapidly to intraosseous access.
   - Initial intravenous bolus of 20 ml/kg of isotonic crystalloid (normal saline or Ringer's lactate) or colloid must be followed by reassessment of each of the 6 therapeutic goals (Box 29.5). If some but not all goals have been met, re-bolus up to a total of 60 ml/kg in the first hour of resuscitation.
   - Rate of fluid bolus depends on the patient's BP.
   - If the patient is in hypotensive shock, rapidly bolus normal saline or RL until the SBP/MAP is normal for age.
   - If the patient is in compensated shock with a normal SBP/MAP for age, each 20 ml/kg bolus may be administered over 20 minutes, titrated to indices of perfusion.
   - If underlying cardiac dysfunction suspected, use smaller fluid aliquots of 10 ml/kg over 20-30 minutes.
   - After the initial 40 ml/kg, consider colloid (gelafusin/starch easily available).
   - Correct hypoglycemia by a separate bolus followed by dextrose infusion titrated to normoglycemia.
   - Cease/slow down fluid rates if shock resolves or features of fluid intolerance develop (tachypnea, WOB, ↑ O_2 requirement, new onset rales, hepatomegaly), see below.
   - Some patients require additional volumes of fluid up to a total of 100 to 200 ml/kg over the first few hours of resuscitation.
   - This large fluid requirement is more common

in patients with wide pulse pressures where the capillary leak combined with increased vascular capacitance lead to large volume deficits.

- Continue to titrate fluids at a slower rate (10-20 ml/kg/hr) even after the first hour till shock resolves. Extra isotonic fluids may be required for initial 6-12 hours.
- It is important to remember that ARDS and multi-organ failure may be more common in patients with uncorrected hypovolaemia and shock

Box 29.2 Initial interventions

1. Assess and maintain airway.
2. O_2 by NRM, capillary glucose (correct if low)
3. Insert 2 large bore peripheral IV cannulae (or intra-osseous)
4. One IV line for rapid fluid boluses: 20 ml/kg boluses of NS/RL until goals achieved (Box 29.5)
   - If SBP/MAP low for age, infuse each bolus by push-pull technique/pressure bag over 5-10 min
   - If SBP or MAP normal for age, infuse by free flow over 20 min (No pediatric burette)
5. Insert 2nd line with aseptic precautions (sterile gloves, skin prep); send cultures x 2 sets (each 5-10 ml) at least 10 min apart; send CBC, ABG, lactate.
6. Administer 1st dose antibiotic
7. Insert urinary catheter

10. **Therapeutic goals (Box 29.6)**
   - Early recognition of shock and initiation of early goal directed resuscitation fluid and inotropic therapy is the best way to optimize outcomes.
   - The caregiver must attempt to meet all 6 therapeutic goals by the initial 6 hours of presentation.
   - However, in a few patients, some goals may not be met even though shock may have resolved.
   - Tachycardia may persist due to persistent SIRS, pain, anxiety, drug effect.
   - Mental status may not normalize in patients with a primary CNS focus.

Box 29.3 CVP in septic shock

Indications for CVP
- To measure cardiac filling pressures and assess need for volume if shock unresoved despite 60 ml/kg
- Patient develops signs of fluid intolerance
- Need for inotropes/pressors
- Need for reliable IV access
- Facilitates blood sampling
   - A CVP is most useful if low in the presence of shock. Ventilated patients and patients with a myocardial dysfunction may require a higher CVP.
   - CVP goals: 10-12 mmHg (non-ventilated) /12-15 mmHg (ventilated).

   - In these patients, following trends in clinical signs may be useful to determine shock resolution. For example some tachycardia may be acceptable provided metabolic acidosis and elevated lactate have resolved, extremities are warm with a normal CFT and a mixed venous saturation between 70 and 75%.
   - Continuous close monitoring in the ICU is essential to detect recurrence of shock.

11. **Fluid intolerance (Box 29.4)**
   - Patients frequently show features of fluid overload/pulmonary edema during fluid resuscitation.
   - These may be in the form of new-onset or worsening rales/creps, hepatomegaly and ↑ O_2 requirement or work of breathing (WOB).
   - Causes of fluid intolerance
     - Capillary leak into lungs
     - Cardiogenic pulmonary edema (due to septic myocardial dysfunction). The CVP may be variable, depending on myocardial compliance.
     - ARDS.
     - Fluid overload.

Box 29.4 Fluid resuscitation

- Administration of > 40 ml/kg fluid in the 1st hr is associated with significant reduction of mortality
- If BP low, infuse each bolus rapidly over 5-10 min
- For compensated shock, infuse 20 ml/kg over 20 min
- Consider 3:1 crystalloid/colloid (starch) administration.
- Continue to titrate fluids after initial bolus (maintain CVP 10-12 mmHg)
- Slower filling better for myocardial dysfunction

Fluid refractory shock

Shock that persists despite adequate volume resuscitation documented by CVP > 12 mmHg ± adequate IVC filling on echo.

Fluid Intolerance

Worsening respiratory status (tachypnea, ↑ WOB, ↑ O_2 requirement), hepatomegaly

- Capillary leak
- Myocardial dysfunction
- Fluid overload
- ARDS

Remember fluid over resuscitation also harmful!!

- Hepatomegaly is a useful indicator
- Insert early CVP (within 1st hr, goal 10-12 mmHg)
- If signs of shock reversed, lower CVP acceptable
- Early echo for IVC filling and respiratory variation if shock not reversed with 60 ml/kg fluid

- Capillary leak is the commonest reason for fluid intolerance in septic shock.
  - This may be seen even with uncorrected hypovolemia and normal cardiac function.
  - Both crystalloids and colloids may leak from the vascular compartment.
  - Uncorrected hypovolemia may be documented by low CVP/echo features of underfilling.
- Management of fluid intolerance
  - Slow down fluid rate, consider colloids.

Box 29.5 Interventions if shock not reversed after 60 ml/kg fluid

- Consider intubation and ventilation (see below)
- Insert CVP and arterial line
- Commence inotrope/vasopressor (see choice below)
- Check central venous saturation

  - Consider inotrope/pressor depending on mean BP.
  - Positive pressure ventilation (CPAP/ invasive ventilation) is usually necessary.
- An early CVP ± ECHO will clarify if hypovlemia corrected. A normal/high CVP in patients with uncorrected shock suggests need for inotrope ± vasodilator. If CVP < 8 mmHg, continue colloids at slower rates with positive pressure.
- If therapeutic goals of shock met, lower CVPs may be acceptable.

12. **Fluid refractory shock (Box 29.4)**

    This is shock that persists despite restoration of normovolemia as documented by a CVP of > 12-15 mmHg or by ECHO demonstrating adequate IVC and cardiac chamber filling.
    - Causes are co-existing myocardial function or other morbidities (see below).
    - An early CVP and expert bedside echocardiographic evaluation will help to clarify if hypovolemia has been corrected and if co-existing right or left heart dysfunction is present.

13. **When to stop/slow down fluids: Patient condition better or worse**
    - Fluids may be ceased if all therapeutic goals met. A lower CVP is acceptable if shock has resolved.
    - Fluids may be ceased if features of pulmonary edema and hepatomegaly occur without further hemodynamic improvement OR a CVP (if present) is > 12-15 mmHg.

- After the initial rapid fluid boluses, a slower background rate of NS/RL should be continued at 10-20 ml/kg/hour until hemodynamics have stabilized.
- Maintenance fluids can be continued, or preferably, early enteral feeds may be commenced as soon as pulses return and perfusion improves.

Box 29.6 Therapeutic Goals: All must be achieved within 1st 6 hr

1. Achieve threshold heart rate for age
2. Maintain MAP/SBP for age
3. Urine output > 1 ml/kg/hr
4. Warm peripheries with CFT =/< 3 sec
5. Normal mental status
6. Improving metabolic acidosis or decreasing lactate.

- **Systolic BP**
  - Minimally acceptable SBP (> 5th centile) = 70 + age x 2
  - Acceptable SBP (> 50th centile) = 90 + age x 2
- Mean Arterial Pressure (MAP): Better indicator of organ perfusion than SBP
  1-6 mo: > 40-45 mmHg; 7 mo-5 yr: > 45-55 mmHg
  > 5-12 yr: >50-60 mmHg; > 12 yr: > 60–65 mm Hg
- Determine if pulse pressure (PP) normal/narrow or wide
  - Narrow PP: PP < ½ of SBP
  - Wide PP: PP > ½ of SBP or > 40 mmHg

14. **Intubation and ventilation (Box 29.7)**

- Early intubation is an important component of therapy for some children in septic shock.
- Indications for intubation: Increased work of breathing, pulmonary edema, hypoventilation, altered mental status (GCS < 8), refractory shock, severe hypoxemia ± hypercapnia and a moribund state.
- Anticipate worsening of hemodynamics when positive pressure ventilation is initiated.
- Continue fluid boluses at 10-20 ml/kg during and after intubation.
- Commence an inotrope/vasopressor infusion prior to intubation.
- Pre-oxygenatate with 100% O_2 via NRM if not already initiated. A PEEP device with an anesthetic flow inflating device or Ambu bag will help to maintain oxygenation in a child with hypoxemia.
- Drugs: Sedative agents used for intubation can precipitate cardiovascular collapse.
- Drug regimen for intubation in shock: Ketamine 1 mg/kg, atropine 0.01 mg/kg, muscle relaxation with succinylcholine 1 mg/kg or vecuronium 0.1-0.2 mg/kg
- If patient is moribund or has severe hypoxemia or decompensated shock, any IV sedation can precipitate cardiac arrest and no drugs are necessary except topical anesthetics. On occasion, low dose fentanyl at titrated boluses of 0.05 mcg/kg may be used. Even sub-therapeutic doses of midazolam can worsen the shock state.
- Consider cuffed endotracheal tubes even in younger children and infants as lung mechanics are frequently abnormal and peri-tubal leak may be significant. Cuff inflation pressures should not exceed 25 mmHg.
- If shock is not reversed despite 60 ml/kg of fluid, an inotrope and/or vasopressor infusion may be necessary (See Fig. 29.1).

Box 29.7 Intubation in shock

- Pre-oxygenate with Bain's circuit/Ambu with PEEP valve
- Consider cuffed tubes
- Set up dopamine @10 mcg/kg/min or noradrenaline 0.1 mcg/kg/min prior to intubation
- Drugs: Ketamine 1mg/kg, atropine 0.01 mg/kg, sux 1 mg/kg or vecuronium 0.01 mg/kg
- If moribund, no drugs OR low dose fentanyl 0.05 mcg/kg

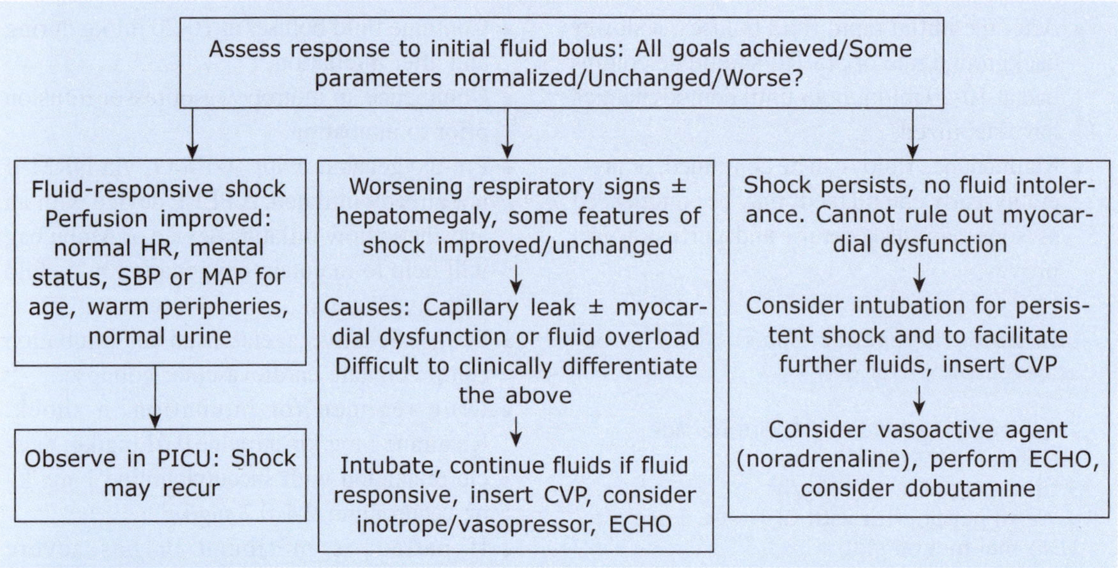

Fig. 29.1 Response to fluid resuscitation determines next line of therapy

- *When to use vasopressor inotrope infusions ?* Children with septic shock who remain hypotensive after 60 ml/kg fluid typically require early vasopressor support after the first 60 ml/kg of fluid loading, usually within the first 1-2 hours.
- *Choice of vasopressor-inotrope infusions* In order to select the most appropriate inotrope/vasoactive agent, the patient may be categorized into one of 4 patterns of shock:
  a. Cold shock with narrow pulse pressure with *low MAP* for age
  b. Cold shock with narrow pulse pressure with *normal MAP* for age
  c. Warm shock with wide pulse pressures and a *low MAP* for age
  d. Warm shock with wide pulse pressures and a *normal MAP* for age

a) *Cold shock with narrow pulse pressure with low MAP for age*
- Choices: dopamine or adrenaline
- Dopamine at a starting infusion rate of 10 μg/kg/min is a usual first line agent.
- At this dose, dopamine improves both cardiac contractility (inotrope) and raises abnormally low SVR (pressor).
- If the hypotension is profound and the patient is unstable, initiate adrenaline (rather than dopamine) at 0.3-0.5 mcg/kg/minute. This is a more efficient inotrope and can also increase MAP due to its pressor effect.
- If the MAP remains low despite dopamine of 10 mcg/kg/min or adrenaline at 0.5-0.6 mcg/kg/min, the addition of noradrenaline (NA) may be preferred rather than escalating the dose of dopamine/adrenaline in order to avoid undesirable tachycardia. NA will effectively increase the SVR along with modest inotropy and minimal chronotropy.
- If MAP normalizes, but the patient remains in cold shock with hypoperfusion and persistent acidosis, add further inotropy with dobutamine at 5-10 mcg/kg/min. Assess cardiac function with early ECHO.
- A continuous background rate of isotonic fluid must be titrated so as to maintain ad-

equate intravascular volume. Over-reliance on pressors in patients with uncorrected hypovolemia can cause multiorgan failure.

b) *Cold normotensive shock: MAP normal or high with narrow pulse pressure*

- Dobutamine at 7.5-10 μg/kg/min is a reasonable initial agent.
- Dobutamine will provide inotropy with moderate vasodilatation, both of which are beneficial for myocardial dysfunction, which is common.
- Alternatives are adrenaline at inotropic doses (0.1-0.3 μg/kg/min).
- Consider milrinone for documented myocardial dysfunction or pulmonary hypertension and/or if shock is unresolved despite standard inotropes such as dobutamine.
- Milrinone, a phosphodiesterase inhibitor, has synergistic effect with catecholamines such as dobutamine. It is also effective when shock is catecholamine refractory.
  - Milrinone is especially effective for 2 groups of patients.
  - Those with right ventricular dysfunction ± pulmonary hypertension: a situation that may be common in patients with pneumonia and septic shock.
  - Presence of diastolic dysfunction: milrinone has unique lusitropic effects (improved ventricular relaxation).
- Milrinone is a potent vasodilator with a relatively long half-life and can cause hypotension especially if the patient is hypovolemic.
  - If the MAP falls with milrinone, consider fluid bolus (10-20 ml/kg). If hypotension not corrected, commence and low dose noradrenaline (0.05 mcg/kg/min) x 2-3 hr until BP stable.

c) *Warm shock with hypotension: Wide pulse pressures and a low MAP for age*

- These patients typically require very large volumes of fluid and vasopressor infusions. Some require inotrope as well.
- Initial therapy after patient has received at least 60 ml/kg fluid is a vasopressor infusion. The best agent is noradrenaline (NA) at 0.05-0.5 mcg/kg/min, titrated to achieve normal MAP for age.
- If the low MAP is refractory to NA at maximum doses (0.5-1 mcg/kg/min), consider adding vasopressin (VP) or terlipressin infusion. VP infusion doses range from 0.0005-0.001 units/kg/min. Higher doses may result in significant splanchnic ischemia.
- If vasopressor infusions result in worsening indices of perfusion (cold extremities with poor peripheral pulses etc) despite improving MAP, underlying left ventricular dysfunction is likely: Consider the addition of an inotrope such as dobutamine. Early ECHO is helpful.
- Other indications for dobutamine in warm shock are persisting metabolic/lactic acidosis or a low central venous saturation ($ScvO_2 < 70\%$). Dobutamine may also be useful in a patient with abnormally high $ScvO_2$ who may have poor O_2 extraction at the tissue level despite a high CO.
- The combination of noradrenaline and dobutamine is useful in restoring splanchnic and vulnerable organ perfusion in hyperdynamic shock.
- A continuous background rate of isotonic fluid must be titrated so as to maintain adequate intravascular volume. Over-reliance on pressors in patients with uncorrected hypovolemia can cause multiorgan failure.

d) *Warm shock with normal/high MAP for age*

- The mainstay of therapy in these patients is continuous aggressive fluid titration therapy as capillary leaks and vasodilatation/vasoplegia are ongoing.
- A continuous background rate of isotonic

Box 29.8 Choice of inotrope vasopressor

Cold shock with narrow/normal pulse pressure

(Usually indicative of myocardial dysfunction with high SVR)

- Titrate fluids 10-20 ml/kg/hr (aim CVP 10-12)
- Mean BP normal/high for age: commence dobutamine @ 10 μg/kg/min
- Mean BP low for age: commence dopamine @10 μg/kg/min OR adrenaline @ 0.1-0.3 μg/kg/min
- Add noradrenaline if MAP remains low despite adrenaline up to 0.5 μg/kg/min/ dopamine @10 μg/kg/min
- Add dobutamine 10 μg OR milrinone 0.25 μg/kg/min if MAP better but shock not reversed OR ECHO evidence of impaired LV/RV function

Warm shock with wide pulse pressure

- Hyperdynamic circulation with low SVR. Some have myocardial dysfunction.
- Fluid intolerance may not occur despite underlying myocardial dysfunction.
- Most need large volume fluid + pressor, some may need inotrope
  - Titrate fluids (aim CVP 10-12 mmHg), get echo early
  - Mean BP low for age: Commence noradrenaline @ 0.1 mcg/kg/min, titrate up to 0.5-1.0 μg/kg/min to normal MAP
  - Add dobutamine if: Extremity perfusion worsens with noradrenaline, acidosis persists OR $ScvO_2$ < 70% or > 80% despite adequate CVP/MAP/HCT, OR ECHO evidence of impaired LV function

fluid (20-30 ml/kg/hr) must be titrated so as to maintain adequate intravascular volume.

- Pressors or inotropes usually not required. However, if the diastolic BP is excessively low, NA may be requred.
- Indications for dobutamine: Signs of tissue hypoperfusion, persisting metabolic or lactic acidosis or a low central venous saturation ($ScvO_2$ < 70%) despite adequate filling.
- The combination of noradrenaline and dobutamine may be useful in restoring splanchnic and vulnerable organ perfusion. However, if the addition of NA or dobutamine worsens tachycardia or acidosis, consider discontinuing the infusion.

15. **Blood transfusion**
   - Although there are increasing reports of transfusion related morbidities and higher immunosuppression risks, a higher hematocrit may be desirable for a patient with shock that is uncorrected despite adequate filling and vasopressor/inotrope treatment.
   - Tissue oxygen delivery may be optimized by maintaining a HCT of 30%. Indications for RBC transfusion include persistent shock, metabolic acidosis (BE > -5), elevated lactate or a central venous saturation ($ScvO_2$) of < 70%, indicating excessive tissue extraction of oxygen in the face of reduced cardiac output.
   - Other blood components (FFP, platelets, cryoprecipitate) may be indicated depending on the clinical circumstance.
16. **Steroids**
   - While studies have indicated that severe septic shock may be associated with relative adrenal insufficiency or resistance to glucocorticoids, the role of steroids in septic shock remains controversial.
   - Low dose steroids may be useful in patients with fluid refractory, vasodilatory shock who are pressor dependant.
   - Other indications are previous steroid use in the preceding 6 months, purpura fulminans, persistent hypoglycemia in association with hyponatremia and hyperkalemia.
   - Dose recommendations vary from a bolus of 1 to 2 mg/kg of hydrocortisone followed by 1 mg/kg Q6-8H.
17. **Acid base and electrolyte abnormalities**
   - Hypoglycemia may develop rapidly in the septic child. Serum glucose should be monitored

Table 29.1 Preparation of inotrope vasopressor infusions

Drug (dose range in μg/kg/min)	Central line (mg/kg to be added in 50 ml NS)	Peripheral line (mg/kg to be added in 50 ml NS)
Dobutamine (7.5-15)	15 mg/kg, 1 ml/hr = 5 μg/kg/min	Same as central line
Dopamine (7.5-15)	15 mg/kg, 1 ml/hr = 5 μg/kg/min	3 mg/kg, 1 ml/hr = 1 μg/kg/min
Adrenaline (0.1-1.0)	0.3 mg/kg, 1 ml/hr = 0.1 μg/kg/min	0.1 mg/kg, 3 ml/hr = 0.1 μg/kg/min
Noradrenaline (0.1-1.0)	0.3 mg/kg, 1 ml/hr = 0.1 μg/kg/min	Note: 5% dextrose preferred to NS for noradrenaline infusion
Milrinone (0.25-0.75)	1.5 mg/kg, 1 ml/hr = 0.25 μg/kg/min	Same as central line
Vasopressin (0.0005-0.001 Units/kg/min)	1.5 Units/kg, 1 ml/hr = 0.0005 U/kg/min	Not recommended

and hypoglycemia promptly treated. If persistent, consider early steroids and 10% dextrose in saline as maintenance fluid.

- Hyperglycemia may occur due to the stress of sepsis. Initial therapy involves dextrose-free fluids. If persistent, the resultant osmotic diuresis may render correction of volume deficits difficult.
- If hyperglycemia persists, a low-dose insulin infusion may be initiated (0.05-0.1 units/kg/hour) with hourly monitoring of capillary blood glucose. It is important to prevent hypoglycemia. When the elevated blood glucose demonstrates a normalizing trend, the insulin may be discontinued.
- Low ionized calcium levels (<0.8 mmol/L) must be corrected in a patient with refractory shock. Mild hypocalcemia may not need correction as calcium related myocardial apoptosis has been reported.
- Patients in septic shock usually have a wide anion gap acidosis from lactic acid. This is a marker of tissue ischemia and does not need bicarbonate correction. The best therapy is to restore normal perfusion.
- Previously sodium bicarbonate was routinely used to correct this acidosis as it was thought that the response to catecholamines was poor and myocardial performance impaired in acidotic patients. However, it is now known that bicarbonate may be unnecessary as undesirable hypernatremia and hyperosmolality may occur with no significant advantages in shock resolution. The acidosis is best corrected by aggressive attempts to restore hemodynamics with fluids, pressor/inotrope and assisted ventilation as indicated.

18. **Monitoring**

Continuous cardio-respiratory and neurological monitoring in the ICU is essential.

- Hourly urine output, intake output monitoring and neurological monitoring.
- Early central venous and invasive arterial monitoring will facilitate rapid and appropriate therapeutic responses to any hemodynamic changes.
- Laboratory monitoring:
  - At admission: ABG, lactate, capillary blood glucose, complete blood count, coagulation profile, electrolytes including ionized calcium, magnesium, renal and liver function tests, blood and suspected source culture.
  - Continue to check blood sugars hourly if labile.
  - ABG, central venous saturations and lactate Q4–6H until patient is stable.
  - Repeat other laboratory testing as clinically indicated.
- Central venous saturation monitoring
  - Serial $ScvO_2$ and lactate levels are an important component of ICU monitoring of septic shock in conjunction with hemodynamic and perfusion indices.
  - Monitoring of the central venous saturation ($ScvO_2$) provides an indirect indicator of the adequacy of the cardiac output (CO).
  - The $ScvO_2$ may be measured from an appropriate sited CVC (SVC-RA junction or IVC-RA junction).
  - Normally, the tissues extract 25% of oxygen from the arterial blood such that, if the arterial saturation is 100%, the central venous saturation should be ≈ 75%.
  - When the CO falls, the tissues will extract a greater percentage of oxygen in order to maintain the same level of O_2 consumption.
  - Thus, provided the O_2 consumption and O_2 content remain constant, a fall in the $ScvO_2$ may indicate an inadequate CO, pointing to the need for further inotropy.
  - In septic shock, the reverse may sometimes occur. The hyperdynamic circulation and high CO in conjunction with maldistribution of blood flow and impaired O_2 extraction at the tissue level result in a higher than normal $ScvO_2$. The high $ScvO_2$ may be associated with lactic acidosis indicating cellular hypoxemia.

19. **Source control**

A specific anatomic site/focus of infection should be established as rapidly as possible and within the first 6 hours of presentation. Investigations such as chest/abdominal ultrasound or CT may be necessary to determine location of abscess/necrotic tissue.

- Remove central and arterial lines if potentially infected or no other focus found.
- Formally evaluate patient for a focus of infection amenable to source control measures as soon as possible following successful initial resuscitation. For example, abscess drainage, tissue debridement. Choose source control measure with maximum efficacy and minimal physiologic upset.

20. **Refractory shock**

- If shock persists despite adequate filling, inotrope/pressor, initiation of steroids and hematocrit of > 30%, consider unrecognized morbidities including pulmonary hypertension, pericardial effusion, tension pneumothorax, hypoadren alism, hypothyroidism, ongoing blood loss, intra-abdominal catastrophe and intra-abdominal hypertension.

21. **Care in the ICU**

- As with all PICU patients, initiate early enteral feeds as soon as hemodynamic stability achieved.
- Nurse in semi-recumbent position with head of bed elevated 30–45° to prevent aspiration.
- If ventilated, employ lung-protective strategies:
  - Target a tidal volume of 6 ml/kg (predicted) body weight

Initial Interventions

- Assess and maintain airway.
- O_2 by NRM, check capillary glucose (correct if low)
- Insert 2 large bore IV cannulae (or intra-osseous)
- 1st IV line for rapid fluid boluses: 20 ml/kg boluses of NS/RL until goals achieved
- If SBP/MBP *low*, infuse each bolus over 5-10 min (push-pull technique/pressure bag)
- If SBP or MBP *normal* for age, infuse by free flow over 20 min (*No pediatric burrette*)
- Insert 2nd line with aseptic precautions; send 2 sets of blood cultures (each 5-10 ml), send CBC, ABG, lactate.
- Administer 1st dose antibiotic
- Insert urinary catheter

↓

Most need 40-60 ml/kg fluid in 1st hr, some require more (upto 100-120 ml/kg in 1st hour)
Assess response to initial fluid bolus: All goals achieved/some parameters normalized/unchanged/worse?

↓

Fluid responsive shock
Normal HR, mental status, SBP or MBP for age, warm peripheries, urine output > 1 ml/kg/hr

↓

Observe in PICU: Shock may recur

Some features of shock improved but respiratory signs worsen ± hepatomegaly
Causes: Capillary leak ± myocardial dysfunction or fluid overload
Difficult to clinically differentiate the above
Intubate, continue fluids if fluid responsive, commence inotrope/vasopressor, CVP, ECHO

Shock persists, no fluid intolerance
Some may have myocardial dysfunction

↓

If shock unresolved after 60 ml/kg fluids, commence inotrope/pressor (see below), insert central line and arterial line, consider intubation (ketamine/atropine/sux)
Aim for CVP of 10-12 mmHg, normal MAP for age.
Check lactate and central venous saturation ($ScvO_2$), aim for 70-80%, transfuse to HCT 30% if $ScvO_2$ <70%.
Consider early ECHO

↓

Initiate inotrope/vasopressor: Choice depends on MAP, pulse pressure (PP), extremity perfusion

↓

Cold shock with narrow pulse pressure
(Usually indicative of myocardial dysfunction with high SVR)
- Titrate fluids 10-20 ml/kg/hr (aim CVP 10-12)
- **Mean BP normal/high for age**: commence dobutamine @ 10 μg/kg/min
- **Mean BP low for age**: commence adrenaline @ 0.1-0.3 μg/kg/min OR dopamine @10 μg/kg/min
- Add noradrenaline if MAP low despite adrenaline upto 0.5 μg/kg/min
- Add dobutamine 10 μg OR milrinone 0.25-05 μg/kg/min if MAP better but shock not reversed OR Echo evidence of impaired LV function

Warm shock with wide pulse pressure
- *Hyperdynamic circulation with low SVR. Some have myocardial dysfunction*
- *Fluid intolerance may not occur despite underlying myocardial dysfunction.*
- Titrate fluids (aim CVP 10-12 mmHg), Echo helpful
- **MAP low for age** or shock unresolved: Commence noradrenaline @ 0.1 mcg/kg/min, titrate upto 0.5-1.0 μg/kg/min
- **Add dobutamine if**: Extremity perfusion worsens with noradrenaline, *OR* acidosis persists OR $ScvO_2$ < 70% or > 80% despite adequate CVP/MAP/HCT, *OR* Echo evidence of impaired LV function

↓

Persistent shock:
" Hydrocortisone 1 mg/kg Q6H
" If MAP still low, add Vasopressin 0.0003-0.002 U/kg/min
" If acidosis persists, $ScvO_2$< 70% OR ↓RV function on Echo, consider milrinone (+ pressor to maintain MAP)

↓

If SHOCK REFRACTORY: Early source control mandatory.
Rule out unrecognized morbidities including pulmonary hypertension, abscess, necrotic tissue, pericardial effusion, tension pneumothorax, hypoadrenalism, hypothyroidism, ongoing blood loss, intra-abdominal catastrophe, intra-abdominal hypertension, etc.
May require U/S or CT chest and abdomen to locate source.

Fig. 29.2 ER and ICU management of Septic Shock

- The upper limit of PIP/plateau pressure should be < 30 cmH_2O.
- Allow permissive hypercapnia, if needed to minimize plateau pressures and tidal volumes.
- Positive end expiratory pressure (PEEP) should be set to avoid extensive lung collapse at end expiration.

- Fluid removal strategies:
  - When hemodynamically stable, fluid overloaded patients who are not spontaneously diuresing may be initiated on a furosemide infusion at 2-5 mg/kg/day so as to hasten weaning from ventilation.
  - Monitor for perfusion and hypokalemia, metabolic alkalosis.
  - If in renal failure or refractory to furosemide, consider peritoneal dialysis.

22. **Adjunctive therapy**

- Agents such IV immunoglobulin may be useful in children with septic shock and Infection Associated Hemophagocytosis (IAHS) where the triad of fever, cytopenia and organomegaly may be present along with elevated ferritin, triglycerides and LDH. Bone marrow aspiration may be diagnostic.
- May also be considered in severe disease (Box 29.9).

Box 29.9 Indicators of severe disease

- Low or falling WBC count
- Low or falling platelet count
- High requirement for fluid
- Short history (<12 hrs)
- Rapid progress of multi-organ failure (renal/ARDS/coagulopathy/liver)

REFERENCES

1. Carcillo JA, Fields AI, Task Force Committee Members. Clinical practice parameters for hemodynamic support of pediatric and neonatal patients in septic shock. Crit Care Med 2002; 30:1363-1378.
2. Dellinger RP, Levy MM, International Surviving Sepsis Campaign Guidelines Committee. Surviving Sepsis Campaign: International guidelines for management of severe sepsis and septic shock. Crit Care Med 2008; 36(1) :296-327.

30

Dengue Fever and Shock Syndromes

Dengue fever, a very old disease, has re-emerged in the past 20 years with an expanded geographic distribution of both the viruses and the mosquito vectors, increased epidemic activity, the development of hyper-endemicity (the co-circulation of multiple serotypes), and the emergence of dengue fever in new geographic regions). There are four closely related, but serologically distinct dengue viruses, the Flaviviridae, called DEN-1, DEN-2, DEN-3, and DEN-4. Life time immunity follows infection by one serotype, but immunity to the other serotypes is short-lived. Dengue virus is spread by Aedes egyptii mosquito and has varied manifestations as described below.

Dengue viral infections affect all age groups and produce a spectrum of clinical illness ranging from asymptomatic to a mild or nonspecific viral syndrome to a severe and occasionally fatal disease characterized by shock and hemorrhage.

Controversies regarding the WHO classification and the 2009 classification system

The traditional WHO classification that has been widely used since 1997 has been phased out and a new system has been introduced since December 2009. The reasons for adopting the new classification system are:

- Although the WHO differentiates between the various categories of dengue virus infections, there is considerable overlap and it is entirely likely that dengue infections exist as a continuum rather than distinct entities .
- The term "DHF" puts undue emphasis on hemorrhage: however, the hallmark of severe dengue (and the manifestation that should be addressed early) is not hemorrhage but increased vascular permeability leading to shock. Hemorrhage may or may not be present in severe dengue and, conversely, may occur in children with otherwise uncomplicated dengue.
- The Tropical Disease Research (TDR) section of WHO have suggested that, rather than differentiating between DF and DHF, it may probably be better to use the terms 'Dengue' and 'Severe Dengue' as shown in Fig. 30.1, with no emphasis on bleeding or on a specific platelet count cut-off.

STAGES AND PHASES OF DENGUE

The three phases are (Fig. 30.2):

1. Febrile phase
2. Phase of plasma leakage or Critical phase
3. Recovery phase

1. **Febrile phase**
   - Usually lasts 2-7 days
   - Progressive leucopenia without clear localization may be a clue of dengue as the diagnosis
   - Monitoring for defervescence and warning signs are crucial to recognize the progression to the phase of leakage or Critical phase

- Defervescence occurs on day 3-7 of illness

2. **Critical phase (Phase of plasma leakage)**
   - Around the time of defervescence, most patients improve, a few deteriorate.
   - Those who improve after defervescence have "dengue without warning signs"
   - Those that deteriorate will manifest warning signs: "dengue with warning signs" and if treatment is delayed or inappropriate, can progress to "severe dengue."
3. **Recovery phase**
   - A gradual reabsorption of leaked fluid takes place in the next 48-72 hours
   - General well being improves, hemodynamic status stabilizes and diuresis ensues.
   - May have a classical rash of "isles of white in the sea of red"

Table. 30.1 Elements of new dengue classification

Probable dengue	Warning signs	Severe dengue
▪ Lives in/travel to dengue endemic area. ▪ Fever and 2 of the following criteria: - Nausea, vomiting - Rash - Aches and pains - Tourniquet test positive - Leukopenia - Any warning sign ▪ Laboratory-confirmed dengue (important when no sign of plasma leakage)	▪ Intense abdominal pain or tenderness ▪ Persistent vomiting ▪ Clinical fluid accumulation ▪ Mucosal bleed ▪ Lethargy, restlessness ▪ Liver enlargement >2 cm ▪ Laboratory: Increase in hematocrit with concurrent rapid decrease in platelet count	▪ Severe plasma leakage with rising hematocrit leading to: - Shock - Fluid accumulation (pleural, ascitic) - Respiratory distress ▪ Severe bleeding ▪ Severe organ involvement - Liver: Elevated transaminases (AST or ALT >=1000) - CNS: Impaired consciousness, seizures - Cardiac or other organ dysfunction

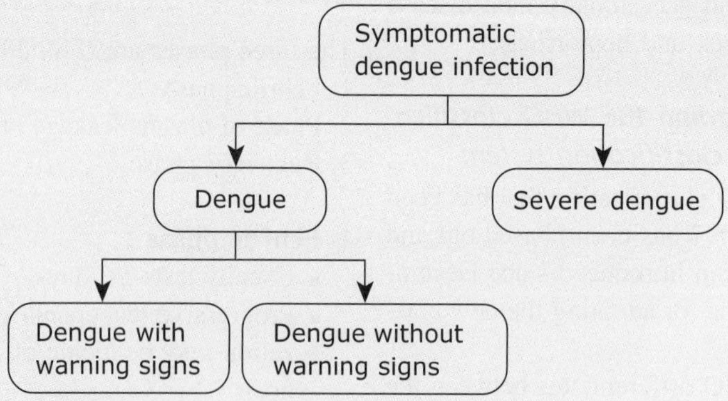

Fig. 30.1 New classification of dengue (TDR, WHO 2009)

- HCT stabilizes or may be lower due to the dilution effect of reabsorbed fluid.
- WBC usually starts to rise soon after defervescence.
- Recovery of platelet count is typically later than that of WBC.

MANAGEMENT OF PATIENTS WITH DENGUE

- Severe dengue is a systemic disease with a complex, dynamic and unpredictable progression. However, successful outcomes with mortality rates of < 1% can be achieved in the vast majority with surprisingly simple and inexpensive interventions, provided they are early, appropriate and are continually targeted to keep pace with the disease evolution.
- Conversely, once the window of opportunity of early treatment is missed or inappropriately addressed, the disease can progress extremely rapidly and can result in refractory shock, relentless hemorrhage and florid multi-organ failure where even expensive and sophisticated intensive care resources may be futile
- Most patients with dengue can be managed without hospitalization provided they are alert, there are no warning signs or evidence of abnormal bleeding, their oral intake and urine output are satisfactory and the caregiver is educated regarding the course of illness, fever control and avoiding non-steroidal anti-inflammatory agents.
- A dengue information card emphasizing and danger/warning signs is useful.

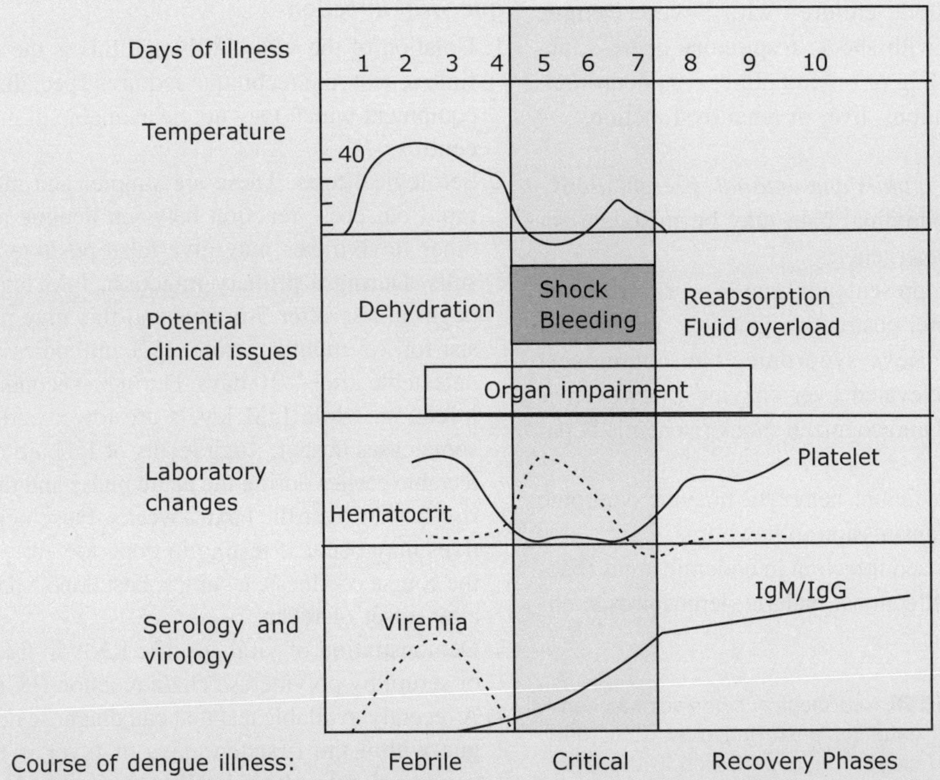

Fig. 30.2 Course of dengue illness and phases of disease (Dengue Hemorrhagic Fever: Diagnosis, Treatment, Prevention and Control, 3rd ed, WHO 2009)

- These patients need daily clinical ± laboratory assessment by trained doctors or nurses until the danger period has past.

Indications for hospitalization and intravenous fluids include "Warning Signs" of significant plasma leak of which severe, intense abdominal pain is considered the most important; other warning signs are persistent vomiting, restlessness or lethargy, clinical fluid accumulation, mucosal bleeds or other significant bleeds, lethargy or restlessness and laboratory feature of rise in HCT along with rapid fall in platelet count. Infants and patients with co-morbid conditions such as diabetes, renal failure and obesity may also require admission.

Indications for intensive care unit (ICU) admission include children with Severe Dengue manifesting with shock, respiratory distress, abnormal bleeding or organ failure, e.g., neurological complications, liver or renal dysfunction

Be aware of pitfalls and unusual presentations.

- Severe abdominal pain may be mistaken for surgical emergencies
- A hepatic presentation may occur with acute liver failure, obstructive jaundice, raised liver enzymes, Reye syndrome. The commonest cause of elevated liver enzymes, however, is prolonged unrecognized shock (ischemic hepatitis).
- Acute renal failure, hemolytic uraemic syndrome
- Vertical transmission in newborns.
- Superimposed infection in endemic areas (bacterial co-infections, malaria, leptospirosis, enteric fever).

☞ **REMEMBER** Neurological signs such as convulsions and extensor posturing may occur due to shock and cerebral hypoperfusion in the critical phase and due to fluid overload during recovery.

Making a diagnosis of dengue viral infections

- The diagnosis of acute dengue virus infection is mainly a clinical one.
- In a patient with suspected dengue fever, an early diagnosis of the progress to DHF can be greatly assisted by close clinical examination for the onset of circulatory instability in conjunction with studies such as serial WBC and platelet counts, trends in hematocrit and bedside ultrasound studies.
- Typical early constellation of imaging finding of DHF is thickening of the gallbladder wall and fluid collections in the pleural and ascitic cavities. Ultrasound findings may precede clinical signs of plasma leakage.

Laboratory methods for confirmation of dengue viral infection

1. Isolation of the virus. Although this is the definitive test, the technique requires specialized equipment which may not be available in most centres.
2. Serological tests. These are simpler and more rapid but cross-reaction between dengue and other flaviviruses may give false positive results. During a primary infection, IgM levels begin to rise after 5-6 days and this may persist for 2-3 months, while IgG antibodies are detectable after 7-10 days. During a secondary infection, while IgM levels are lower and in some cases absent, high levels of IgG are detectable earlier during the acute phase and they rise further over the next 2 weeks. False negatives may occur if testing in done too early in the course of illness; testing is best done 5 days after onset of fever.
3. Demonstration of viral specific RNA in tissue or serum by polymerase chain reaction (PCR).
4. A recently available test that can diagnose dengue within the first few days of fever is the non-structural protein 1 (NS1) monoclonal antibody in an ELISA format that can detect dengue NS1 antigen in blood.

It is crucial to be aware of the temporal sequence of events so as to choose the most appropriate test. The choice of test depends on which of the two stages the patient might be in, viz, stage I where fever and viremia are present *(virological and molecular diagnosis most appropriate)*; or stage II, the post-pyrexial period lasting a few weeks *(serological tests appropriate)*.

Monitoring of patients with dengue shock

- Pulse, blood pressure and respiration should be recorded continuously until stable.
- Record hematocrit Q 2-4thhourly in unstable patients for the first 12 hrs, then Q 6-8th hourly
- A fluid balance sheet should be kept, recording the type of fluid and the rate and volume of its administration in order to evaluate the adequacy of fluid replacement.
- Urinary catheter in all patients with shock.
- Infusion pump will help in precise regulation of fluid input.

The four major priorities of management of a child with DHF in the ICU

A. Controlled reversal of shock by replacement of plasma losses

B. Detection and treatment of overt/occult hemorrhage

C. Prevention of fluid overload

D. Avoiding complications of unnecessary interventions such as invasive lines, nasal tubes, etc

A. **Reversal of shock with titrated rehydration**

Isotonic non-dextrose containing crystalloids such as normal saline, Ringer's lactate are effective in the majority. In severe/refractory shock, colloids such as plasma substitutes (6% hetastarch/5% albumin) may be preferred.

- In dengue shock, slow fluid filling at rates of 25 ml/kg of NS/RL or hetastarch over the first 2 hours may be sufficient unless the patient is in severe shock. These smaller volumes are sufficient in not only reversing shock, but also help to minimize complications of fluid overload including the need for assisted ventilation.

☞ **REMEMBER** *Reversal of shock in a patient with dengue shock is different from septic shock resuscitation.*

- Dengue shock patients need smaller volumes of fluids at slower rates as compared to septic shock (who frequently need greater than 60 ml/kg fluid in the first hour).
- Moreover, in septic shock, early inotropes/pressors are useful in fluid refractory shock, whereas in dengue shock, the cardiac function is usually normal and the commonest cause of fluid refractory shock is unrecognized hemorrhage. Inotropes are usually not necessary as they can worsen the shock state.

- However, patients with severe shock with hypotension need initial rapid fluid boluses until the pulses are palpable and the BP is recordable. As soon as clinical improvement begins, fluid administration rates must be slowed down.
- The significant differences in fluid resuscitation volumes for septic versus dengue shock may probably relate to the fact that DSS patients are vasoconstricted with a narrow pulse pressure as opposed to the predominantly vasodilated states in septic shock.
- Differentiating dengue shock from septic shock at the time of presentation is therefore of prime importance in order to customize fluid resuscitation: Compared to patients with septic shock, DSS patients are more likely to have hemoconcentration, a narrow pulse pressure and better preserved mental status.
- However, it must be emphasized that in the event that the 2 entities cannot be clearly differentiated, treating with larger volumes of fluid at the rates recommended for septic shock may be necessary.

End-points/goals of fluid administration

- As clinical signs of hydration are misleading in dengue (even patient with shock can appear overhydrated with hepatomegaly and lung crackles), more objective guides to guide fluid titration are valuable.
- In this respect, aiming for a minimal urine output of 0.8-1 ml/kg/hr is a valuable end-point. The kidneys receive the second highest blood flow in the body. If the urine output is adequate in the absence of glycosuria or recent diuretic use, then it may be safely inferred that the rest of the body is being adequately perfused.
- Furthermore, an hourly urine output of > 1.5-2 ml/kg/hr may be the earliest sign of overhydration and should prompt reduction of IV fluid rates, even if oral intake is insufficient (routine "maintenance fluids" not necessary).

Measurement of hourly urine output serves 3 important functions:

- Indicates adequacy of shock resuscitation if greater than 0.8-1.0 ml/kg/hr
- Early indicator of fluid overload if > 2 ml/kg/hr (provided no glycosuria/diuretic use)
- Indicates onset of recovery phase if urine output increases despite minimal IV fluids (in conjunction with stable HCT and vitals)

- Other end-points are minimal acceptable mean pressures, normalization of the narrow pulse pressure and a fall in hematocrit of approximately 20% of admission values (in the non-bleeding patient).
- *Using hematocrit as a monitoring tool*
  - Assessing 2-4th hourly HCT in conjunction with the circulatory status will provide valuable clues.
  - A high or rising HCT + unstable hemodynamics →Increase volumes of crystalloids.
  - A high or rising HCT + stable hemodynamics with adequate urine output →do not increase fluid rates, but continue close monitoring.
  - A low or "normal" HCT + unstable hemodynamics →important indicator of occult hemorrhage and the need for urgent blood transfusion.
  - A low or "normal" HCT + stable patient → prompt cessation of IV fluids is the most important action indicated.
- *Continued rehydration to match ongoing plasma loss:* A variable degree of plasma loss may continue for 24-36 hrs requiring necessitating constant, careful titration of fluid administration tailored to the vitals, clinical status, hematocrit, urine output.

☞ **REMEMBER** Dextrose containing fluids such as "Isolyte P" or 5% dextrose in ½ normal saline should not be administered for rehydration.

- Rapidly administered dextrose may result in hyperglycemia and osmotic diuresis, delaying correction of hypovolemia.
- Secondly, dextrose is rapidly metabolized resulting in a hypotonic solution that is inappropriate for shock correction.
- Hypotonic fluids may contribute to fluid overload.

Indications for inotropes/vasopressor in dengue

- Caregivers must desist from over-zealous prescriptions of inotropes as these agents can paradoxically worsen the shock state especially if hypovolemia is sill uncorrected.
- Inotrope/pressor support may *occasionally* be indicated in late presenters with dengue shock when features of low cardiac output persist despite having received 40-60 ml/kg of fluid and correction of blood loss, i.e., patients with fluid/ blood transfusion refractory shock in whom myocardial dysfunction is suspected or confirmed by echocardiography.

- Inotropes must be ceased if tachycardia or the shock state worsens after initiation.
- Pressors may also be indicated prior to intubation of a patient with dengue shock as some patients may have catastrophic decompensation during this period.

Indications for central venous pressure (CVP) monitoring

- Most patients may be managed extremely well with 2 reliable peripheral lines. CVP monitoring has limited utility in DSS and is seldom indicated except in late presenters, see below and Fig. 30.3.
- The risks of central venous line insertion are usually greater than the benefits, but if shock persists despite 40-60 ml/kg fluids and correction of suspected hemorrhage, an experienced operator may consider insertion of a central venous catheter (CVC). Ultrasound guided placement, if available, will minimize complications.

B. **Detection and treatment of hemorrhage**

> ☞ **REMEMBER** While patients with severe dengue have significant coagulation abnormalities, these are not severe enough to cause major bleeding. Major risk factors for significant DIC with uncontrollable bleeds in dengue are profound shock (most important), acidosis, hypoxemia and thrombocytopenia.

- Clinical features of significant hemorrhage may be subtle and include increase in tachycardia, abdominal distension and/or tenderness, stress induced leukocytosis (instead of the characteristic leucopenia), agitation/lethargy, acidosis and evidence of worsening organ function.
- Other features suggestive of occult hemorrhage include:
  - Hypotensive shock at presentation
  - HCT not as high as expected for the degree of shock
  - Persistent shock despite restoration of fluid volume
  - Inappropriate fall in hematocrit post resuscitation.
- The most important intervention in a patient with dengue shock and life-threatening bleeds is restoration of oxygen carrying capacity with fresh whole blood (WB) or packed red blood cell (PRBC) transfusions; this must be done emergently rather than waiting for the hematocrit to fall significantly.
- The 2009 WHO Dengue Guidelines emphasize that in a bleeding dengue patient, the threshold for PRBC/whole blood must be higher than that suggested for septic shock (where a hematocrit < 30% is the usual transfusion threshold).
- This is because hemorrhage in dengue is most often preceded by a background of protracted shock due to plasma leak resulting in the characteristic elevated hematocrit. Uncorrected shock sets the stage for hemorrhagic hypovolemic shock, and when a significant blood loss does occur, the final post hemorrhage hematocrit may not be as low as expected.
- Correction of shock with two or more aliquots of fresh WB/PRBC usually breaks the vicious cycle of acidosis, hypoperfusion and DIC by restoring circulating volume and improving tissue oxygen delivery. This will arrest the abnormal bleeding in most cases, but should be administered in a controlled fashion to prevent fluid overload.
- Administration of other blood components such as platelets, fresh frozen plasma (FFP) or cryoprecipitate may contribute to volume overload and are not as important as fresh WB or PRBC, unless the bleeding is ongoing despite 2-3 aliquots of blood transfusion.
- It is also important to remember that preventive platelet transfusion is unlikely to decrease the incidence of significant bleeds.

C. **Prevention and therapy of fluid overload**

- While shock reversal with fluid resuscitation is vital, it is equally important to try to minimize fluid overload and the need for assisted ventilation.
- Shock in DSS occurs due to capillary leak. During fluid resuscitation, further capillary leak will occur and some degree of generalized edema including pulmonary edema is inevitable.
- Edema may be minimized by administering just sufficient fluid to restore a circulating volume that is sufficient to perfuse organs and tissues.

☞ **REMEMBER** A urine output in excess of 1.5-2 ml/kg/hr (in the absence of glycosuria/diuretics) may be indicative of excess circulating volume and should prompt reduction of intravenous fluid.

- Re-absorption of extravasated fluid may cause hypervolemia with a fall in hematocrit and can progress to pulmonary edema if concurrent IV fluid are continued.

Other strategies to prevent fluid overload

- Avoid hypotonic fluids for rehydration/maintenance
- Avoid prophylactic blood product transfusions in non-bleeding patients (even if thrombocytopenia and coagulopathy are significant), as it has been well described that early and adequate shock correction remains the best way to prevent hemorrhagic complications. Conversely, failure to recognize occult hemorrhage as a cause of shock and administering boluses of isotonic crystalloids rather than whole blood/PRBC can worsen both shock and fluid overload.
- Also important is prompt cessation of IV fluids during the recovery phase as reabsorption of the leaked plasma occurs during this period, and extraneous IV fluid can easily worsen fluid overload, precipitate pulmonary edema and large pleural ± ascitic collections.
- In symptomatic patients with fluid overload and respiratory distress, diuretics such as furosemide as a continuous bolus may be useful.
  - The decision to administer diuretics in a patient with dengue and fluid overload requires considerable judgment as diuretics can easily worsen the circulatory status in children who are still in the critical phase of plasma leakage.
  - If the critical period has passed as evidenced by a stable hematocrit, stable hemodynamics and a good urine output despite minimal IV fluids, a patient with significant respiratory symptoms may be

Table 30.2 Volume replacement flow chart for patients with dengue with "warning signs"

- Assess airway, breathing, obtain baseline hematocrit (HCT)
- Commence fluid resuscitation with normal saline/Ringer's Lactate at 5-7 ml/kg over 1-2 hours
- If hemodynamics and hematocrit are stable, plan a gradually reducing IV fluid regimen.
- Titrate fluids based on vitals, clinical exam, urine output (aim for 0.5-1 ml/kg/hr) and serial HCT.
- IV fluids (IVF) 5–7 ml/kg/hr for 1–2 hours, then:
- Reduce IVF to 3–5 ml/kg/hr for 2–4 hours;
- Reduce IVF to 2–3 ml/kg/hr for 2–4 hours
- Continue serial close clinical monitoring and Q6-8 hourly HCT
- Oral rehydration solutions may suffice when vomiting subsides and hemodynamics stable
- A monitored fluid regimen may be required for 24-48 hours, until danger period subsides

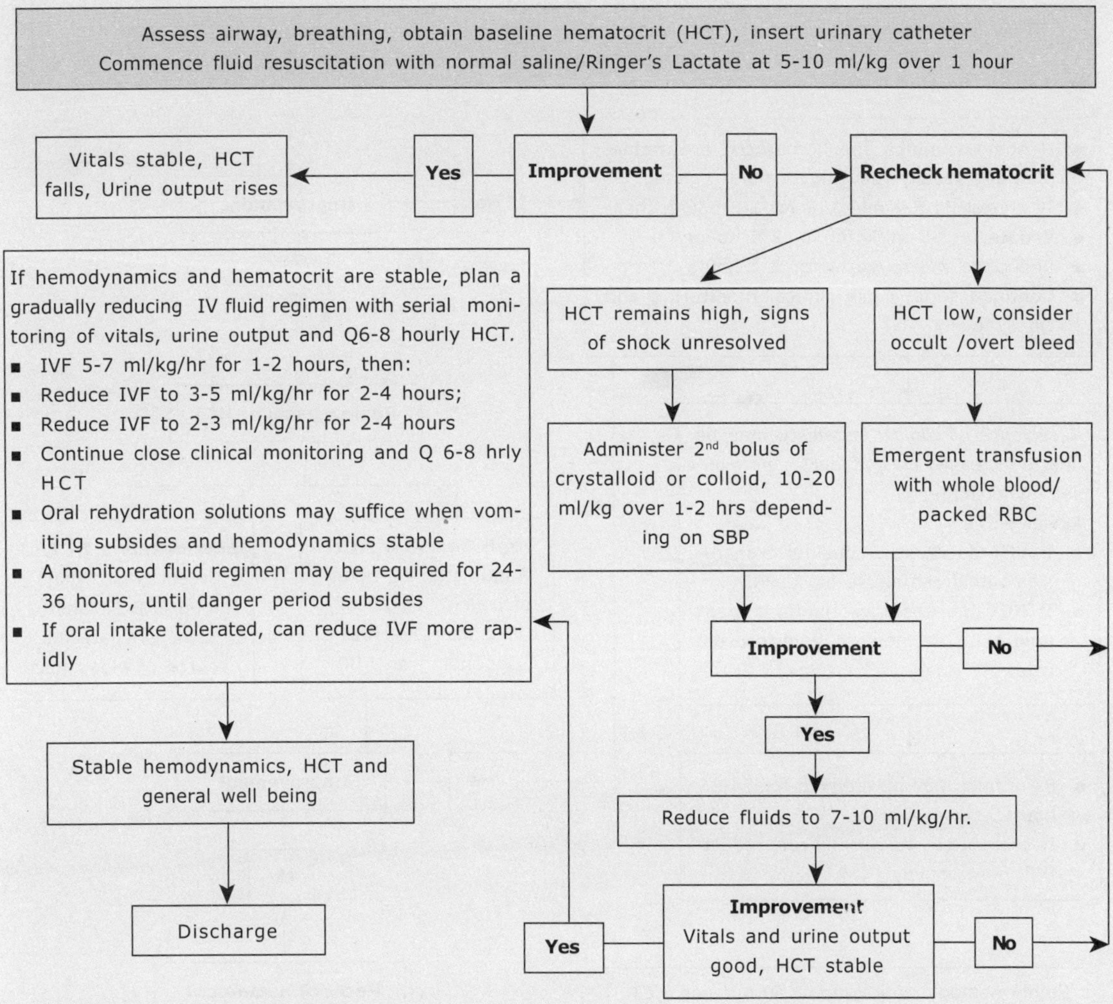

Note

Recurrence of clinical instability may be due to increased plasma leak or new onset hemorrhage:

Review HCT

- If HCT decreases, consider transfusion with fresh whole blood/PRBC.
- If HCT increases, consider repeat fluid bolus or increase fluid infusion rate

Fig. 30.3 Volume replacement flow chart for patients with severe dengue and compensated shock

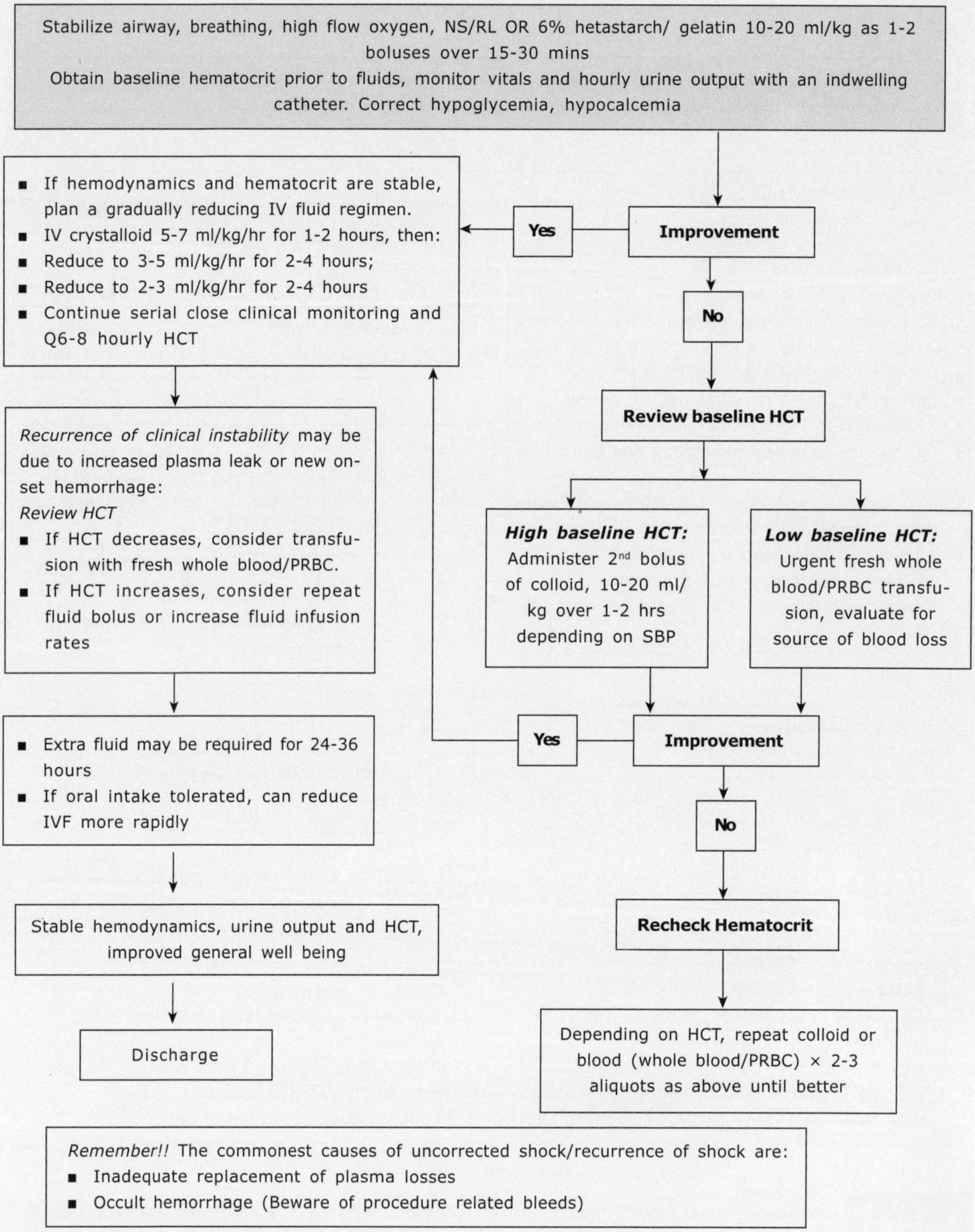

Fig. 30.4 Suggested approach to a patient with Severe Dengue and hypotension at presentation

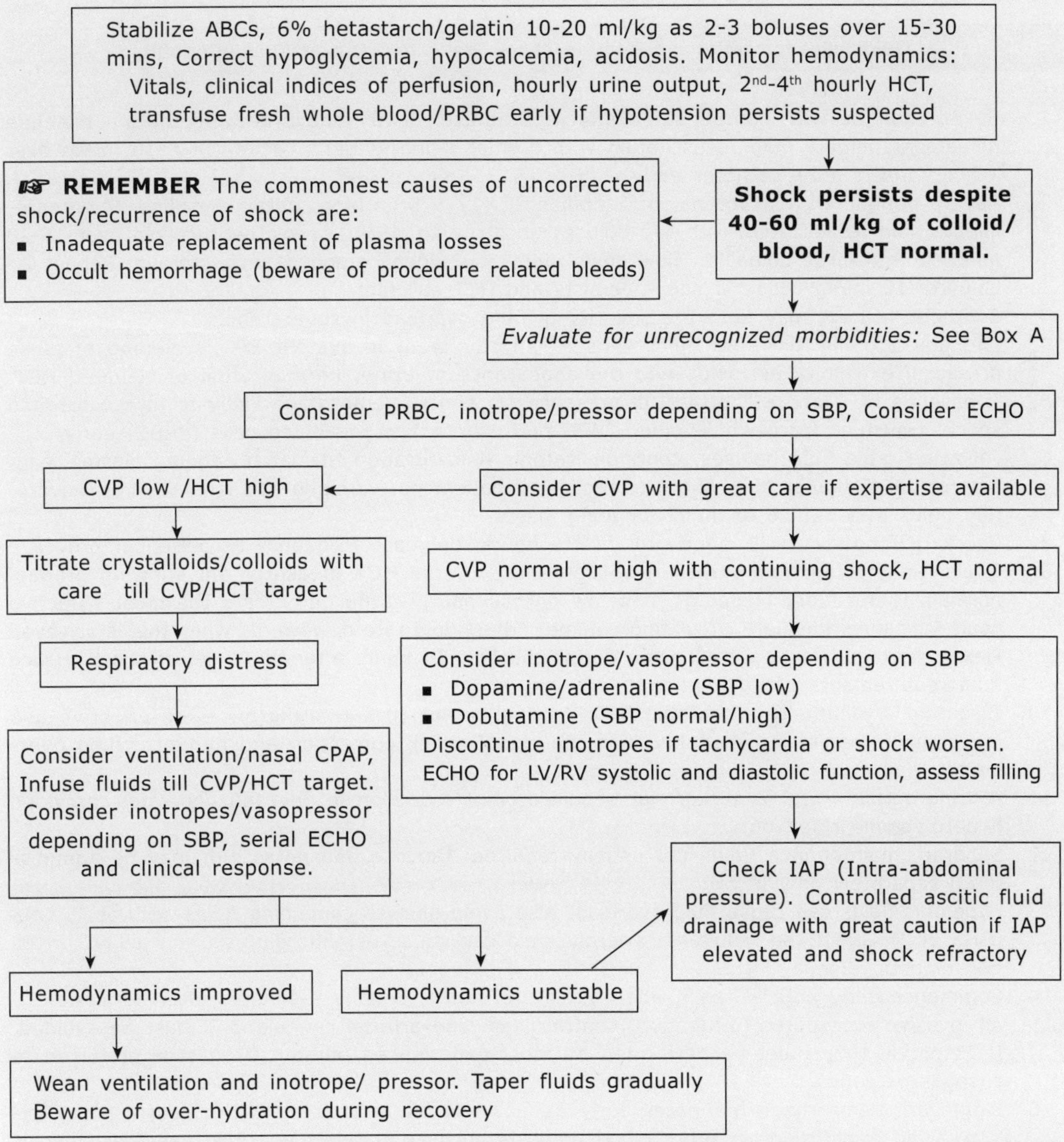

BOX A: Unrecognized morbidities that may contribute to refractory dengue shock

1. Occult bleeds – Rx: Whole blood/PRBC transfusion
2. Co-existing bacterial septic shock/malaria – Rx: antibiotics/antimalarials, cardiovascular support, blood transfusion
3. Myocardial dysfunction (systolic or diastolic) – Rx: Cardiovascular support, evaluate with ECHO if available
4. Positive pressure ventilation contributing to poor cardiac output – Rx: Titrated fluid and cardiovascular support
5. Elevated intra-abdominal pressure (IAP) – Rx: Cautious drainage
6. Wide-spread hypoxic-ischemic injury with terminal vasoplegic shock – No treatment effective

Fig. 30.5 Suggested approach to Severe Dengue and refractory shock (late presenters)

Table 30.3 Guidelines for reversing dengue shock while minimizing fluid overload

1. Severe dengue with compensated shock: Stabilize airway and breathing, obtain baseline hematocrit, initiate fluid resuscitation with normal saline/Ringer's Lactate at 5-10 ml/kg over 1 hour. Insert urine catheter early.
2. Severe dengue with hypotension: Stabilize airway & breathing, obtain baseline hematocrit, initiate fluid resuscitation with 1-2 boluses of 20 ml/kg NS/RL or synthetic colloid over 15-20 minutes until pulse palpable. Slow down fluid rates when hemodynamics improve. Repeat 2nd bolus of 10 ml/kg colloid if shock persists and HCT still high.
3. Synthetic colloids may limit the severity of fluid overload in severe shock
4. End points/goals for rapid fluid boluses: Improvement in systolic BP , widening of pulse pressure, extremity perfusion and the appearance of urine, normalization of elevated HCT
5. If baseline HCT low or "normal" in presence of shock, hemorrhage likely to have worsened shock, transfuse fresh whole blood (WB) or fresh packed red blood cells (PRBC) early.
6. Following rapid fluid boluses, continue isotonic fluid titration to match ongoing plasma leakage for 24-48 hours. After shock correction, if patient not vomiting and is alert, oral rehydration fluids may suffice to match ongoing losses.
7. Check HCT hourly to 2nd hourly for first 6 hours, decrease frequency as patient improves.
8. Goals for ongoing fluid titration: Stable vitals, serial HCT measurement showing gradual normalization (if not bleeding), and low normal hourly urine output are the most objective goals indicating adequate circulating volume. Adjust fluid rate downwards when this is achieved
9. Plasma leakage is intermittent even during the first 24 hours after the onset of shock. Hence fluid requirements are dynamic.
10. Targeting a minimally acceptable hourly urine output (0.5-1 ml/kg/hr) is an effective and inexpensive monitoring modality that can signal shock correction and minimize fluid overload.
11. A urine output > 1.5-2 ml/kg/hour should prompt reduction in fluid infusion rates, provided hyperglycemia ruled out.
12. Separate maintenance fluids not usually required. Glucose and potassium may be administered separately only if low.
13. Hypotonic fluids can cause fluid overload. Also avoid glucose containing fluids such as ½ GNS (GNS or ½ GNS): the resultant hyperglycemia can cause osmotic diuresis and delay correction of hypovolemia
14. Commence early enteral feeds when vitals are stable, usually 4-8 hours after admission.
15. All invasive procedures (intubation, central lines, and arterial cannulation) must be avoided. If essential, they must be performed by most experienced person. Orogastric preferred to nasogastric tubes.
16. Significant hemorrhage mandates early fresh whole blood or fresh PRBC transfusion. Minimize/avoid transfusions of other blood products such as platelets and FFP unless bleeding is uncontrolled despite 2-3 aliquots of fresh WB or PRBC.

cautiously commenced on a furosemide infusion at 0.1 mg/kg/hour.

- Meticulous monitoring whilst on diuretics cannot be over-emphasized and, if the circulatory status remains stable, the dose may be cautiously increased.

D. **Avoiding complications of ICU therapy**

- Complications of aggressive invasive ICU interventions may lead to significant morbidity and mortality in sick, bleeding children with dengue although these are seldom reported.
- Catastrophic bleeding may result from ICU

practices such as insertion of invasive central and arterial lines and intubation.

- Other potentially risky invasive care practices are rapid drainage of large volume pleural and ascitic fluid collections during the critical phase of plasma leakage: these can often result in sudden worsening of the hemodynamic status and catastrophic hemorrhage.
- As stated previously, judicious IV hydration will minimize large volume effusions and may completely obviate the need for the thoracic and/or abdominal paracentesis with its attendant complications

Other supportive therapies in dengue

- *Correction of electrolytes and acidosis*
  - Electrolyte and metabolic disturbances include hypoglycemia, metabolic acidosis, hyponatremia, and hypocalcemia (particularly in cases in which massive blood products transfusions are given).
  - Acidosis in particular, if uncorrected, may worsen DIC.
- *Sedatives*
  - Agitation may be a sign of shock, hepatic failure, metabolic derangement, encephalopathy or cerebral edema. Address the above issues, if present.
  - Avoid long acting and hepatotoxic sedatives. Chloral hydrate may be preferred.
- *Antibiotics:* Not indicated unless co-infections suspected
- *Oxygen therapy*
  - All children in shock should be given oxygen in the highest concentration in the least invasive mode as possible.
  - Nasal CPAP applied non-invasively by mask may help to improve respiratory distress and hypoxemia.

Therapies that are not useful and are not indicated

- Steroids. A Cochrane database review states that there is no good quality evidence that corticosteroids are helpful as serum cortisol levels are frequently elevated in dengue shock.
- IV Immunoglobulins

Criteria for discharge

- Return of appetite.
- Clinical improvement.
- Good urine output.
- Stable hematocrit.
- 2 days after recovery from shock.
- No respiratory distress from pleural effusion and ascites.

In the recovery phase, it is common to see persisting thrombocytopenia even in some otherwise stable patients. However, provided that the patient is otherwise stable, alert, able to take fluids by mouth and has a good urine output, he/she may be discharged. No specific therapy is indicated.

REFERENCES

1. Dengue Hemorrhagic Fever: Diagnosis, Treatment, Prevention and Control, 3rd ed. A joint publication of the World Health Organization (WHO) and the Special Programme for Research and Training in Tropical Diseases (TDR), Geneva, 2009
2. Wills BA, Nguyen M. Dung, MD, Loan H T et al. Comparison of Three Fluid Solutions for Resuscitation in Dengue Shock Syndrome. NEJM 2005; 9(353):877-889

31

Cardiogenic Shock

- **Definition**: A pathophysiologic state in which an abnormality of cardiac function is responsible for the failure to meet the metabolic needs of the tissue.
- Cardiogenic shock occurs when the heart muscle is unable to pump blood effectively. This may arise when myocarditis or congenital heart disease decreases cardiac contractility, when tachycardia causes ineffective filling or when bradycardia causes insufficient forward blood flow.
- *Myocardial dysfunction is frequently a common final event seen as a late manifestation of shock of any etiology.*

Table 31.1 Etiology of cardiogenic shock

- Cardiomyopathy/myocarditis
- Sepsis
- Myocardial stunning: Transient myocardial dysfunction following a hypoxic-ischemic event
- Trauma (myocardial contusion)
- Congenital/acquired heart disease
- Tachy- or bradyarrhythmias
- Post cardiac surgery/bypass

PATHOPHYSIOLOGY

Compensatory responses to decreased stroke volume/cardiac output (CO)

- Tachycardia.
- ↑ Systemic vascular resistance (SVR) in an attempt to maintain blood pressure.
- Hypotension is always a late sign in cardiogenic shock.
- These compensatory responses may be counterproductive as tachycardia and ↑ SVR will further increase cardiac work.

Table 31.2 Myocardial dysfunction in sepsis

- May involve the left ventricle and/or right ventricle
- Can result in systolic or diastolic dysfunction

Causes
- Myocardial depressant factor
- Reduced coronary blood flow due to low diastolic BP
- Adrenergic receptor dysfunction
- Impaired sarcolemmal calcium flux
- Iatrogenic: High dose inotrope/pressor

Congestive cardiac failure (CCF) vs cardiogenic shock

- CCF is a chronic process where the body adapts to low ejection fraction (EF) by increasing heart rate and augmenting the preload and afterload.
- These patients are usually well compensated, although they may be symptomatic in terms of edema, low blood pressure, respiratory distress or fatiguability.
- Symptoms improve with oral decongestive therapy and correction of aggravating factors.

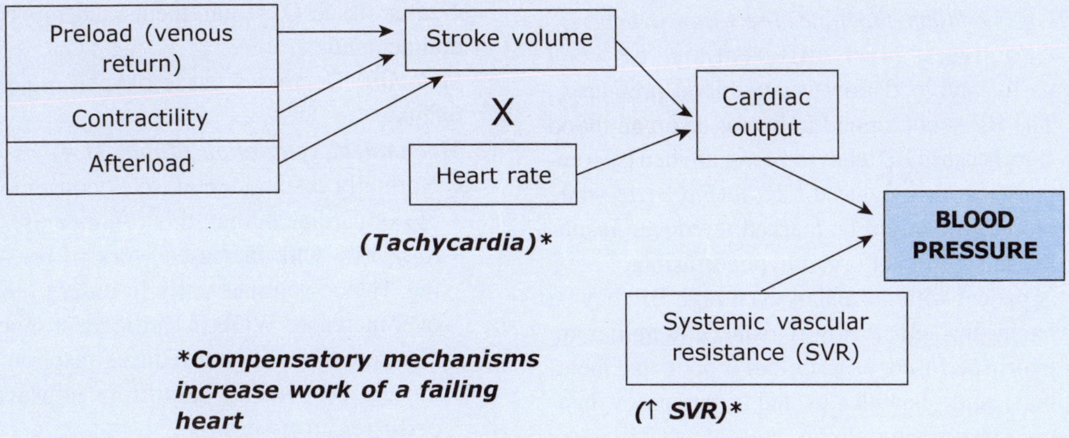

Fig. 31.1 Determinants of blood pressure

- *In cardiogenic shock*, the decreased CO occurs more abruptly and there is acute decompensation with features of shock, tissue hypoperfusion and acidosis.
- Blood pressure may be normal or low.
- These patients need rapid, more intensive therapeutic measures to re-establish adequate perfusion and oxygen delivery to end organs.

Systolic and diastolic dysfunction

- *Systolic dysfunction:* Impaired contractility
- *Diastolic dysfunction:* Stiff, non-compliant ventricles with impaired diastolic relaxation.
- Both can coexist. It is important to recognize the presence of diastolic dysfunction because therapy aimed to improve systolic function (catecholamines) can worsen diastolic dysfunction.
- *When to suspect diastolic dysfunction*
  - If shock persists despite adequate filling and ECHO shows preserved ejection fraction (EF).
  - Features of pulmonary edema occur even with small volume resuscitation.
  - The CVP is usually high and large increments occur with filling.
  - ECHO with Doppler studies is confirmatory.

Table 31.3 Diagnosis of cardiogenic shock

1. **Clinical features**
   - Predominant LV dysfunction: Pulmonary edema, shock with narrow pulse pressure, tachycardia, gallop rhythm
   - Predominant RV dysfunction: Tachycardia, dyspnea, increased work of breathing, hepatomegaly, raised JVP/CVP
2. **CXR**: Cardiomegaly ± pulmonary edema
3. **ECG**: Look for abnormal rhythms, features of ALCAPA (Anomalous left coronary artery from pulmonary artery)
4. **Rapid echocardiography**
   - Assess preload, contractility, RV and LV systolic & diastolic function
   - Pulmonary artery pressures
   - Coronary anatomy (Kawasaki, ALCAPA)
   - Structural problems, tamponade

MANAGEMENT OF CARDIOGENIC SHOCK

"Target perfusion (flow) and not pressure (numbers)"

- Caregivers must differentiate between perfusion/blood flow versus blood pressure.
- The BP is not a good indicator of organ blood flow because BP tends to be maintained by compensatory/drug induced ↑ SVR (Fig. 31.1), while blood flow might be markedly reduced resulting in significant organ hypoperfusion.
- A patient with normal or even high BP may be having inadequate flow if his/her extremities are poorly perfused, urine output is poor, and metabolic acidosis with elevated lactate or low central venous saturation is present.

Table 31.4 Intubation of cardiogenic shock is a high risk procedure!!

- Beware and anticipate hypotension during intubation
- Give isotonic fluids 5-10 ml per kg slowly
- Commence inotropes prior to intubation (adrenaline 0.1-0.2 mcg/kg/min or dopamine 10 mcg/kg/min).
- Low dose fentanyl usually has a safe hemodynamic profile.
- Ketamine usually maintains BP well, but can have negative inotropy when low CO has been present > 48 hr
- Midazolam, even at low doses, can cause hypotension due to its negative inotropy.
- *Awake intubation may be the safest option in a moribund patient as any/all agent(s) may cause deterioration*

General goals of management of cardiogenic shock

3 pronged approach

A. Minimize demands on a failing heart.
B. Maximize performance of myocardium.
C. Improve tissue oxygen delivery.

A. Minimize demands on a failing heart

1. ***Control elevated temperature***: Fever increases tissue O_2 requirements and myocardial demands.
2. ***Sedation:*** Decreases tissue oxygen requirements
3. ***Mechanical ventilation (Table 31.4)***
   - Normally respiratory muscles consume < 5% of cardiac output; this can increase up to > 50% with increased work of breathing. Hence ventilate early in order to take over increased WOB in cardiogenic shock.
   - Controlled ventilation reduces respiratory muscle O_2 demand permitting improved perfusion to tissues.
   - In a normal heart, PEEP reduces cardiac output by reducing preload. However, in a failing heart, reduced preload is beneficial.
   - PEEP also improves stroke volume by reducing LV afterload.
   - PEEP opens alveoli, improves oxygenation.
   - Ventilation permits sedation, thereby reducing metabolic demand.
   - Non-invasive ventilation (NIV) may suffice if the patient is not very sick. However, in a child with significant low cardiac output, NIV may not be ideal as the caregiver cannot take over the work of breathing completely and full sedation may be impossible.
   - Administer oxygen even if saturations are stable to improve tissue oxygen delivery. O_2 is also a pulmonary vasodilator.

B. Maximizing the performance of a failing heart: Optimize the 4 determinants of CO, viz, heart rate, preload, contractility and afterload.

1. ***Tachycardia control***
   - In cardiogenic shock, tachycardia is a compensatory response to ↓ stroke volume (SV).
   - Measures to improve SV (judicious filling, inotropy) will reduce tachycardia.

- Other measures include sedation, correction of anaemia and dysrhythmias.
- A low normal heart rate in the face of shock needs a chronotropic drug (dobutamine, adrenaline) to improve cardiac output. Also correct hypothermia, if present.

2. ***Optimize preload***
- The decision to infuse fluids in cardiogenic shock is not straightforward.
- Volume administration may not be necessary in most patients with cardiac failure/ cardiogenic shock who already have fluid retention and congestive features; however, some patients may need fluid due to overdiuresis or fluid losses (vomiting, ↓intake).
- Stretching of cardiac muscle fibres with fluid improves stroke volume (Frank- Starling principle).
- Hence, in a hypotensive patient with cardiogenic shock, a titrated, small volume fluid challenge (5-10 ml/kg colloid over 60-120 minutes) may be given and the hemodynamic response including CVP carefully assessed (Table 31.5).
- A *"bedside Frank Starling test"* may be performed during the fluid bolus and clinical features assessed in conjunction with the CVP. Evaluate whether the HR, BP, respiratory distress, liver span, extremity perfusion is better or worse.
- A favourable response (Table 31.5) indicates that the fluid is helping. Fluids must be ceased if the patient appears to be deteriorating either in terms of hemodynamics or pulmonary edema or hepatomegaly develops.
- Guidelines regarding exact volume of fluid are not easy; one can also assess preload responsiveness by pressure on the liver or performing a reverse Trendelenburg test.
- *Drugs to reduce preload/ congestive features.*

Table 31.5 CVP interpretation may not be straightforward

- A low CVP in a patient with shock indicates hypovolemia
- A high CVP reflects ↑ preload, ↓contractility (systolic dysfunction), ↓ compliance of ventricle (diastolic dysfunction) and ↑ afterload.
- A high CVP does not reliably rule out hypovolemia.
- Failing hearts require a higher CVP

Favourable response to fluid challenge
- Decreased tachycardia
- Improved peripheral perfusion
- Increased BP
- Improved urine output
- Rise of CVP > 3 mmHg but < 5 mmHg followed by a gradual fall.

a. Venodilators increase vascular capacitance and decrease congestive features by decreasing filling pressures.
   Drugs such as such as nitroglycerine may be commenced as an infusion at 1-5 mcg/kg/min. Start at low doses and increase gradually if tolerated. Hypotension is more common in volume depleted patients.
b. Diuretics: Frusemide may be administered after BP is reasonably stabilised *preferably as a 24 hr continuous infusion* (1-2 mg/kg/day, max 0.1-0.5 mg/kg/hr) in order to cause steady diuresis and prevent sudden large swings in intravascular volume.

☞ **REMEMBER** Avoid diuretics in a hypotensive patient even if the patient has pulmonary edema as it will further reduce stroke volume and can cause catastrophic hypotension

3. ***Improve contractility***
- Usual options are inotropes with pressor effects (adrenaline, dopamine) or inodilators (dobutamine, milrinone).
- Digitalis glycosides augment myocardial contractility and control tachycardia, but because of a narrow therapeutic to toxic ratio, long half-life and dependence for clearance on renal function, it is rarely useful in the acute phase of cardiogenic shock.
- In cardiogenic shock, intravenous and not oral inotropes are the mainstay of treatment.
- Correct hypocalcemia, hypomagnesemia. Calcium is an inotrope: Infuse 10% calcium gluconate 0.1-0.4 ml/kg/hour. Monitor ionized Ca^{++} levels; cease if levels >1.3 mmol/L.
- Correct acidosis: Administer bicarbonate only if pH < 7.1-7.2.

☞ **REMEMBER** *The role of inotropes in cardiogenic shock*
- Inotropes improve stroke volume by increasing contractility while concurrently increasing myocardial oxygen demands ("whipping a tired horse").
- Hence use the minimal possible dose and accept the lowest BP that results in adequate perfusion and resolving acidosis.
- Use of inotropes is a short term temporizing measure for a patient in cardiogenic shock. When the cardiac output improves and the patient's condition stabilizes, the caregiver must wean inotropes and concentrate more on preload and afterload reduction (diuretics and ACE inhibitors): a strategy that improves long term cardiac function without increasing myocardial work demands.

Choice of inotropes

This depends on whether the mean blood pressure is normal or low.

a) *Cardiogenic shock with moderate/severe hypotension: Use inotropes with pressor effects*
- Inotropes with associated pressor effects may worsen cardiac function by increasing afterload and myocardial work and must be avoided as far as possible.
- However, in a hypotensive patient, the associated low diastolic blood pressures may reduce coronary blood flow and cause myocardial ischemia, worsening the shock state.
- Such patients may benefit from pressors or inotrope-pressor agents such as dopamine at 7-10 mcg/kg/min or adrenaline in doses 0.2-0.5 mcg/kg/min.
- Adrenaline > 0.3 mcg/kg/min and high dose dopamine > 10 mcg/kg/min can cause undesirable increase in afterload, cause supply-demand mismatch, unfavourably increase myocardial oxygen consumption, worsen tachycardia with decreased time for filling and increase the tendency for dysrhythmias.
- Dopamine has become unpopular due to various reasons, including decreased efficacy due to depleted catecholamine stores in shock and adverse endocrine effects.
- In a hypotensive patient with cardiogenic shock, commence adrenaline at 0.2-0.5 mcg/kg/min. Start at lowest dose in range, titrate to acceptable MAP.
- Once the BP has stabilized, inodilators may be added and the dose of adrenaline may be gradually tapered.

b) *Cardiogenic shock with normal BP or mild hypotension: Inodilators are the key.*
- Preferred agents in this setting are dobutamine at 5-10 mcg/kg/min or milrinone at 0.25-0.75 mcg/kg/min.
- In the unstable patient with cardiogenic shock, dobutamine is the preferred initial agent because of its shorter half-life of 1-2 minutes and less propensity to cause hypotension.
- If perfusion and acidosis do not improve in 3-4 hours, consider the addition of milrinone.

- Both inodilator drugs act through different pathways and are synergistic with extremely favorable effects in cardiogenic shock.
- Combining dobutamine and milrinone may permit the practitioner to avoid complications that may be seen with higher doses of a single agent.
- *Milrinone has potent inotropy as well as vasodilatory effects and can result in impressive afterload reduction without tachycardia.* Thus, it is an extremely useful agent in cardiogenic shock.
- Its main disadvantage is its ability to cause hypotension in volume depleted patients.
- Other side effects are thrombocytopenia (dose and duration dependent) and accumulation in renal failure.
- Loading dose of milrinone may be withheld in order to prevent hypotension. Pretreatment with 5-10 ml/kg colloid will also improve tolerance to this agent. If hematocrit < 30-35%, a red cell transfusion may be administered.
- Milrinone does not have chronotropic effects and, if tachycardia occurs during its use, it indicates excess vasodilatation that has been exacerbated by volume deficits.
- If tachycardia and hypotension occur, the dose of milrinone may be either decreased or ceased and fluid resuscitation commenced. Some patients may need a brief period of low dose noradrenaline (0.05-0.1 mcg/kg/min) for 2-3 hours until the milrinone induced hypotension has resolved.

4. ***Afterload reduction (Figs. 31.2 and 31.3).***

☞ **REMEMBER** Afterload reduction is the best way to improve CO without increasing myocardial work and is the sheet anchor of management of cardiogenic shock.

- Afterload may be reduced by non-pharmacologic measures and by vasodilators/inodilators.
- *Non pharmacologic reduction of afterload* may be achieved by reversing conditions which increase SVR such as hypothermia, hypoxemia, pain and anxiety: it is important that these are adequately addressed before initiating vasodilators.
- Arterial relaxation results in increased ejection fraction while venous relaxation shifts blood to the peripheries and decreases pulmonary edema.
- Intravenous vasodilators with a rapid onset of action and short half-life such as the nitrovasodilators (nitroglycerine and sodium nitroprusside) are preferred in the acute setting and are used in situations where myocardial dysfunction is associated with elevated filling pressures and the BP is normal or near normal. The combination of inotropy + afterload reduction results in hemodynamic improvement not possible with either agent alone (Fig. 31.2).
- *Pure vasodilators* (also see chapter on inotropes and vasoactive agents)
  - Sodium nitroprusside (SNP): 0.5-5 mcg/kg/min.
  - Nitroglycerine (NTG): 1-10 mcg/kg/min. Higher dose ranges are needed for arterial vasodilatation.

☞ **REMEMBER** With the widespread availability of an effective inodilator such as milrinone which has the dual advantages of vasodilatation with inotropy, pure vasodilators are used less frequently.

☞ **REMEMBER** While vasodilators are extremely useful to reduce afterload and improve the function of a failing heart, they can cause precipitous fall in BP and must be titrated carefully.

- Measures to mitigate the hypotensive effects of afterload reducers.

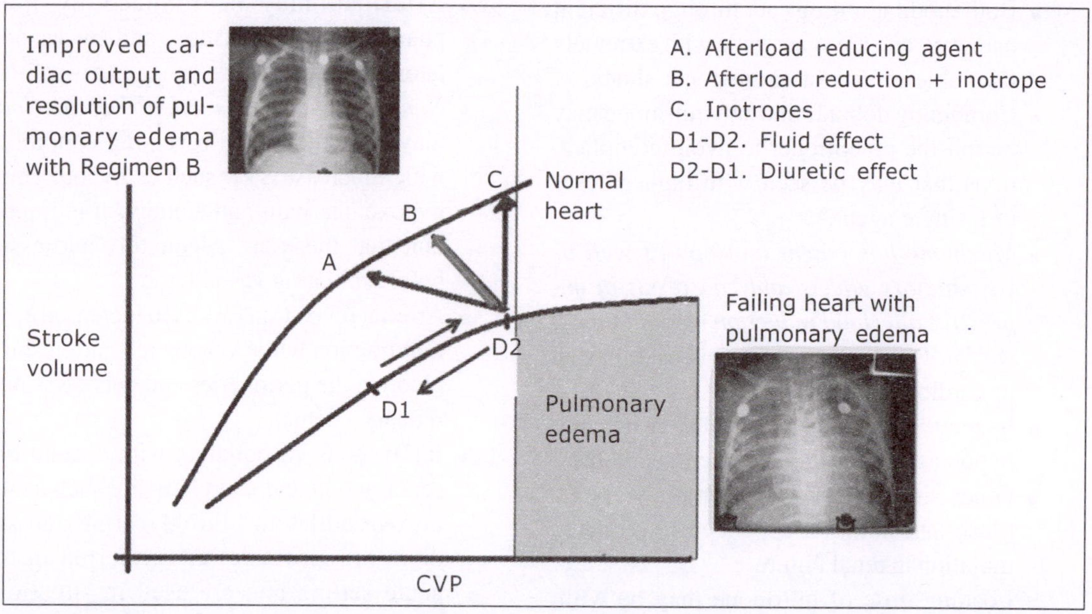

Fig. 31.2 Aims of therapy in cardiogenic shock are to improve cardiac output and decrease congestive symptoms with a combination of inotropes and afterload reducers.

- Hypotension can be precipitated by even minor degrees of hypovolemia. Pre-treatment with 5-10 ml/kg colloid may pre-empt the fall in BP.
- Always start at the lowest doses and very gradually titrate upwards.

- If hypotension occurs, cease the infusion immediately and resuscitate with fluids.
- Fortunately, SNP/NTG have a short half-life (1-2 min) and the BP will rapidly recover.

C. **Improve tissue oxygen delivery**

1. Correct anemia in order to increase oxygen carrying capacity. Maintain hematocrit between 30 nad 35%.

2. Improve oxygenation: Administer high flow oxygen, consider early ventilation (NIV or invasive ventilation).

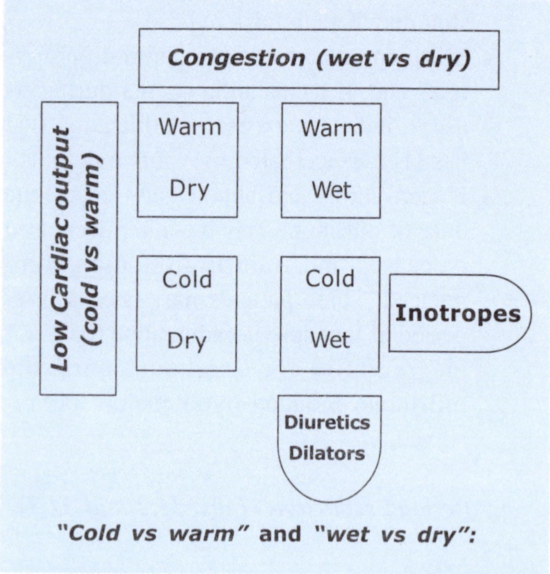

Fig. 31.3 Current classification into low CO +/- congestive features will help in selecting the appropriate therapeutic approach

MONITORING HEMODYNAMIC VARIABLES IN A PATIENT WITH CARDIOGENIC SHOCK

- Remember that a low normal BP is perfectly acceptable if a patient's perfusion parameters are adequate.
- Continuous monitoring of the following is essential with the following end-points:
  - Achieve threshold heart rate for age
  - Maintain minimal acceptable MAP/SBP for age (See below). Invasive arterial monitoring highly recommended.
  - Urine output > 1 ml/kg/hr.
  - Warm peripheries with normal CFT .
  - Central venous saturations ($ScvO_2$) > 70-75%
  - Normal mental status
  - Improving metabolic acidosis or decreasing lactate.
- *Systolic BP goals:*
  - Minimally acceptable SBP (> 5th centile) = 70 + age x 2
  - Acceptable SBP (> 50th centile) = 90 + age x 2
- *Mean Arterial Pressure (MAP) goals:* MAP is better than SBP as an indicator of organ perfusion
  - 1-6 mo: > 40-45 mmHg; 7 mo-5 yr: > 45-55 mmHg
  - 5-12 yr: > 50-60 mmHg; > *12 yr*: > 60-65 mmHg
- *Arterial or venous lactate trends:*
  - Follow either venous or arterial lactate trends consistently.
  - A rising trend of lactate is good indicator of tissue hypoperfusion that may be seen in either patients with low CO, excess metabolic demands or those receiving excess pressors/inotropes.
- *Central venous saturations ($ScvO_2$):*
  - The $ScvO_2$ is a sensitive surrogate indicator of the adequacy of whole body tissue oxygenation.
  - Mixed venous saturations (MvO_2) require placement of pulmonary artery catheter that is not practical: However, the $ScvO_2$ requires only a central line placed close to the right atrium.
  - O_2 delivery to tissues is dependent on cardiac output, Hb and O_2 saturations. Assuming that latter two are maintained, changes in $ScvO_2$ will reflect the cardiac output.
  - Normal value of central venous saturations is 70–75%, i.e., in a patient with a good CO, if the arterial saturation is 100%, a tissue O_2 extraction of 25% will result in a $ScvO_2$ of 75%.
  - When the CO falls, a greater proportion of O_2 will be extracted resulting in a $ScvO_2$ of < 70%.

CARDIOGENIC SHOCK IN SPECIAL SITUATIONS

A. *Cardiogenic shock in the setting of septic shock*

- Approximately 1/3rd to 50% of patients with septic shock will have decreased LV ± RV function.
- The clinical diagnosis of cardiogenic shock may not be straightforward as septic patients with a normal heart may also show signs of fluid intolerance due to capillary leak (non-cardiogenic pulmonary edema).
- Conversely, patients with ↓LVEF may tolerate large volume filling well because of the dilated vasculature and normal myocardial compliance.
- Suspect underlying myocardial dysfunction if the following are noted:
  - Peripheral pulses and perfusion worsen when pressors such as noradrenaline are added for vasodilatory shock.
  - Metabolic acidosis, lactic acidosis or low $ScvO_2$ persists despite adequate filling, establishment of a normal MAP and a hematocrit >30%.

- Presence of tachycardia with gallop.
- Treatment of septic shock with myocardial dysfunction is 3 pronged and includes:
  - Slow and steady filling to keep filling pressures high normal (CVP 10-12 mmHg), colloids are preferred.
  - Inotropes such as dobutamine.
  - Vasopressors at the lowest dose that results in an acceptable MAP.
- Severe decompensated shock mandates adrenaline infusion.
  - Add dobutamine after MAP improves.

B. *Treatment of diastolic dysfunction*

- Tachycardia control is important: The first step is to minimize/avoid chronotropic agents such as catecholamines as a lower HR will improve diastolic relaxation time.
- Lusitropic drugs (milrinone) will help diastolic relaxation.
- Slow filling with colloids.
- Use low dose diuretics with care in a patient with pulmonary edema.

C. *Treatment of right ventricular (RV) failure/pulmonary hypertension:*

- Assiduously avoid hypotension which will worsen RV myocardial perfusion. This is especially relevant as the RV is perfused both during systole and diastole.
- Institute measures to reduce pulmonary vascular resistance (PVR). Ensure adequate sedation (especially during procedures and suctioning), maintain low normal pCO_2, avoid hyperinflation, hypoxemia, acidosis.

Summary/Pearls

- Cardiogenic shock occurs when the heart muscle is unable to pump blood effectively.
- Compensatory responses to ↓CO such as tachycardia and ↑ SVR may be counterproductive and further worsen cardiac function.
- *The blood pressure is not a good indicator of organ blood flow* because the BP tends to be maintained by compensatory/drug induced ↑ SVR even when blood flow is markedly reduced. Focus on perfusion and not on pressure.
- A low normal BP may be acceptable if organ perfusion and blood flow are good.
- The principles of management are:
  - *Decrease demands* by sedation and early ventilation and temperature control.
  - *Improve myocardial efficiency* by optimizing preload, improving contractility, afterload reduction and tachycardia control
  - Inodilators such as dobutamine and milrinone are useful as they provide both inotropy and afterload reduction without undue tachycardia.
  - *Reduction in afterload* is the best way to improve CO without increasing myocardial work.
  - *Improve tissue oxygen delivery by* correcting anemia and providing high flow oxygen.
- Indication for adrenaline in cardiogenic shock:
  - Avoid if possible as it can result in unfavourable oxygen consumption, worsen tachycardia, increase afterload, increase lactic acidosis.
  - Use only in a patient with significant hypotension.
  - Use minimal doses that will improve BP without excess tachycardia, reduce dose if metabolic acidosis worsens or central venous saturations fall.
  - Use concominant inodilator.
- Explore all correctable causes including surgical options where applicable.

- Use pulmonary vasodilators (dobutamine is mainstay), NTG, magnesium, prostacyclins, sildenafil, nitric oxide. Milrinone once MAP stable.
- Use low dose pressor such as noradrenaline. This will increase afterload of LV and prevent leftward shift of interventricular septum.

D. *Myocarditis*: Intravenous immunoglobulin 1 g/kg over 24 hours may be useful.

E. *Rheumatic carditis*: Steroids, aspirin, penicillin.

F. *Surgical management for*: ALCAPA, other CHD, rheumatic valve disease.

NEWER TREATMENT OPTIONS

- Levosimendan (inodilator) is a new calcium sensitizer for the treatment of acutely decompensated chronic heart failure. It differs from classic inotropes because of its ability to improve myocardial efficiency without increasing myocardial oxygen demand, its anti-stunning properties, its effects on coronary blood flow, and its lusitropic effects.
- Ventricular assist device (VAD)/ECMO may be useful in severe myocardial dysfunction.

ONGOING CHRONIC THERAPY OF CCF/ CARDIOGENIC SHOCK

- Once the acute phase of the treatment has resulted in cardiovascular stabilization, low dose oral afterload reducing agents with a longer half-life may be initiated and inotrope/vasodilator infusion can be gradually weaned as tolerated.
- Serial echocardiographic evaluation may be helpful during weaning.
- Inotropes can be safely weaned even if the LV ejection fraction remains low in an otherwise stable child who is well compensated.
- Oral agents such as angiotensin converting enzyme (ACE) inhibitors cause vasodilatation by blocking the renin-angiotensin system and the use of diuretics can prevent or reverse abnormal fluid retention. The oral agents can be steadily escalated to full dose under supervision.
- Digoxin/beta-blockers can be used for reduction in heart rate and ventricular remodelling.

REFERENCES

1. Treatment of Heart Failure in Infants and Children: Medical Management. In: Nichols DG, ed: Rogers' Textbook of Pediatric Intensive Care, 4th ed. Lippincot Williams and Wilkins, Baltimore:2008; 584-599
2. Pharmacology of the cardiovascular system. In: Pediatric Critical Care. Fuhrman and Zimmerman (Eds). 3rd ed. Philadelphia, PA, 2006, Mosby Elsevier, 300-331.

32

Inotropes and Vasoactive Agents

Shock and inadequate perfusion are a frequent occurrence in critically ill children.

There are various strategies to reverse the hemodynamic instability including fluid administration, positive pressure ventilation and administration of inotrope/vasoactive agents. In general, vasoactive agents should only be used after correcting fluid deficits.

Choosing the appropriate agent is crucial to the success of therapy. The choice depends on proper understanding of both the disordered pathophysiology and an understanding of the selected agent's properties.

CLASSIFICATION

- Inotropes and vasoactive drugs may be classified based on the receptor that they act on and their physiologic response (Table 32.1 and 32.2) and whether they are direct or indirectly acting. Many agents have overlapping effects.
  - Direct acting agents act by stimulating the noradrenergic receptor, e.g., adrenaline, noradrenaline
  - Indirect acting agents cause the release of noradrenaline from the receptor which is responsible for the effect, e.g., dopamine, dobutamine.
- Inotropes may be further classified based on the class of drugs and mechanism of action
  - Catecholamines: Effects mediated by various adrenergic receptors that use cAMP dependent signaling cascade.
    E.g., dopamine, dobutamine, adrenaline, noradrenaline
  - Phosphodiesterase (PDE) III inhibitors: Non-sympathomimetic agents. PDE inhibition results in ↑ cellular concentrations of cAMP by inhibiting its destruction.
    E.g., milrinone, amrinone
  - Calcium sensitizers: New class of agents that ↑ sensitivity of cardiac myofilament to calcium, e.g., levosimendan
  - Cardiac glycosides, e.g., digoxin. This drug is best reserved for chronic therapy.

INDIVIDUAL AGENTS

- Catecholamines: Dopamine, dobutamine, adrenaline, noradrenaline
- Phosphodiesterase inhibitors: Milrinone, amrinone
- Vasopressors: Vasopressin, phenylephrine
- Vasodilators: Nitroglycerine, sodium nitroprusside

Dopamine

Hemodynamic effects: Dose dependent, acts at D, β_1, β_2 and α_1 receptors (Table 32.1).

- Low dose (2-5 mcg/kg/min): Acts on D receptors usually increasing urine output, although clinically not significant. Has no role in preventing renal failure as previously thought.
- Moderate dose (5-10 mcg/kg/min): Inotrope. Acts on β_1 receptors to increase cardiac output.

Table 32.1 Types of receptor and expected physiologic response

Receptor	Physiologic response	Agent
α_1 (Alpha-1)	Systemic and pulmonary arteriolar vasoconstriction	Adr, NA, Dop
β_1 (Beta-1)	Increased contractility and heart rate	Adr ≥ Dop, Dobut ≥ NA
β_2 (Beta-2)	Systemic vasodilatation, bronchodilation, hypokalemia	Adr, Dobut
D (Dopaminergic)	Increased renal and splanchnic blood flow	Dopamine

Dop = Dopamine, Dobut = Dobutamine, Adr = Adrenaline, NA = Noradrenaline.

Table 32.2 Classification based on main hemodynamic response

Agent class	Physiologic response	Usual end result	Examples
Inotrope	↑ Cardiac contraction	↑ CO, BP unchanged or ↑	Dop, dobut, milrin, adr, NA
Chronotrope	↑ HR	Tachycardia, ↑ CO	Isoprenaline, dop, adr, dobut (high dose)
Vasopressor	↑ Vascular tone, ↑ SVR, ↑ PVR	↑ BP, CO unchanged or ↓	Adr, NA, vasopressin dopamine (high dose)
Vasodilator	↓ Arterial + venous tone, ↓ SVR, ↓ PVR	BP unchanged or ↓, CO↑	Nitroprusside, nitroglycerin, milrinone
Inodilator	↑ Cardiac contraction, ↓ SVR, ↓ PVR	↑ CO, BP unchanged or ↑ (hypotension can occur if hypovolemic)	Milrinone, amrinone, dobutamine, levosimendan
Lusitrope	Diastolic relaxation of ventricles	↑ CO (if diastolic dysfunction present)	Milrinone, amrinone

Cardiac output: CO, Systemic vascular resistance (SVR), pulmonary vascular resistance (PVR), Dop =Dopamine, Dobut = Dobutamine, Adr = Adrenaline, NA = Noradrenaline, Milrin= Milrinone.

- High dose (>10 mcg/kg/min): Predominant pressor with minimal inotropy due to α_1 mediated vasoconstriction.

Indications

- Fluid refractory septic shock.
- Cardiogenic shock with moderate hypotension. In a normotensive patient with cardiogenic shock, dobutamine or milrinone may be preferred.
- Many critically unwell patients with hypotensive shock/hypoperfusion that persists after fluid resuscitation (e.g., ARDS) may improve with dopamine. If the shock fails to resolve with dopamine, a more detailed hemodynamic assessment may be necessary.

Side effects

- At higher doses (>10 mcg/kg/min), vasoconstriction can cause tissue hypoperfusion, increased myocardial oxygen consumption, arrhythmias, tachycardia.
- Extravasation causes tissue necrosis by releasing noradrenaline.
- Tachyphylaxis if used for more than 48 hr.
- Some reports suggest that prolonged use of dopamine can cause immunosuppression and endocrine disturbances.

Dose

- 5-20 mcg/kg/min.
- Avoid higher doses, i.e., > 10 mcg/kg/min as it has greater pressor effect than inotropy.
- If hypotension still a problem despite 10 mcg/kg/min, consider fluid or alternative agents such as adrenaline or NA.

Dobutamine

Hemodynamic effects: Dobutamine is a synthetic catecholamine that acts on β_1 and β_2 receptors with minimal action on α_1 receptors resulting in inotropy, chronotropy, vasodilatation. In a patient with impaired cardiac function, dobutamine improves cardiac output by improving stroke volume and decreasing afterload with minimal tachycardia (unless infusion rates exceed 10 mcg/kg/min).

Indications

- Cardiogenic shock with normal blood pressure, e.g., myocarditis with compensated shock. However, dobutamine may also be effective in patients with borderline low BP (provided the patient is normovolemic) as its inotropic effect will improve CO and blood pressure.
- Many critically unwell patients with normotensive shock/hypoperfusion that persists after fluid resuscitation (e.g., ARDS, post arrest) may be treated with dobutamine. If improvement fails to occur, a more detailed hemodynamic assessment may be necessary.
- Fluid refractory septic shock with normal blood pressure and impaired extremity perfusion. In a hypotensive patient, dopamine or adrenaline is preferred.
- In children with warm, vasodilated septic shock, the initial treatment approach is aggressive fluid resuscitation followed by the addition of a pressor such as noradrenaline in order to raise abnormally low SVR. Dobutamine may be added if metabolic acidosis (or low central venous saturation) persists or worsens after the addition of pressor in order to address possible co-existing myocardial impairment and improve micro-circulatory blood flow to vulnerable regions (gut, splanchnic, renal perfusion).

Side effects

- Dobutamine increases myocardial O_2 consumption and can cause supply-demand mismatch. Thus if tachycardia worsens after initiating dobutamine, the patient may be better off without it and other correctable causes of shock should explored (e.g., uncorrected hypovolemia).

- Tachycardia and arrhythmias that may be more frequent in patient with myocarditis, electrolyte abnormality or at higher doses (> 10-15 mcg/kg/min).

Dose

- 5-20 mcg/kg/min.
- Commence infusion at 5-10 mcg/kg/min, can increase infusion rates to 15 mcg/kg/min if hemodynamics do not improve.
- If shock still not reversed, re-evaluate hemodynamics, consider supplemental fluids or other agents.

Adrenaline/epinephrine

- Adrenaline is the principal stress hormone and produces extensive metabolic and hemodynamic effects.
- Depending on the infusion dose, adrenaline acts at the α_1, β_1 and β_2 receptors to produce varying hemodynamic effects.

Note

- At infusion rates > 0.5 mcg/kg/min, adrenaline can increase BP but CO and organ perfusion can worsen with a potential for vulnerable organ (gut, kidneys) ischemia and failure. (Numbers look better but patient's perfusion may be worse).
- ↑ myocardial O_2 consumption can worsen supply-demand mismatch. Ischemic changes may be seen on ECG at higher doses.

Indications and doses (Table 32.3)

- Cardiogenic shock with decompensated shock despite standard inotropes (e.g., severe myocarditis). With significant hypotension, coronary pressures may be inadequate to perfuse the myocardium: in this situation, adrenaline improves the diastolic BP resulting in better coronary perfusion and improved myocardial function.
- Myocardial dysfunction is common after cardiac arrest and may be associated with ↑ SVR and PVR. Hypotensive shock following cardiac arrest may be treated with adrenaline infusion. Normotensive shock may be treated with dobutamine.
- Cold septic shock refractory to fluids and dobutamine/dopamine, where a co-existing cardiogenic element is suspected. In addition to inotropy, adrenaline infusion at rates 0.3-0.4 µg/kg/min normalizes SVR if low.
- Severe shock of any etiology unresponsive to fluids and standard inotropes.

Table 32.3 Hemodynamic effects of adrenaline are dose dependent

Low dose (0.05-0.3 mcg/kg/min): - Potent inotropy, chronotropy, vasodilatation	↑ Systolic BP, ↓or ⇔ diastolic BP, ↑ /⇔ MAP, ↑ Cardiac output (CO), ↑ Myocardial O_2 demands.
High dose (0.5-1.0 mcg/kg/min): - Predominantly pressor (no increase in inotropy)	↑ ↑HR, ↑ ↑SBP, ↑ DBP, ↑ ↑MAP, ⇓CO, ↑ ↑PVR ↑ ↑Myocardial O_2 demands

SBP: Systolic BP, DBP: Diastolic BP, MAP: Mean arterial pressure, CO: Cardiac output, PVR: Pulmonary vascular resistance

How to start and titrate adrenaline infusion

- Start infusion at 0.1-0.3 mcg/kg/min (depending on BP) and titrate to target minimal MAP that re-establishes perfusion. Great inter-patient variability exists.
- If the BP improves but perfusion worsens (cold peripheries, thready pulses, increasing metabolic acidosis), add inodilators such as dobutamine or milrinone to improve perfusion and flow.
- Doses > 0.6 mcg/kg/min are rarely useful as ensuing organ ischemia may lead to MODS.
- If hypotension persists despite infusion rates of > 0.5 to 0.6 mcg/kg/min, consider adding a predominant pressor with less chronotropic effect such as noradrenaline, rather than increasing adrenaline doses further.
- Max dose is toxicity limited; doses up to 1 mcg/kg/min have been used; however, rarely clinically useful.

Side effects

- CVS: High dose increases afterload, myocardial O_2 consumption, undesirable tachycardia (less time for diastolic filling) and subendocardial ischemia. Risk of atrial and ventricular tachyarrhythmias, hypertension.
- Metabolic: Hyperglycemia, hypokalemia, hypophosphatemia, metabolic acidosis due to elevated lactate.
- CNS: Excitability, tremor.
- Skin: Local extravasation can cause skin necrosis, ulceration and gangrene. Hence best infused via a central line.
- When patients on beta blocker (e.g., prophylaxis for esophageal varices, tetralogy of Fallot, hypertension etc) receive adrenaline, the β-effect is blunted and α-effect predominates with severe hypertension and pressor effect without much inotropy.

Noradrenaline (NA)

NA is a predominant pressor (α effect), with mild/moderate inotropy (β_1), but no chronotropy.

Hemodynamic effects: Increases blood pressure by vasoconstriction. It is an attractive agent because it effectively raises the BP with minimal tachycardia and also has mild inotropy.

Indications

- NA is a useful agent in vasodilatory shock as it increases SVR, MAP and perfusion pressures without excessive tachycardia.
- Warm septic shock with low SVR and low MAPs despite fluid resuscitation is a typical and common PICU scenario where NA is useful.
- Raised ICP. This agent is used to target optimum CPP by maintaining high normal MAP for age.

Dose

0.05-1 mcg/kg/min.

Side effects

- NA mediated increased afterload may worsen a failing heart, therefore NA is not an appropriate agent in cardiogenic shock.
- NA can elevate MAP to the desired range but causes worse perfusion (cold extremities with feeble pulses, delayed CFT, decreased urine output) culminating in multi-organ failure. Evaluate cardiac function, consider fluids ± inotropes if pulses disappear after commencing NA.
- Extravasation can cause tissue necrosis. Infuse via dedicated central line.

Vasopressin

Hemodynamic effects: Potent pressor due to its actions at the $V_1\alpha$ receptor

Indications

- Catecholamine-resistant, vasodilatory septic shock. Vasopressin should only be used if adequate fluids and noradrenaline (NA) at maximal doses (0.5-1 mcg/kg/min) have failed in improving MAPs in vasodilatory septic shock.

Vasopressin should not be used as a 1st line agent or as a substitute for NA. In this setting, vasopressin is used at a replacement dose for possible relative vasopressin insufficiency in septic shock. Hence the suggested dose range should not be exceeded even if the patient remains hypotensive because of the risk of organ ischemia.

- Vasoplegic shock following cardiopulmonary bypass.
- Care of the potential organ donor after brain death: These patients can have catastrophic loss of vascular tone requiring careful titration of pressors in order to optimally preserve organ function.
- Central diabetes insipidus (DI): DI is common after resection of craniopharyngiomas and also in patients after brain death.
- Note: $V_1\alpha$ receptors are absent in cerebral and pulmonary circulation. Hence vasopressin does not cause cerebral or pulmonary vasoconstriction. It is a useful agent in patients with pulmonary hypertension and hypotension.

Side effects

- Potent vasoconstriction can cause widespread organ, tissue and digit ischemia. Distal limb ischemia is a greater risk at higher doses or in volume depleted individuals.
- Extravasation causes skin necrosis

Dose range

- 0.0005-0.001 Units/kg/min.
- How to prepare vasopressin infusion: Add 1.5 units/kg in 50 ml 5% dextrose or NS, infuse at 1-2 ml/hr (1 ml/hr = 0.0005 u/kg/min).

Phenylephrine

- *Effects*: Potent pressor that acts directly on alpha-1 receptors to produce hypertension and a reflex decrease in heart rate.
- *Indications*: Emergency stat dose for sudden hypotension due to vasodilation, e.g., following sedative drugs, rapid sequence intubation or epidural infusion overdose while fluid resuscitation is on flow.
- *Side effect*: Severe vasoconstriction can cause tissue hypoperfusion.
- *Dose*: 2-10 mcg/kg IV, 0.1-0.2 mg/kg IM.

The phosphodiesterase inhibitors/the bipyridines: Milrinone, amrinone

- These agents increase cytosolic cAMP levels by inhibiting its breakdown.
- Amrinone is used less frequently than milrinone because of its longer ½ life and toxicity (thrombocytopenia).
- Note: Sildenafil is a phosphodiesterase-5 inhibitor that may be administered orally.

Milrinone

- Milrinone has inotropy, lusitropy and vasodilatory effects (independent of beta-adrenergic receptor stimulation) without chronotropy, resulting in improved contractility, decreased preload and afterload.
- It is useful in a patient with cardiogenic shock as cardiac output (CO) will improve and associated congestive symptoms (pulmonary edema, hepatomegaly) will decrease.
- Despite the reduction in SVR, the BP may improve because of ↑ contractility, stroke volume and CO.
- It has synergistic effects with catecholamines and will result in an even greater improvement in CO in patients who have responded to dobutamine.
- Milrinone can also produce an improvement in CO in patients with inadequate/no response to dobutamine (catecholamine refractory).
- Its lusitropic effect is responsible for improved diastolic relaxation and ↑ CO in patients with stiff ventricles (diastolic dysfunction).
- Precipitous hypotension and tachycardia may occur in volume depleted patients.

Indications

- Catecholamine refractory cold shock with normal blood pressure
- Cardiogenic shock with normal blood pressure (reverses low CO with high SVR)
- Pulmonary hypertension (↓PVR, improves RV function)
- Diastolic dysfunction (lusitropy)
- Low CO following cardiopulmonary bypass in patients with inadequate response to dobutamine, provided residual lesions have been ruled out.

Side effects

- Potent arterial and venodilatory effects can result in hypotension particularly if a loading dose has been given in hypovolemic patients. May be prevented by cautious volume infusion prior to initiation and/or avoiding a loading dose, particularly if the BP is borderline low.
- Hypotension may be addressed by discontinuation of the drug, volume resuscitation and a brief, low dose infusion of a pressor such as NA (0.05 mcg/kg/min x 1-2 hours).
- As milrinone has a relatively longer half-life (1.5 hours) it may be best avoided in the acute stage when an unstable patient presents with precarious hemodynamics. At this juncture, catecholamines ± nitro-vasodilators that have half-life of 1-2 minutes are preferred as, if hypotension worsens, the effect may be rapidly reversed by cessation of the agent. After the patient is somewhat more stable, milrinone infusion may be commenced, usually after 12-24 hrs.
- Thrombocytopenia is more common with amrinone but can also occur with prolonged use (> 5 days at high infusion rates).
- Toxicity (hypotension, thrombocytopenia) can occur more frequently in renal failure due to drug accumulation.

Dose

- 50 mcg/kg loading dose over 60 minutes.
- Maintenance infusion rates: 0.25-0.75 mcg/kg/min, usual infusion rate is 0.5 mcg/kg/min.
- If a loading dose is not given, an infusion may be expected to start acting 2-3 hours after commencing the infusion.
- In renal failure (creatinine clearance < 20 ml/min/1.73 m^2), infusion rates must not exceed 0.25 mcg/kg/min.

The vasodilators: Nitroglycerin (NTG)

- NTG has dose dependent effects: it is predominantly a venodilator that also produces systemic and pulmonary arterial dilation at higher doses.

Hemodynamic effects

- Low dose (< 3 mcg/kg/min): NTG ↑ venous capacitance and reduces elevated left and right sided filling pressures. Thus, congestive features such as pulmonary edema may decrease without significant changes in CO or BP.
- Moderate to high dose (3-10 mcg/kg/min): NTG reduces SVR and PVR. CO may increase. Hypotension can occur if volume depleted.

Clinical role and indications

- Acute pulmonary edema, pulmonary hypertension.
  - Nitrates can relieve pulmonary congestion without compromising stroke volume or increasing myocardial oxygen demand
- Cardiogenic shock with precarious hemodynamics.
  - Low dose NTG may more safely reduce afterload in an unstable patient where more potent vasodilators may be risky.

Side effects

- As with all vasodilators, hypotension can occur at higher doses, especially if patient is volume depleted.
- Rapid development of tolerance, limiting their effectiveness to 24-48 hr.

Dose range

- 0.05-10 mcg/kg/min

The vasodilators: Sodium nitroprusside (SNP)

SNP produces potent arterial dilatation and ↑ vascular capacitance by acting directly on vascular smooth muscles.

Hemodynamic effects

- Dose dependent arterial vasodilatation by ↓ SVR, ↓PVR resulting in decreased preload and afterload.
- Rapid half-life of 2 minutes permits effective titration of dose to desired response.

Indications

- Severe hypertension, hypertensive emergency.
- To reduce afterload in hypertensive heart failure or mitral regurgitation.
- Cardiogenic shock/acute LV failure:
  - At appropriate doses, nitrates produce balanced vasodilation of the venous and arterial sides of the circulation, thereby reducing LV preload and afterload, and improving CO with consequent improved tissue perfusion.
  - Continuous monitoring of CVP and intra-arterial pressures is mandatory to prevent catastrophic consequences.

Side effects

- Hypotension. If the infusion is ceased as soon as hypotension develops, the BP usually recovers rapidly. Some patients may require volume resuscitation.
- Cyanide toxicity can occur at higher doses (rare if doses < 3 mcg/kg/min are infused for < 3 days). Toxicity can occur even at low doses in the presence of renal failure.

> - ☞ **REMEMBER** SNP should be titrated carefully and usually requires invasive arterial monitoring and close supervision.
> - Photosensitive, hence cover the entire infusion system with silver foil.
> - SNP should be tapered gradually to avoid rebound effects.

Dose

- Infusion range: 0.3-10 mcg/kg/min.
- Cardiogenic shock with normal BP and normovolemia. Initiate infusion cautiously at 0.05 mcg/kg/min and titrate carefully to 1-2 mcg/kg/min.
- In patients with hypertensive crisis, SNP can be initiated at 1 mcg/kg/min and increased up to 3-5 mcg/kg/min.

CARE AND MONITORING OF A PATIENT RECEIVING AN INOTROPE/VASOACTIVE INFUSION

- Each drug and dose must be tailored to the desired hemodynamic endpoints because great inter-patient variability means that the clinical response may be highly variable.
- Monitoring in the ICU
  - All patients who need cardiovascular support should be placed on a continuous cardio-respiratory monitor in the ICU.
  - Continuous invasive arterial and central venous (CVP) monitoring is highly desirable in these patients. This permits early, more accurate titration of fluid and vasoactive agents, with minimal side effects and optimizes the chances for a good outcome.
- *Side effects may be greater if:*
  - The patient is hypovolemic. Pressors have a greater risk of organ hypoperfusion and multiorgan failure; hypotension is more likely if the agent has vasodilatory effects.
  - A patient with normal cardiac function is more likely to exhibit side effects such as tachycardia and increased O_2 consumption.
- *Infusion pumps and priming:*
  - Syringe infusion pumps are preferred over volumetric infusion pumps, as the latter have

Table 32.4 Summary of hemodynamic effects of vasoactive agents

	Inotropy	Chronotropy	Lusitropy	Vasodilator	Pressor
Dopamine	++	++	-	-	++ (>7.5-10 μg/kg/min)
Dobutamine	++	++	-	+	-
Adrenaline	+++	+++	-	+ (0.05-0.3 μg/kg/min)	++ (> 0.3-0.5 μg/kg/min)
Noradrenaline	+	-	-	-	+++
Milrinone	++	-	+++	++	-
NTG	-	-	-	+ (high dose)	-
SNP	-	-	-	+++	-

Table 32.5 Choice of vasoactive agent depends on underlying pathophysiology

	Normal BP		Low BP	
	First line	Second line	First line	Second line
Cardiogenic shock (myocardial dysfunction +↑ SVR)	Dobutamine	Milrinone	Adrenaline	Low dose milrinone + Noradr, Calcium
Anaphylactic shock (⇓ SVR)		Adrenaline	Adrenaline	Adrenaline + Noradr
Warm septic shock (⇓ SVR ± myocardial dysfunction)	Noradrenaline (*preferred*) OR dopamine with aggressive fluid resuscitation. Add dobutamine if shock not reversed		NA	Vasopressin
Cold septic shock (myocardial dysfunction, SVR ↓ or↑)	Dobutamine	Milrinone	Adrenaline	Add NA if MAP remains low Add dobut if more inotropy required.

Dop = Dopamine, Dobut = Dobutamine, Adr = Adrenaline, NA = Noradrenaline.

Table 32.6 Drug dose range and formulation of infusions

Drug	Diluent	Peripheral line	Peripheral line dilution	Central line	Central line dilution
Dopamine	NS/D5	6 mg/kg in 100 ml	1 ml/hr= 1 μg/kg/min* Short term use only	15 mg/kg in 50 ml	1 ml/hr = 5 μg/kg/min, Range: 5-15 μg/kg/min
Dobutamine	NS	6 mg/kg in 100 ml	1 ml/hr=1 μg/kg/min	15 mg/kg in 50 ml	1 ml/hr =5 μg/kg/min Range: 5-15 μg/kg/min
Adrenaline	NS/D5	0.6 mg/kg in 100 ml	1 ml/hr=1 μg/kg/min* Short term use only	0.3 mg/kg in 50 ml	1 ml/hr =0.1 μg/kg/min Range: 0.1-1.0 μg/kg/min
Nordrenaline	D5	0.6 mg/kg in 100 ml	1 ml/hr=1 μg/kg/min* Short term use only	0.3 mg/kg in 50 ml	1 ml/hr = 0.1 μg /kg/min Range: 0.1-1.0 μg/kg/min
Milrinone	NS/D5	0.75 mg/kg in 50 ml	1 ml=0.25 μg/kg/min	0.75 mg/kg in 50 ml	1 ml/hr =0.25 μg /kg/min Range: 0.25-0.75 μg/kg/min
NTG	D5	6 mg/kg in 100 ml	1 ml=1 μg/kg/min	3 mg/kg in 50 ml	1 ml/hr =1 μg /kg/min Range: 0.5-10 μg/kg/min
SNP	D5	6 mg/kg in 100 ml	1 ml=1 μg/kg/min	3 mg/kg in 50 ml	1 ml/hr =1 μg/kg/min Range: 0.5-6 μg/kg/min

* Central line preferred because of high skin necrosis risk with peripheral line extravasations

less accurate delivery rates at low volumes. Even with a syringe pump, infusion rates of < 1 ml/hr may be somewhat erratic.

- When a new inotrope is being initiated, a brief "rapid purge" of 0.2-0.3 ml may be given in order to enable the drug to quickly reach the circulation: Cease the "purge" at the onset of tachycardia.
- Since even brief discontinuation of vasocative therapy in a patient with severe underlying hemodynamic impairment can lead to catastrophic low output states, ensure that a freshly prepared infusion of the same inotrope is ready even before the previous infusion has been completed.

■ *Central vs peripheral lines*

- Vasoactive agents must be infused through a dedicated port/catheter in order to prevent fluctuations or interruptions in infusion rates when other medications are infused through the same line. Several inotropes may be "piggy-backed" into the same lumen and infused undisturbed. Other drugs (antibiotics, sedatives, fluid boluses) should be administered via a separate lumen or IV line in order to prevent sudden surges in HR and BP. Likewise, blood sampling must not be carried out via the inotrope line.
- In an emergency, if a central line is not immediately available for inotrope use, infuse through a wide bore cannula that is placed as

proximally as possible. Use lower dilution solutions for peripheral route so that it reaches the systemic circulation faster and minimizes tissue injury in the event of extravasation.
- Dopamine, noradrenaline, adrenaline and vasopressin should preferably be given only via a central line as skin necrosis and gangrene can occur when extravasations occur in a peripheral line. Tissue injury may be worse if the patient is hypoperfused, acidotic or on multiple high dose pressors.
- An external jugular line is a good interim access in an emergency until central lines are secured.

- *Combining agents*
  - It is often necessary to combine two or more agents in order to achieve the desired end points.
  - Warm vasodilated shock: Large volume fluids + pressor are the mainstay of therapy. However, dobutamine may be added if extremity perfusion worsens or metabolic acidosis or low central venous saturations are present.
  - Cardiogenic shock: Inodilators such as milrinone will dramatically improve cardiac output but can produce hypotension despite volume resuscitation. The addition of low dose noradrenaline (0.05 mcg/kg/min) will maintain MAP and diastolic BP (important for coronary perfusion) without unduly increasing afterload.

PREPARING THE INFUSION

- The following are highly irritant and have a high risk of skin necrosis if extravasation occurs:
  - Dopamine adrenaline, noradrenaline and vasopressin
- The following do not have skin necrosis risk and may be given via a dedicated peripheral line:
  - Dobutamine, milrinone, nitroglycerin and SNP.
  - However, central line infusions ensure more reliable delivery into the circulation.

REFERENCES

1. Kelly M, Sturgill M, Notterman D. Pharmacology of the cardiovascular system. In: Pediatric Critical Care. Fuhrman and Zimmerman (Eds). 3rd ed. Philadelphia, PA, 2006, Mosby Elsevier, 300-331.

33

Arrhythmias in Critically Ill Children

- Abnormal rhythms are not uncommon in children and may be detected in both critically ill children and otherwise healthy children.
- The management is individualized depending on the following:
  a) Presence of symptoms
  b) History of heart disease, drug history
  c) In symptomatic patients, the diagnostic and management approach may be simplified by clarifying the following questions-
    - Hemodynamically stable or unstable?
    - Regular or irregular?
    - Rhythm fast or slow?
    - If fast, is the tachycardia narrow complex or broad complex?
- This chapter will cover important rhythms that care givers of critically ill children are required to be familiar with. A complete overview of all pediatric arrhythmias may be provided in the excellent references.

RHYTHMS ORIGINATING IN THE SINUS NODE

All rhythms that originate in the sinoatrial (SA) node (sinus rhythm) have two important characteristics. Both are required for a rhythm to be called sinus rhythm.

- P waves precede each QRS complex with a regular PR interval that may be normal, prolonged or short.
- The P axis falls between 0 and +90 degrees, an often neglected criterion. This produces upright P waves in lead II and inverted P waves in aVR.

1. Sinus arrhythmia

- This is the most common irregularity of heart rhythm seen in children.
- This is a normal variant where there is a phasic variation in the heart rate, increasing during inspiration and decreasing during expiration.
- The characteristics of sinus rhythm are maintained.

Table 33.1 In all abnormal rhythms, think of and correct contributing factors (5 Hs and 4 Ts)

5Hs	4Ts
▪ Hypoxia	▪ Tension pneumothorax
▪ Hypovolemia	▪ Tamponade
▪ Hydrogen ion (Acidosis)	▪ Toxic or toxicity overdose
▪ Hyper- or hypokalemia and metabolic causes	▪ Thromboembolism (pulmonary or cardiac)
▪ Hypothermia	

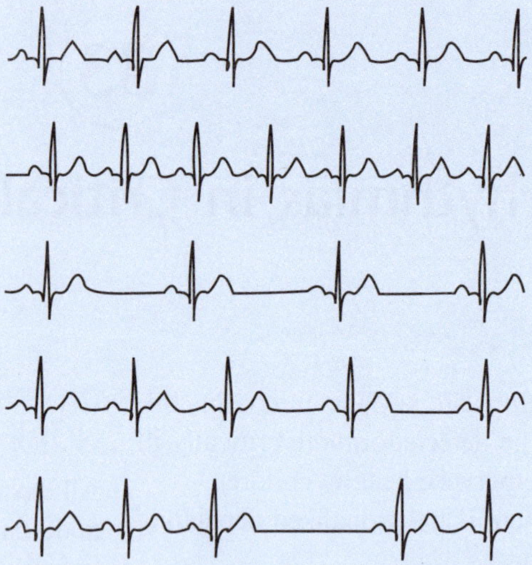

Fig. 33.1 Normal and abnormal rhythms originating in the sinoatrial node. (From Park MK, Guntheroth WG: How to Read Pediatric ECGs, 4th ed. Philadelphia, Mosby, 2006).

- The rhythm reflects a healthy interaction between autonomic respiratory and cardiac control activity in CNS.
- *Significance.* Sinus arrhythmia has no significance because it is a normal finding in children and a sign of good cardiac reserve.
- *Management.* No treatment is indicated.

2. Atrial flutter

Description

- The pacemaker lies in an ectopic focus, and a "circus movement" in the atrium is the mechanism of this arrhythmia.
- Atrial flutter is characterized by an atrial rate (F wave with "sawtooth" configuration) of about 300 (range 240 to 360) beats/minute, a ventricular response with varying degrees of block (e.g., 2:1, 3:1, 4:1), and normal QRS complexes (Fig. 33.2).

Causes

- Atrial flutter usually *suggests a significant cardiac pathology,* although neonates with atrial flutter may have no structural heart disease.
- Structural heart disease with dilated atria, acute infectious illness, myocarditis or pericarditis, previous surgery involving atria (the Senning procedure, Fontan operation or atrial septal defect repair), digitalis toxicity, and thyrotoxicosis are possible causes.

Significance

- The ventricular rate determines eventual cardiac output; very rapid ventricular rates may decrease cardiac output.
- Thrombus formation can cause embolic events.
- Uncontrolled atrial flutter lead to CCF, syncope or chest pain.

3. Atrial Fibrillation (A-Fib)

Description

- Atrial fibrillation is less common than atrial flutter in children.
- The mechanism of this arrhythmia is circus movement, as in atrial flutter. Atrial fibrillation is characterized by an extremely fast atrial rate (f wave at a rate of 350 to 600

Table 33.2 Management of atrial flutter and atrial fibrillation

	Atrial flutter	Atrial fibrillation
Acute conversion	Short duration or presence of CCF: - Synchronized DC conversion *(best)* - IV amiodarone or procainamide - *Adenosine not useful* in conversion to sinus rhythm, useful to confirm diagnosis	Short duration or presence of significant symptoms: - Synchronized DC conversion - *Adenosine not useful* in conversion to sinus rhythm, useful to confirm diagnosis
Chronic suppression	- If rhythm present > 48 hr, beware risk of atrial thrombus that can embolize - Perform ECHO (TEE most sensitive) - Anticoagulate with warfarin - Cardioversion after 2-3 weeks - Continue warfarin 4 weeks more	- If rhythm present > 48 hr, echo for atrial thrombus - Depending on urgency of cardioversion, use heparin (more rapid) or warfarin (2-3 weeks) prior to cardioversion - Continue warfarin 4 weeks more
Ventricular rate control	β-blockers or calcium channel blockers	β-blockers, verapamil or digoxin
Prevention of recurrences	β-blockers, verapamil or digoxin	Amiodarone or procainamide
Refractory cases	Antitachycardia pacing or radiofrequency ablation	Rate control preferred to cardioversion for chronic cases

beats/minute) and an irregularly irregular ventricular response with normal QRS complexes (FIg. 33.2).

Causes

- Atrial fibrillation may be present in CHD associated with dilated atria, such as seen with rheumatic disease, Ebstein's anomaly, tricuspid atresia, AV valve regurgitation.
- Suspect thyrotoxicosis, pulmonary emboli and pericarditis in a previously normal child with acute A-fib.

Significance of A-fib

- Loss of coordinated contraction of the atria and ventricles and rapid atrial rates leads to decreased cardiac output, as occurs in atrial tachycardia.
- Atrial fibrillation usually suggests a significant cardiac pathology.

Management of A-fib

- Management for atrial fibrillation is similar to that described under atrial flutter (see Table 33.2).
- *In chronic cases, ventricular rate control rather than conversion is increasingly used.*

4. Conduction abnormalities (FIg. 33.3)

a) First degree heart block occurs when all atrial impulses are conducted to the ventricles but with a prolonged PR interval. Rhythm is regular.

b) Second degree heart block occurs when not all impulses are transmitted to the ventricles.

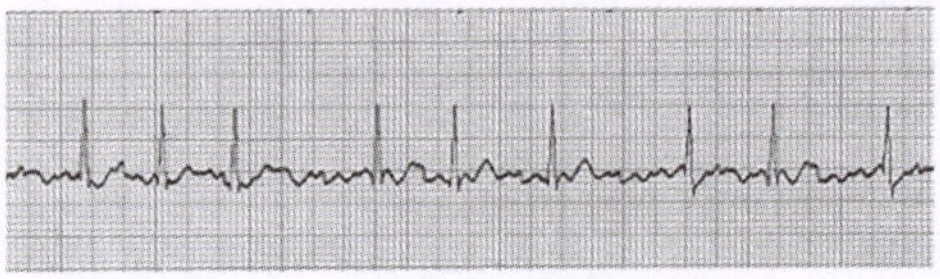

A. Atrial flutter

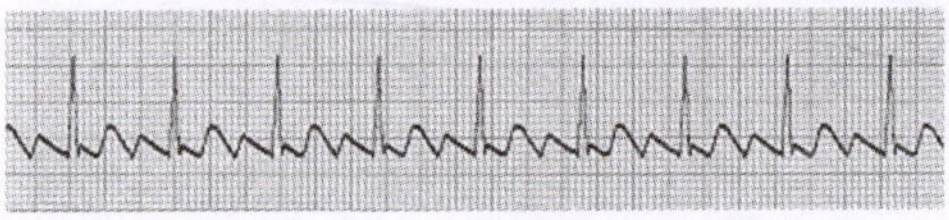

B. Atrial Fibrillation

Fig. 33.2 Atrial flutter and Atrial Fibrillation

These are divided into:

- Mobitz Type I block (Wenckebach phenomenon). The PR interval gradually increases until an impulse is not conducted and a ventricular complex does not occur.This is due to a conduction delay within the AV node.
- Mobitz Type II block. This is characterized by the sudden drop of an atrial impulse without the increasing length of the PR interval. QRS morphology may vary. Usually due to a conduction defect in the His conduction system. May progress to complete heart block.

c) *Third degree AV block/ Complete heart block*

- Most common cause of abnormal bradycardia in infants and children. Complete dissociation between P waves and QRS complexes (Fig. 33.3).
- Can be congenital – in this case it is *strongly associated* with maternal SLE.
- Mother of an affected infant should be worked up.
- Most common structural heart defect associated is corrected transposition of great vessels

Management of complete heart block

- May be asymptomatic – follow clinically
- Slower the heart rate and wider the QRS escape rhythms, the higher the risk.
- Acute treatment: isoproterenol infusion, atropine.
- Indications for implantable pacemaker: Symptomatic bradycardia. Presence of syncope, exercise intolerance, ventricular arrhythmias, structural disease

VENTRICULAR ARRHYTHMIAS

Ventricular arrhythmias are uncommon in children but may have life-threatening consequences. The following will be briefly discussed.

- Premature ventricular complexes (PVC)
- Ventricular tachycardia
- Ventricular fibrillation

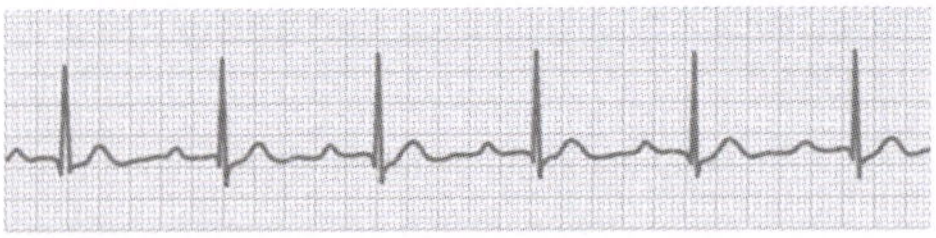

a. First degree heart block

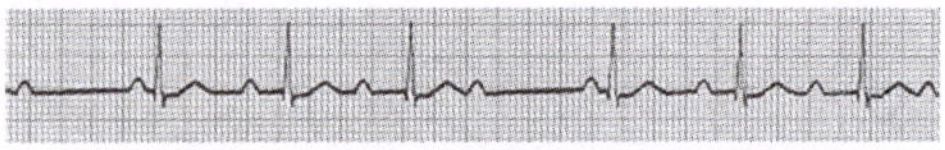

b. Second degree Mobitz Type I block (Wenckebach phenomenon).

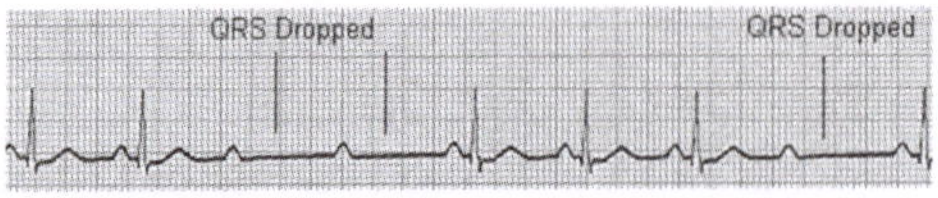

c. Second degree Mobitz Type II block

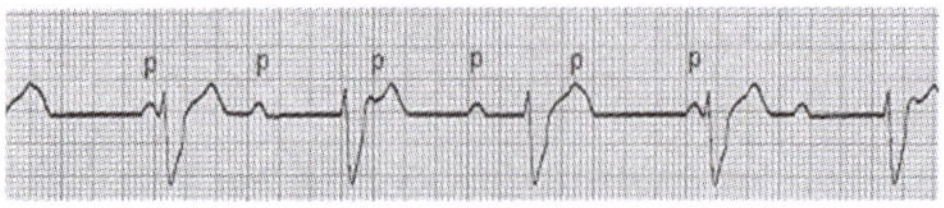

d. Third degree AV block

Fig. 33.3 Conduction abnormalities

Ventricular arrhythmias are characterized by the following (Fig. 33.4)

- Bizarre and wide QRS complexes.
- T waves pointing in directions opposite to QRS complexes.
- QRS complexes randomly related to P waves, if visible.

1. Premature Ventricular Contractions (PVC)

- Not very commonly seen in children, incidence of 0.3 to 2.2%
- Early, wide QRS complexes
- T waves in opposite direction of QRS
- A full compensatory pause usually appears; that is, the length of two cycles, including the premature beat, is the same as that of two normal cycles (Fig. 33.4).
- The following forms of PVCs may be seen:
  - *Bigeminy* (sinus beat followed by PVC, repeating as a pattern) *vs couplets* (two abnormal QRS complexes appear in sequence).
  - Ventricular *trigeminy* (each abnormal QRS complex regularly follows two normal QRS complexes) *vs triplets* (three abnormal QRS complexes appear in sequence).
  - Three or more successive PVCs are arbitrarily termed *ventricular tachycardia.*
  - *Unifocal (monomorphic or uniform) PVCs (Fig. 33.4)*: Abnormal QRS complexes have the same configuration in a single lead and are assumed to originate from a single focus. Most common type of PVC encountered.
- *Multifocal (polymorphic or multi-form) PVCs:* Abnormal QRS complexes have different configurations in a single lead and are assumed to originate from different foci.

Causes of PVCs

- PVC may appear in otherwise healthy children. Up to 50% to 70% of normal children may show PVCs on 24-hour ambulatory ECGs.
- PVCs may be a marker of the following significant disorders:
  - Myocarditis, myocardial injury or infarction, cardiomyopathy and cardiac tumors.
  - Congenital or acquired heart disease, may be seen in preoperative or postoperative periods.
  - Long QT syndrome, mitral valve prolapse (MVP).
  - Drug induced: Digitalis, catecholamines, theophylline, caffeine, amphetamines, and some anesthetic agents.

Significance

- Occasional PVCs are benign in children, particularly if they are uniform and disappear or become less frequent with exercise.
- PVCs are more significant if the following are true:
  - They are associated with underlying heart disease (pre- or postoperative status, MVP, cardiomyopathy).
  - There is a history of syncope or a family history of sudden death.
  - They are precipitated by, or become more frequent with, activity.

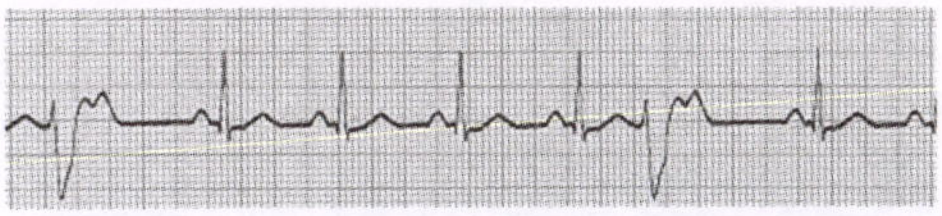

a. Monomorphic PVC

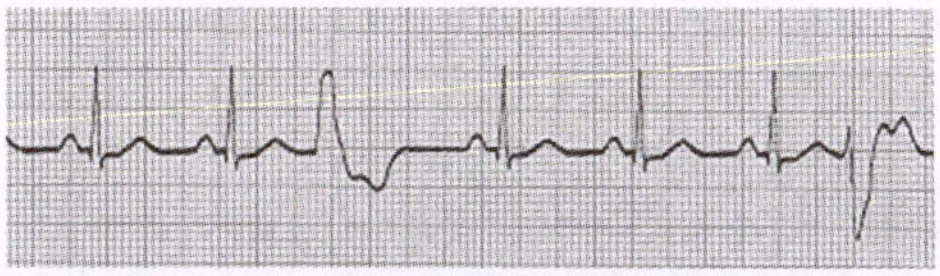

b. Polymorphic PVC

Fig. 33.4 Premature ventricular contractions

- They are multiform, particularly couplets.
- There are runs of PVCs with symptoms or PVCs are incessant or frequent.

Management approach

- ECG: Assess corrected QT interval (QTc) prolongation, ST-T changes, and other abnormalities.
- Echo: To detect structural heart disease or functional abnormalities.
- 24-hour ambulatory ECG (Holter monitoring): To detect the frequency and severity of the arrhythmia.
- Exercise stress testing: Benign PVCs disappear with exercise, significant PVCs are induced or exacerbated with exercise.
- Cardiac catheterization if arrhythmogenic RV dysplasia is suspected.

Therapy

- Unifocal PVC, including ventricular bigeminy and trigeminy, which disappear with exercise and are associated with a structurally and functionally normal heart are considered benign, no therapy needed
- All children with symptomatic ventricular arrhythmias and those with complex PVCs (multiform PVCs, ventricular couplets, unsustained ventricular tachycardia) should be treated
  - Options: β-Blockers, phenytoin sodium and mexiletine
  - *Avoid QT interval prolonging agents* such as amiodarone, bretylium.

2. Ventricular tachycardia

- Ventricular tachycardia (VT) is a series of three or more PVCs with a heart rate of 120 to 200 beats/minute (Fig. 33.5).
- VT is a wide complex tachycardia with:
  - QRS complexes that are regular, wide complex and bizarre
  - Atrioventricular dissociation and
  - T waves pointing in the opposite direction.
- VT may be sustained (lasting more than 30 seconds) or unsustained (lasting less than 30 seconds).
- This is a life threatening arrhythmia that mandates emergent treatment and workup.
- Presenting symptoms may be dizziness, syncope, palpitation, or chest pain. Family history may be positive for ventricular arrhythmia or sudden death.
- Differentiating VT from SVT with aberrant conduction may be difficult. *However, in children, almost all wide QRS tachycardias are VT. They should be treated as such until proved otherwise.*
- *Torsade de pointes* (meaning "twisting of the points") is characterized by a paroxysm of VT with progressive changes in the amplitude and polarity of QRS complexes (Fig. 33.6).

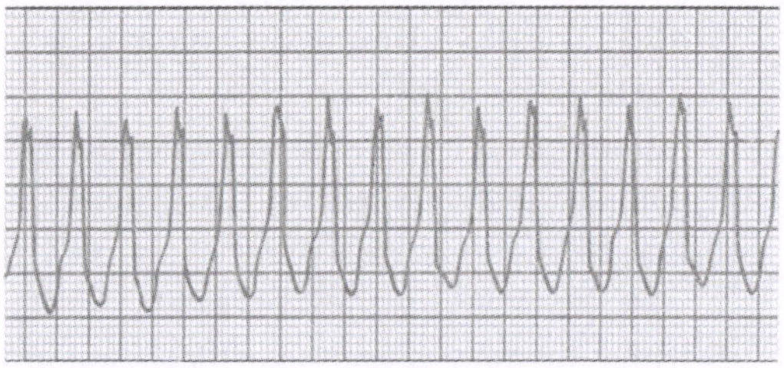

Fig. 33.5 Ventricular tachycardia

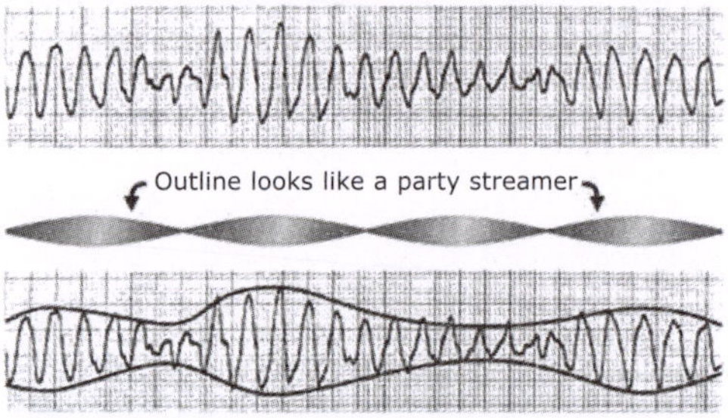

Fig. 33.6 Torsade de pointes, a specific form of VT seen with long QT syndromes

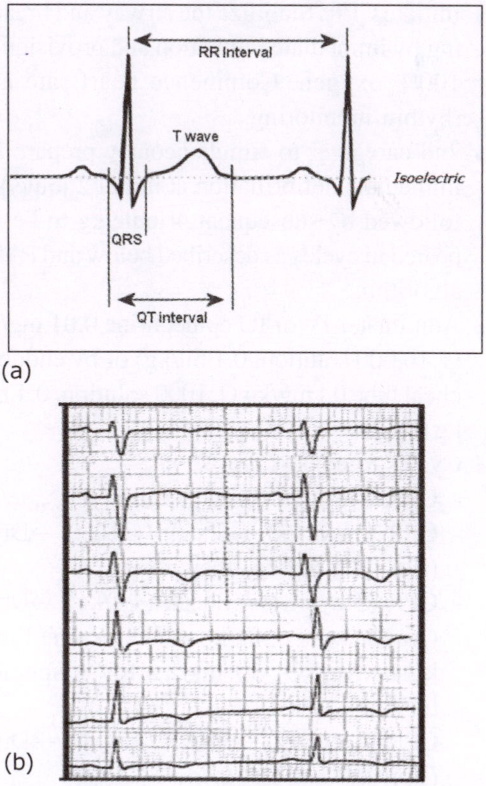

Fig. 33.7 (a) Calculating QT interval; (b) ECG demonstrating Long QT

- It is a distinct form of polymorphic VT, occurring in patients with marked QT prolongation.
- Long QT syndrome may be congenital or acquired (drug induced). Hypomagesemia may cause progression of long QT to VF.

Causes of VT

- Structural heart diseases, pre- and post-operative CHD (TOF, TGA, DORV).
- Myocarditis, pulmonary hypertension, arrhythmogenic RV dysplasia, myocardial tumors, myocardial ischemia, and infarction.
- Drug induced: Catecholamines, digitalis toxicity, organophosphate insecticides. Many antiarrhythmic drugs are proarrhythmic.
- Torsades de pointes may be seen in patients with congenital long QT syndrome.

Significance

- VT usually signifies a serious myocardial pathology and can be a cause of sudden cardiac death.
- With a fast heart rate, cardiac output may decrease abruptly, and the rhythm may deteriorate to ventricular fibrillation and a pulseless rhythm.

Therapy

- *If critically ill with hemodynamic compromise: Immediate electrical therapy indicated*
  - VT with pulse: Synchronized DC cardioversion 0.5 to 1 joule/kg, repeat as needed.
  - Pulseless VT: Defibrillation 2-4 joules /kg. Treat as VF (See PALS algorithm in Appendix)
  - Correct arrhythmogenic factors (e.g., 5 Hs, 4Ts, especially hypokalemia, hypoxemia, acidosis).
- *Drug treatment in conscious patients:*
  - Options are IV lidocaine, procainamide, amiodarone.
  - Lignocaine dose: IV bolus of 1 mg/kg per dose over 1 to 2 mins followed by continuous infusion 20 to 50 μg/kg per minute. If possible, the preservative free form should be used. Lidocaine or procainamide may also be used following cardioversion in order to suppress re-initiation of the tachycardia.
  - Drug-refractory and postoperative VT: IV amiodarone useful.
  - Torsade de pointes: IV injection of magnesium sulfate is effective and safe treatment.
- Prevention of recurrence: Beta blockers (particularly in long QT syndrome), phenytoin.
- Long term: Surgical or radiofrequency ablation or implantable defibrillator.

3. Ventricular fibrillation (VF, V-fib) (Fig. 33.8)

- Rare in children.
- V-fib is usually a degeneration of VT and is a terminal arrhythmia because it results in ineffective circulation. Immediate resuscitation must be provided.
- The ECG in V-fib is characterized by bizarre, disorganized QRS complexes of varying sizes and configurations. The rate is rapid and irregular.

Causes of V-fib

- All causes of VT can also cause VF.
- Long QT syndrome, Brugada syndrome.
- Electrolyte abnormalities.
- Severe hypoxemia.
- Decompensated shock with myocardial ischemia, acidosis.
- Pre- and post-operative CHD repair.
- Myocarditis, cardiomyopathies.
- Severe blunt chest wall trauma can cause abrupt VF (commotio-cordis).

Treatment of VF

(See PALS algorithm in Appendix)

- Resuscitation from VF is successful only if done immediately as an emergency. The longer the myocardium is allowed to fibrillate, the more difficult is conversion to a sinus rhythm.
- Initiate CPR: Stabilize the airway and breathing by immediate intubation and provision of 100% oxygen. Commence heart rate and rhythm monitoring.
- 2nd caregiver to simultaneously prepare for immediate defibrillation at initial 2 joule/kg, followed by subsequent 4 joule/kg to be repeated in cycles as described below and PALS algorithm.
- Administer IV or IO epinephrine 0.01 mg/kg (1:10,000 solution, 0.1 ml/kg) or by endotracheal tube 0.1 mg/kg (1:1000 solution, 0.1 ml/kg).
- Cycles to consist of:
  - CPR →Shock (2 J/kg) then →
  - CPR (5 cycles) →Shock (4 J/kg) →Drug (Epi 0.01 mg/kg) then →
  - CPR (5 cycles) →Shock (4 J/kg) →Drug (Amiodarone 5 mg/kg or Lignocaine 1 mg/kg or $MgSO_4$ 50 mg/kg for suspected torsade)
  - CPR (5 cycles) →Shock (4 J/kg) →Drug (Epi 0.01 mg/kg) then →
  - *Cycles to continue till perfusing rhythm established*
- Search for and treat precipitating cause (5Hs, 4Ts).
- Electrophysiologic studies and implantable defibrillators are often indicated in patients who survive ventricular fibrillation.

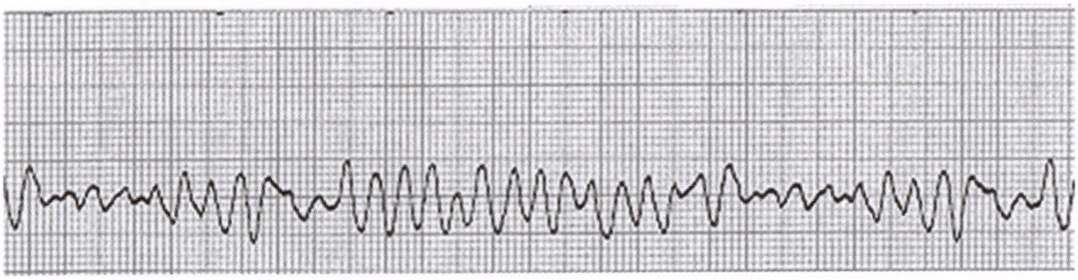

Fig. 33.8 Ventricular fibrillation

REFERENCES

1. Park MK, Guntheroth WG: How to Read Pediatric ECGs, 4th ed. Philadelphia, Mosby, 2006
2. Pediatric Advanced life support (PALS manual). Downloaded from circ.ahajournals.org at VA MED CTR BOISE on November 30, 2008.
3. Pediatric Arrhythmias. From http://www.emedu.org/ecg/givemall.php

34

Supraventricular Tachycardia (SVT)

- Most common abnormal tachycardia seen in pediatric practice.
- Most common arrhythmia requiring treatment in paediatric population.
- Formerly called *paroxysmal atrial tachycardia (PAT)* as the onset and offset were characteristically abrupt.
- Most frequent age at presentation:
  - First 4 months of life (~50%)
  - 2nd peak at 8–10 yr and in adolescence.
  - SVT in children > 5 years: associated with high probability of recurrence
- Wolff-Parkinson-White (WPW) syndrome as cause of SVT may be inherited in an autosomal dominant fashion.

DESCRIPTION

- Rapid, regular, usually narrow QRS rhythm, originating above the ventricles (Fig. 34.1).
- Three groups of tachycardia are included in SVT:
  - AV re-entrant/ reciprocating tachycardia (most common mechanism of SVT)
  - Nodal (or AV junctional) tachycardia.
  - Atrial ectopic tachycardia.
- In SVT caused by reentry, two pathways are involved; at least one of these is the AV node, and the other is an accessory pathway which may be an anatomically separate bypass tract.
- Patients with accessory pathways frequently have Wolff-Parkinson-White (WPW) pre-excitation.

CAUSES

- No heart disease is found in about half of patients. This idiopathic type of SVT occurs more commonly in young infants than in older children.
- WPW pre-excitation is present in 10% to 20% of cases, which is evident only after conversion to sinus rhythm, not during the SVT episode.
- Some congenital heart defects (e.g., Ebstein's anomaly, single ventricle, corrected TGA) are more susceptible to this arrhythmia.
- SVT may occur following cardiac surgeries

PRESENTATION

- Paroxysmal, sudden onset and offset.
- Heart rates of SVT vary with age
  - Infants: Rate is > 220 bpm
  - Older children: Rate is > 180 bpm (180-250).
- P waves difficult to define, but 1:1 with QRS.
- Important to differentiate from sinus tachycardia.

Symptoms

- May be asymptomatic and rapid rates noted incidentally, especially in older children.
- Some older children may describe a sensation of a fast heart rate, palpitations, or chest tightness.
- Hemodynamic compromise/CCF in newborns and those with structural heart disease.

Table 34.1 Differentiating between SVT and sinus tachycardia (ST)

	SVT	Sinus tachycardia (ST)
Compatible history	Vague, non-specific or absent history	Consistent history (e.g., fever, fluid loss, pain)
P waves	Present, normal	Absent or abnormal
Beat to beat variability of heart rate (HR)	No HR variability. Abrupt onset and offset of tachycardia	Variable, gradual normalization of rate to normal when inciting cause of ST resolves
Heart rates	Infants: $\geq$220 bpm Older children: $\geq$ 180 bpm	Infants: $\leq$ 220 bpm Older children: $\leq$ 180 bpm

TREATMENT OF SVT: DEPENDS ON SYMPTOMS

Goals of treatment: Identify unstable patients, differentiate from sinus tachycardia (Table 34.1), and terminate the rhythm.

1. **Treatment of stable SVT**
   - Vagal maneuvers in stable patients (carotid massage, ice-pack to side of face, *NO EYEBALL MASSAGE).*
   - Adenosine if IV access readily available, drug of choice
     - Mechanism: Stops conduction through AV node, interrupts re-entrant circuit and restores sinus rhythm.
     - It is important to get an ECG printout during therapy. During period of AV block, the P wave morphology will help to identify the etiology (abnormal/absent P wave, flutter waves)
     - Adenosine dose: 0.1 mg/kg (max 6 mg), repeat 0.2 mg/kg (max 12 mg) in central line or in a peripheral line closest to central circulation.
     - Extremely short ½ life (≈ 9 seconds), metabolized by RBC.
     - Use 2 syringe technique with 3-way stopcock. One syringe to contain adenosine,

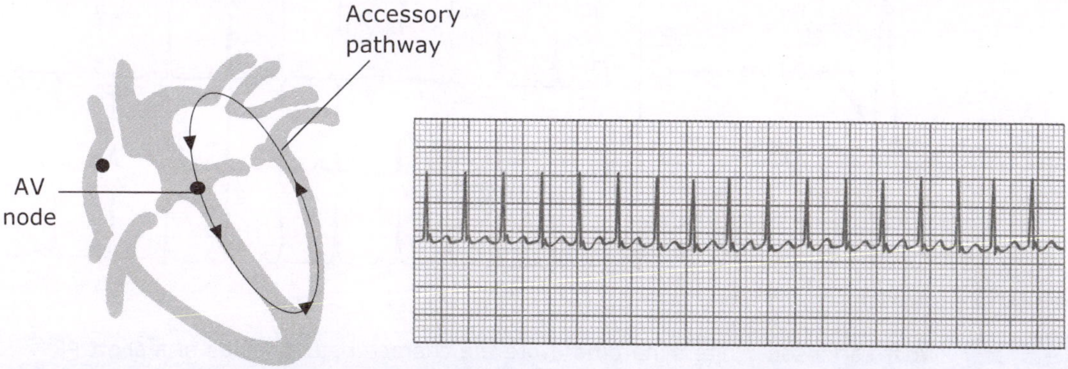

Fig. 34.1 SVT. Note a normal QRS complex tachycardia without visible P waves.

10 ml saline in 2nd syringe. Give adenosine rapidly with one syringe and immediately flush saline with the other in order to ensure that the drug reaches the heart without getting metabolized.
- Can cause chest pain, bronchospasm.
- Less effective if drug refrigerated and in patients on beta-agonists and theophylline.

■ Continuous ECG and BP monitoring required.

2. **Treatment of hemodynamically unstable SVT**
   ■ Evaluate airway and breathing for possible intubation and controlled ventilation.
   ■ Therapeutic options:
   a. IV adenosine as above.
   b. Synchronized cardioversion, 0.5-1.0 joules/kg. Also useful if IV access not available.
   - Consider sedation if possible.
   - If initial shock unsuccessful, repeat using a dose of 2 J/kg.
   - If a second shock is unsuccessful or the tachycardia recurs quickly, consider drug therapy (amiodarone)
   c. Amiodarone
   - Dose: 5 mg/kg IV/IO; repeat up to 15 mg/kg. Maximum: 300 mg.
   - Adjust administration rate to urgency; infusion rates vary over several minutes to an hour (give more slowly when perfusing rhythm present)
   - Continuous ECG and blood pressure monitoring necessary.
   d. If above unsuccessful, obtain expert consultation; options are procainamide, transesophageal atrial pacing.

3. **SVT: Management after conversion to sinus rhythm**
   ■ All patients need post-conversion ECG in order to identify those with WPW syndrome (25% patients with SVT) (Fig. 34.2)
   ■ Digoxin contraindicated in WPW syndrome because of risk of sudden death.
   ■ All patients with SVT will also need an echo to identify structural problems.
   ■ Prevention important if episodes are frequent:
   - Beta blockers and digoxin as first line.
   - Amiodarone, flecainide, sotalol are other options.
   ■ Radiofrequency catheter ablation
   - Very effective, undertaken with increasing frequency as expertise increases.
   - Cutoff points usually are > 5 years and 15 kg, unless severe SVT.

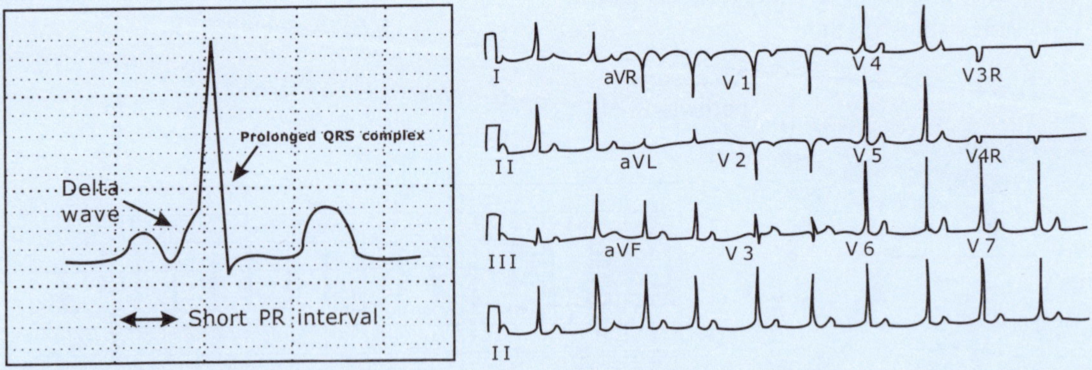

Fig. 34.2 Wolff-Parkinson-White syndrome. Note the characteristic findings of a short PR interval, slurred upstroke of QRS (delta wave), and prolongation of the QRS interval.

OTHER SUPRAVENTRICULAR TACHYCARDIAS

(See chapter on arrhythmias)

- Atrial flutter, atrial fibrillation, ectopic atrial tachycardia, junctional tachycardias.
- Not commonly seen in pediatric patients.
- Adenosine does not terminate these rhythms as they originate above AV node.
- Treatment options depending on cause: Cardioversion, amiodarone, procainamide, or ablation.

REFERENCES

1. Park MK, Guntheroth WG: How to Read Pediatric ECGs, 4th ed. Philadelphia, Mosby, 2006.
2. Pediatric Advanced life support (PALS manual). Downloaded from circ.ahajournals.org at VA MED CTR BOISE on November 30, 2008

35

Cyanotic Spells (Hypercyanotic Spells/Tet Spells)

INTRODUCTION

- Cyanotic spells generally occur in patients with congenital cyanotic heart disease and decreased pulmonary blood flow (e.g., tetralogy of Fallot, DORV with PS, tricuspid atresia etc).
- Cyanotic spells may also be a manifestation of shunt malfunction in patients in whom a systemic-pulmonary palliative procedure (e.g., Blalock-Taussig shunt) has been performed.
- The spells may occasionally be fatal.
- Most respond to medical measures, but *their presence should be considered as an indication for prompt surgical intervention.*

PATHOPHYSIOLOGY

- There is complex interplay of events in a child who presents with a cyanotic spell. The basic pathophysiology is due to:
  - Obstruction to the pulmonary blood flow in the presence of
  - An intra-cardiac communication.
- The three major mechanisms that interact are:
  - A vulnerable respiratory center
  - Infundibular contraction/spasm
  - Tachycardia.
- The ensuing hypoxia and lactic acidosis leads to intense pulmonary vasoconstriction.

CLINICAL FEATURES

- Peak age: 2 to 4 months.
- Initiated by feeding, crying, bowel movement or shortly after the infant wakes up.
- Paroxysm of hyperpnea (deep breathing).
- Irritability and incessant cry.
- Increase in cyanosis and decrease in murmur.
- May lead to seizures, limpness, cerebrovascular accident/stroke or death.

PRINCIPLES IN MANAGEMENT

- Re-establish pulmonary blood flow by measures that decrease pulmonary vascular resistance (PVR) and increase systemic vascular resistance (SVR).
- Improve oxygenation.
- Increase the systemic venous return.
- Correct dehydration.
- Correct acidosis.

MANAGEMENT

- Administer *oxygen* in highest possible concentration in a non-threatening manner.
- *Knee chest position* will increase SVR and improve pulmonary blood flow.
- *Hyperhydrate* with repeated boluses of 20 ml/kg of normal saline/Ringer's lactate. This corrects the shock and acidosis as well as decreases hyperviscosity which improves pulmonary blood flow.
- *Sodium bicarbonate* 1-2 mEq/kg diluted 1:1 with sterile water; infuse over 5-10 minutes; may

be repeated after 10 minutes in refractory spells. Corrects acidosis, causes pulmonary vasodilatation.

- *Morphine* 0.2 mg/kg subcutaneous (SC) or 0.05-0.1 mg/kg IV slowly over 10 minutes. Administer SC if IV route not available; do not attempt IV initially.

  Mechanism of action of morphine:
  - Pulmonary venodilator.
  - Breaks cycle of hypoxia and agitation.
  - Depresses the hyperexcitable respiratory center; hence ↓hyperpnea.
  - Possible negative inotropic effects on infundibulum with decreased spasm.
- *IV Esmolol* is the β-blocker of choice (short acting agent with a half-life of 9 minutes)
  - Mechanism: Negative inotropic effect relaxes infundibular myocardium
  - Dose: 0.5 mg/kg over 1 minute followed by 50 mcg/kg/min x 4 minutes.
  - If no response, continue esmolol as an infusion at doses of 50-200 mcg/kg/min.
  - If esmolol unavailable, administer IV propranolol at 0.01-0.05 mg/kg.
  - Propranolol may be repeated up to a maximum dose of 0.1 mg/kg
- *Packed red cell transfusion:* Maintain PCV > 45%, increases oxygen delivery to tissues
- *Increase SVR with pressors*: Increased SVR will divert blood flow from the systemic to the pulmonary circulation. Options include:
  - Phenylephrine: Dose 0.02 mg/kg IV *or*
  - Noradrenaline infusion at 0.01-0.05 mcg/kg/minute *or*
  - Ketamine infusion at 1-4 mg/kg/hr. Combine with glycopyrrolate 5-20 mcg/kg as an antisialogogue.
- *Correct hypoglycemia*
- *Intubation and controlled ventilation:* For severe and refractory spells in order to enable complete sedation and paralysis (decreased oxygen demands)
- Alert cardiac surgeons for emergency surgical intervention (Blalock-Taussig shunt).

SECTION 8 : CENTRAL NERVOUS SYSTEM

36

Management of Raised ICP Part 1: Pathophysiology and Evaluation

- Raised intracranial pressure (ICP) is a pathological state which occurs in many serious neurological conditions. If not appropriately treated, ICP can rapidly rise to the point where cerebral ischemia or brain herniation occurs, both of which can result in significant morbidity or death.

PATHOPHYSIOLOGY

The intracranial pressure (ICP) volume

- Within the rigid skull, 3 noncompressible compartments contribute to the ICP: The brain parenchyma, the major compartment that is normally responsible for 80% of ICP. The CSF and intracranial blood volume, each account for 10% of the ICP in the physiological state.
- Abnormal increase in any of the 3 compartments initially results in compensatory mechanisms that limit the rise in ICP. If these are insufficient to offset the increase in intracranial volume, then the ICP rises, Figs 36.1 & 36.2.
- In infants and young children (with open sutures and fontanelles), chronically increased intracranial volume may be compensated by the expansion of the intracranial vault. However, these do not provide protection for acute rapid increases in the intracranial volume.
- Acute ICP rises or substantial increase in intracranial volume can cause displacement of the brain resulting in herniation syndromes (uncal, central or medullary herniation, *see Table 36.1*), which, along with hypoxic-ischemic damage from reduced cerebral perfusion pressure (CPP), are the most important causes of death.
- Normal ICP varies with age. In the newborn, ICP averages 4.5 cm H_2O or 6 mmHg, and rises slowly with age.
- In normal adults, ICP is approximately 10-15 mmHg (1 cmH_2O = 1.3 mmHg).

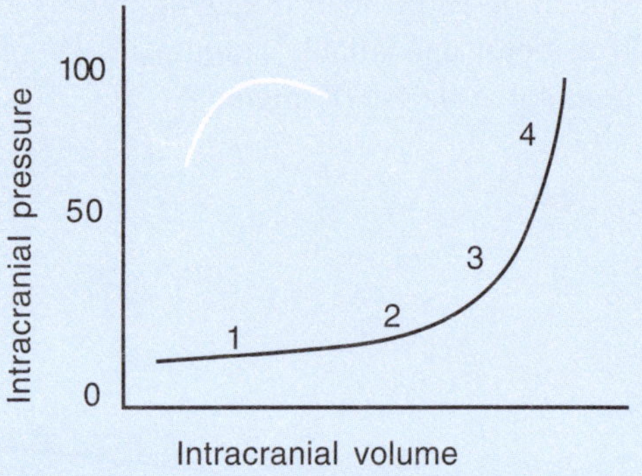

Fig. 36.1 *Intracranial pressure-volume curve.* This curve reflects the compensatory mechanisms of the cranio-spinal axis so that initially, increase in the intracranial volume results in only minor ICP rise (points 1 and 2).

However, when compensatory mechanisms are exhausted, even small increments in the intracranial volumes result in a steep ICP rise (points 3 and 4).

- ICP of 20 mmHg or greater is considered abnormally elevated.

Cerebral Perfusion Pressure (CPP) and Cerebral Blood Flow (CBF)

- The pressure of blood perfusing the brain (CPP) is determined by the difference between the upstream pressure (the mean arterial pressure, MAP) and the downstream pressure (the ICP). CPP = MAP - ICP
- It is important to maintain a normal CPP as this is a critical determinant of cerebral blood flow (CBF) and plays an important role in ICP management.
- Cerebral ischemia may result when CPP is lowered, either from raised ICP or lowered MAP (hypotension) or both.
- The critical CPP for maintaining CBF in adults is approximately 50 mmHg. However, in the presence of intracranial pathology, the goal for CPP should be higher (at approximately 70 mmHg in adults, to avoid ischemia, and below 110 mmHg to avoid hyperemia).
- In children with suspected raised ICP, ensure an adequate CPP by maintaining a *high normal MAP for age* and avoid therapies that can cause systemic hypotension.

Cerebral autoregulation

- Normally CBF is "autoregulated" at a constant level over a wide range of MAP (from 50 to 150 mmHg), Figure 36.3.
- Pressure autoregulation of this type is medi-

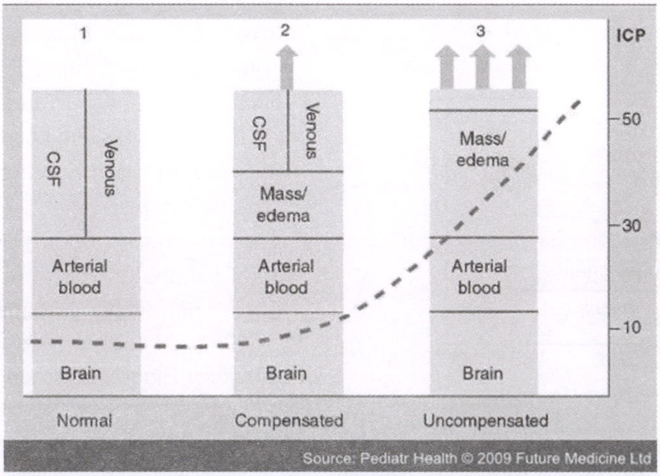

Fig. 36.2 The figure explains the relationship between intracranial volumes and intracranial pressure in physiological and pathophysiological conditions (The Munro-Kellie Doctrine). The volume of the intracranial vault is generally fixed in most children. The contents of the intracranial vault in the normal condition include the brain, arterial blood, venous blood and CSF, and are maintained at a relatively low ICP (panel 1; normal). After an injury, swelling/edema/pathological tissue can increase within the brain (panel 2; compensated). Compensatory mechanisms, including increased CSF absorption, extrusion of CSF into the spinal canal and extrusion of venous blood into the thorax, initially limit any changes in ICP. When these compensatory changes are exhausted (panel 3; uncompensated), any further increases in intracranial volumes are associated with concomitant increases in ICP that eventually can compromise arterial blood flow, ultimately leading to cerebral herniation. CSF: Cerebrospinal fluid; ICP: Intracranial pressure.

ated by changes in arteriolar diameter and cerebrovascular resistance.

- When the MAP falls and the CPP falls, the cerebral arterioles dilate to maintain a constant CBF and ensure a constant delivery of oxygen and nutrients to the brain.
- When the MAP rises and CPP rises, the vessels constrict, maintaining CBF and preventing hyperemia.
- Thus whether a patient is hypotensive or hypertensive, the CBF autoregulates to maintain a constant CPP and neuronal perfusion.
- However, when the MAP/CPP falls below the critical lower limit of autoregulation, the CBF can fall and cerebral ischemia can occur.
- In adults, a fall in CPP < 60 mmHg leads to cerebral ischemia. Thus the CPP is a surrogate marker of CBF.

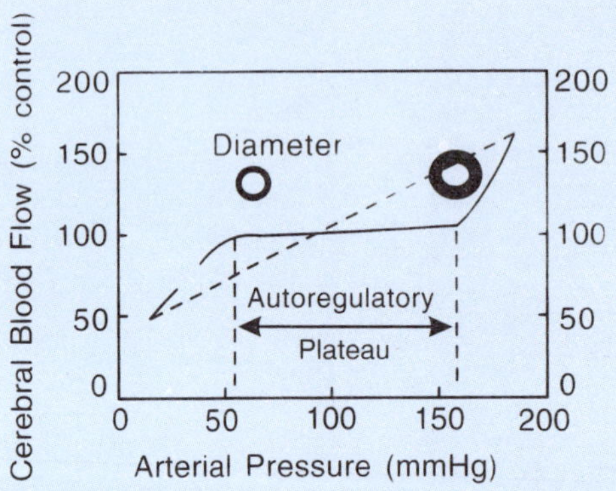

Fig. 36.3 Cerebral autoregulation. Note that within the limits of autoregulation, CBF is kept constant by changes in blood vessel caliber. When mean BP falls or rises, the cerebral blood vessels dilate and constrict respectively.

- The autoregulatory curve is shifted to the left in children and shifted to the right in patients with chronic hypertension.
- Autoregulation may be impaired by intracranial pathology such as head trauma.
- When autoregulation is lost, CBF becomes "*pressure-passive*": i.e., the CBF is at the mercy of the patient's BP. Systemic hypotension can lead to cerebral ischemia and systemic hypertension can lead to hyperemia.
- Accurate CPP monitoring needs an ICP and an invasive arterial monitor.

Physiological variables that affect intracranial pressure

In addition to the MAP, the following physiological variables also regulate CBF and influence acute changes in ICP

- The *$paCO_2$* has a near linear relationship with CBF within the physiological range, producing a 2-6% increase of CBF for each mmHg rise of $paCO_2$. High $paCO_2$ results in ↑ CBF and ↑ ICP. low $paCO_2$ can cause ↓ CBF, ↓ ICP but has potential for ischemia, Figure 36.4.
- Changes in *paO_2* do not produce changes in CBF until the patient becomes hypoxic (paO_2 < 60 mmHg), above which point the CBF increases steeply.
- The *cerebral metabolic rate* (expressed as cerebral metabolic rate for oxygen, $CMRO_2$) has a direct relationship with the CBF. Elevated tem-

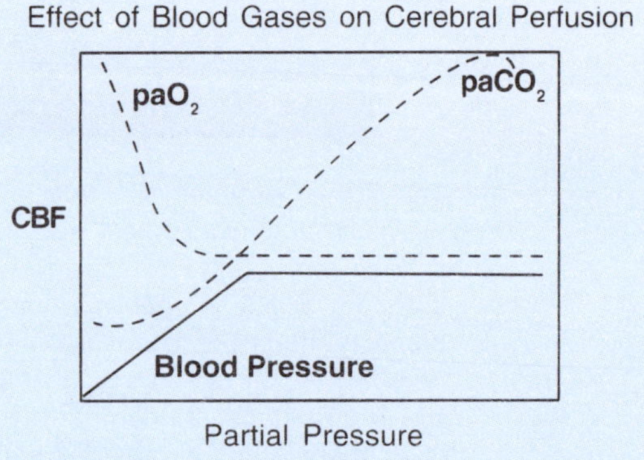

Fig. 36.4 Physiological variables and ICP. (*Downloaded from: homepage.mac.com/tegtmeyer/residents/icp.html, March 2008*)

Table 36.1 Herniation syndromes

Type	Clinical hallmark	Causes
Uncal / lateral transtentorial Uncus of temporal lobe herniates downward medially through tentorium 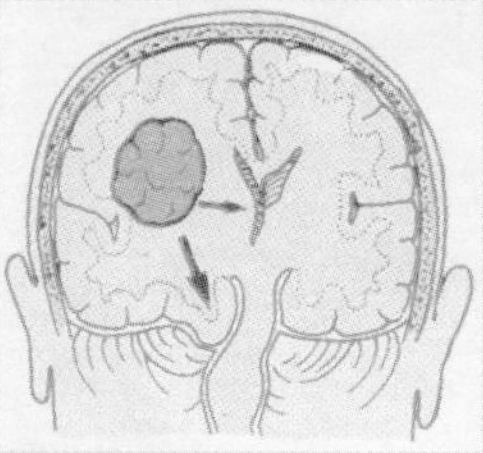	Ipsilateral 3rd CN palsy Contralateral motor posturing	Temporal lobe mass lesion
Central transtentorial Downward displacement of diencephalon through tentorium with pressure on brainstem	Coma with progression from bilateral decorticate to decerebrate posturing, pupils mid position, poorly reactive	Diffuse cerebral edema Acute hydrocephalus
Subfalcine Shift of affected hemisphere to opposite side	Coma with asymmetric (contralateral > ipsilateral) motor posturing	Convexity (frontal or parietal) mass lesion
Tonsillar /cerebellar (upward or downward) 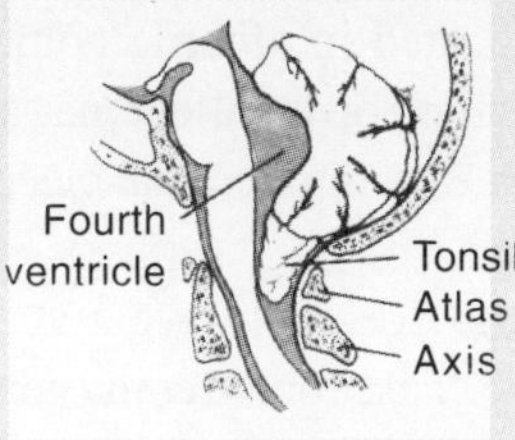	Sudden progression to coma with respiratory arrest and bilateral motor posturing in a patient with cerebellar signs	Posterior fossa / cerebellar mass lesion

(Figures downloaded from nu.kku.ac.th/site/250262/nursing5/27.htm)

perature and seizures can markedly increase the $CMRO_2$ and thus cause massive surges in the CBF (up to 300 times).

CAUSES OF INTRACRANIAL HYPERTENSION

1. **Increased brain mass**
   - Brain tumor
   - Cerebral edema, 3 types

Vasogenic: Blood brain barrier defect which may be inflammatory or traumatic in origin resulting in icreased vascular permeability.

Cytotoxic: Neuronal swelling due to disruption of intracellular machinery and/or cellular membrane function. Cause may be traumatic, inflammatory or hypoxic-ischemic.

PEDIATRIC EMERGENCIES & CRITICAL CARE

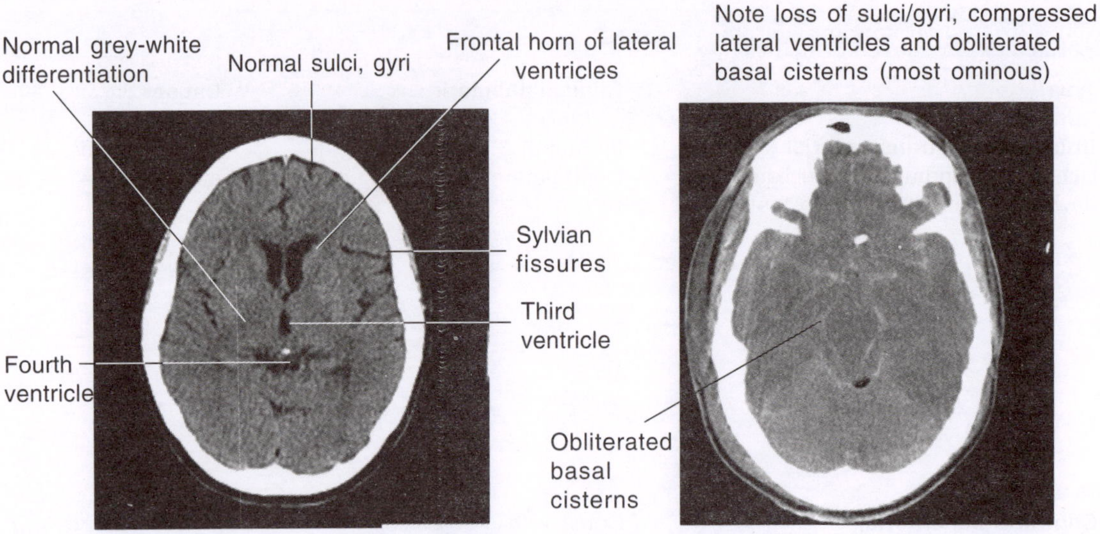

Fig. 36.5 CT scan brain, normal (left), severe cerebral edema (right)

- *Interstitial:* Increased intraventricular pressure due to obstruction of normal CSF pathways.

2. **Increased CSF volume**
   - Decreased absorption
   - Obstructed CSF flow
   - Overproduction of CSF
3. **Increased intracranial blood volume**
   - Cerebral vasodilatation (hypoxia, hypercarbia)
   - Obstructed venous flow

SYMPTOMS AND SIGNS OF INCREASED ICP AND HERNIATION

- Headache
- Vomiting
- Depressed level of consciousness (lethargy, stupor, coma)
- Sixth cranial nerve palsies
- Hypertension, with or without heart rate changes (usually bradycardia, sometimes tachycardia)
- Increased muscle tone with brisk tendon reflexes
- Papilledema is rare in acutely elevated ICP

☞ **REMEMBER** The Cushing's triad consisting of bradycardia, hypertension and apnea is a very late sign of intracranial hypertension.

NEURO-IMAGING IN SUSPECTED ICP

- Urgent imaging is indicated in afebrile coma, the presence of focal signs or papilledema, as the diagnosis includes stroke, intra-cranial bleed, tumor or hydrocephalus.
- However, any child who does not have a very obvious metabolic/toxic cause for the coma generally requires to be imaged.
- A CT scan may provide information about the cause of altered mental status and the presence of intracranial hypertension; however a normal CT scan does not rule out raised ICP.
- *CT scan features of raised ICP* (Fig. 36.5)
  - Obliterated sulci and gyri
  - Poor gray-white differentiation
  - Compressed lateral ventricles
  - Loss of basal cisterns *(indicates imminent / established tentorial herniation)*

- An MRI may be more specific for early changes of herpes simplex encephalitis (where CT may be normal), posterior fossa and white matter pathology.
- A cranial ultrasound may miss subdural collections or even extensive infarcts and a CT or MRI is an essential investigation in a deeply comatose infant even when the anterior fontanelle is open.

REFERENCES

1. Mayer SA, Chong JY: Critical care management of increased intracranial pressure: J Intensive Care Med 2002; 17: 55-67.

37

Management of Raised ICP Part 2: Therapeutic Options

- If intracranial hypertension is not appropriately treated, the ICP can rapidly rise to the point where cerebral ischemia or brain herniation occurs, both of which can result in significant morbidity or death.
- Frequent neurological assessment and targeted therapy is essential to prevent ICP related neurological catastrophe.

Therapy must be rapid and systematic and focus on the following aspects:

A. Immediate stabilization (airway, breathing, circulation)
B. Control of ICP and CPP management
C. Monitoring in the PICU
D. Supportive management
E. Evaluation and treatment of underlying disorder

Stabilization of the Patient's Vitals is the Priority: Assess the Airway, Breathing and Circulation (ABCs)

- Patients with raised ICP will not be able to maintain or protect their airway because of altered mentation and loss of airway tone. Early control of the airway is paramount to prevent airway obstruction and aspiration.
- Even if spontaneously breathing with normal gas exchange, *early intubation, ventilation and deep sedation are often overlooked as key interventions for ICP control.*
- Safe intubation is facilitated by rapid sequence intubation with deep sedation and muscle relaxants. Inadequate sedation during intubation causes more coughing and gagging, thus increasing ICP.
- *Indications for intubation:*
  - GCS $\leq$ 8 or fall in GCS > 3 points
  - Evidence of herniation
  - Airway compromise
  - Irregular respiratory efforts
  - Hypoxemia and/or hypercarbia
- *Drug regimen for intubation:*
  - Premedication with lignocaine 1 mg/kg for cough suppression and prevent ICP surges.
  - Deep sedation with thiopentone (2-5 mg/kg) or propofol (2-3 mg/kg). If hypotensive, use the lower dose range for thiopentone along with rapid fluid resuscitation and vasopressor support.
  - Ketamine was thought to worsen ICP; however, recent literature supports neuroprotective role of ketamine. Hemodynamics are also well maintained with this agent.
  - Muscle paralysis with vecuronium 0.1-0.2 mg/kg
  - Consider mannitol 0.5-1.0 g/kg if BP normal and signs of herniation present.
- *During the process of securing **A**irway and **B**reathing, assess for **C**irculatory status which may be compromised*, especially after sedatives administered and/or the etiology is infectious.

Rapid correction of shock with isotonic fluid resuscitation, followed by inotropic support may be required, aiming for a high normal mean arterial pressure for age

ICP AND CPP MANAGEMENT

Although clear guidelines for CPP targets are unavailable, guidelines suggest the following: Maintain ICP below 20 mmHg and CPP above 60 mmHg in adolescents, CPP between 50-60 mmHg in children (1-12 years) and between 40-50 mmHg in infants.[2]

ICP: Basic level therapy (Fig. 37.1)

- Elevate head end of bed 30° with head in neutral position, avoid jugular compression (promotes venous drainage from brain).
- Maintain deep sedation at all times. Pain, discomfort, agitation and coughing cause ICP elevation. Continuous infusions of midazolam along with opioids (morphine or fentanyl) are effective agents. Also give boluses of fentanyl 1-2 mcg/kg prior to suctioning and other noxious stimuli. Muscle paralysis not routinely used unless critical hypoxemia present.
- Monitor core temperature. Maintain body temperature normal to mildly hypothermic. *Fever is harmful!!* Control fever with paracetamol, tepid sponging and cooling blankets. Monitor for and aggressively treat fever and sepsis.
- Ventilation strategy:
  - Maintain $paCO_2$ 35-40 mmHg, paO_2 > 60 mmHg. Monitor with continuous capnography and pulse oximetry and frequent blood gases.
  - Minimize PEEP. However, if PEEP required for maintenance of oxygenation, then oxygenation takes priority; PEEP up to 15 mmHg has not been shown to increase ICP.
- Hemodynamic management:
  - Maintain euvolemia. Avoid hypotonic fluids *(even RL is hypotonic). See fluid therapy.*
  - Mean arterial pressure (MAP) targets based on CPP goals (see above). If ICP monitoring unavailable in a patient with suspected intracranial hypertension, assume ICP of at least 20 mmHg and maintain MAP high normal with colloids and pressors at needed. E.g., in order to maintain CPP > 60 mmHg in an adolescent, a MAP of at least 80 mmHg is necessary if the ICP is assumed to be 20 mmHg.
  - Noradrenaline can be used (through central line). If associated myocardial dysfunction suspected, an inotrope such as dobutamine should be added.
- CSF drainage via ventricular catheter is extremely effective as it permits both ICP monitoring and drainage.
- Osmotherapy: common agents are mannitol and hypertonic saline

  a) *Mannitol* widely used (Table 37.1)
  - Mannitol is indicated acutely for patients in whom there is a strong clinical suspicion of raised ICP or imminent herniation.
  - Mannitol has two distinct effects.
    i. The immediate effect is related to its rheologic properties (decreased blood viscosity) resulting in a transient increased CBF followed by a more sustained fall in CBF.
    ii. The delayed osmotic effects occur after 15-30 minutes and last for 4-6 hours.
  - Dose: 0.25-1.0 gm/kg/dose. Use high initial dose, provided hemodynamics normal. Subsequent doses may be smaller.
  - Can be used PRN 4-6th hourly for acute increases in ICP.
  - Urinary fluid losses should be replaced with normal saline to avoid volume depletion.
  - Serum osmolality must be maintained < 320 mOsm/L to prevent renal toxicity.
  - With repeated use, mannitol may accumulate in injured brain and cause paradoxical increase in cerebral edema, hence avoid scheduled doses for > 48 hours.
  - Intracranial bleed is not a contraindication for mannitol.

Table 37.1 Mannitol - Concerns and contraindications

Concerns	Effects	How/ when to avoid
Excess diuresis	Hypovolemia, fall in CPP	Lower doses 0.25-0.5 g/kg (1.2-2.5 ml/kg of a 20% solution) repeated 4-6th hourly*
Use in focal pathology with midline shift (e.g., necrotizing encephalitis, edema surrounding intracranial hemorrhage, tumor, infarct)	Mannitol may cause "selective debulking" of normal brain parenchyma with increase in midline shift	Mannitol should be reserved for features of severely increased ICP or impending herniation
Rebound effect	Worsening edema after discontinuation	Limit use to less than 48-72 hours. Use smaller doses. Avoid concurrent hypotonic IV fluid or dilute enteral feeds
Contraindications		Hypotension, renal failure Serum osmolality > 320 mOsm/kg

**Emergency therapy for herniation syndromes: 1.0-1.5 g/kg of 20% mannitol; subsequent doses: 0.2.5-0.5 g/kg q4-6h, measure serum osmolality*

b) *Hypertonic saline:* Acts like mannitol by causing fluid to shift from neurons and interstitial compartment to the intravascular compartment resulting in brain shrinkage. Additional advantage is ability to maintain circulating volume and thus the CPP.
- Maintain serum sodium between 145-160 mEq/L.
- Serum osmolality up to 360 mOsm/L is tolerated with fewer complications as intravascular volume is well maintained.
- Safer than mannitol in patients with unstable or borderline hemodynamic status.
- Dose: Initial bolus of 5-6 mL/kg over 10 minutes followed by continuous infusion at 0.1-1 ml/kg/hr.
- As elevated serum osmolality will result in ADH mediated water retention, restrict fluids to 2/3rd whilst the patient is receiving 3% saline.

- Maintain glucose in the normal range. *Both hypo- and hyperglycemia are detrimental.*
- Steroids: Most useful for vasogenic edema related to tumors, granulomas and abscesses. Not useful for ICP related to infarcts, hemorrhage or trauma.

Escalated therapy for patients who continue to have raised ICP

If despite the above treatments, the patient continues to show evidence of raised ICP, further measures to tackle refractory raised ICP must be instituted. Repeated imaging may be necessary; specific surgically correctible lesions should be attended to.

- Lower pCO_2 targets to 30-35 mmHg. Profound hyperventilation with pCO_2 of 25-30 mmHg may be necessary as a short term temporizing measure for acute neurological deterioration, bearing in mind the risk of inducing cerebral ischemia in the process.
- High-dose barbiturates, preferably with continuous EEG monitoring if available.
  - Thiopentone sodium is widely used in this setting, but has many adverse effects
  - Dose: Bolus 3-5 mg/kg followed by 1-5 mg/kg/hour.

  Side effects of thiopentone sodium
  - Significant hypotension may ensue and invasive hemodynamic monitoring is mandatory (CVP, arterial line). Target high normal mean BP for age. In the event of hypotension, consider inotrope/pressor support.
  - Immunosuppressive, risk of infections.
  - Can cause ileus and feed intolerance.
  - Thiopentone can accumulate with prolonged infusions. Hence, if used > 48-72 hours, the drug can be abruptly ceased.
- Decompressive craniectomy to be considered in refractory intracranial hypertension. *See below*
- Moderate hypothermia (32-34°C) × 24 hours may be useful by decreasing $CMRO_2$ and thus decreasing CBF. Prevent shivering with muscle relaxants, cease feeds, monitor for infections and coagulopathy. Rewarm slowly at 1°C/hour, anticipate hypotension.

Surgical options

- Early decompression of hydrocephalus if present.
- Even when ventricles are not dilated, early insertion of a ventricular drain is useful as a monitoring tool (ICP monitor) and therapeutic modality (permits CSF drainage).
- If ICP due to space occupying lesion, early resection indicated.
- Decompressive craniectomy to be considered in refractory intracranial hypertension. Bilateral removal of skull flaps and lifting dura allows decompression of the underlying brain and can prevent herniation and cerebral ischemia in some cases. Survival and functional outcome are best if performed *early* (with initial 36–48 hours) when medical treatment does not appearing to be working.

Monitoring during therapy of raised ICP

- Heart rate, invasive arterial blood pressure and CVP monitoring
- Intracranial pressure monitoring (ventricular, parenchymal or subdural).
- Precise hourly fluid balance monitoring. An indwelling urinary catheter usually necessary.
- ABG Q4H, continuous capnography and pulse oximetry.
- Blood glucose Q2 -4th hourly, electrolytes every 6-12 hours.
- Serum osmolality Q12H, BUN daily.
- Hemogram, infection screen.
- Cranial imaging as necessary (See neuroimaging features in ICP, part 1).

Supportive therapy in the ICU

- **Fluid management**: *Avoid hypovolemia, hypervolemia, hypotonic fluids. Aim for euglycemia, euvolemia*
  - There is accumulating data that hypovolemia worsens outcome in children with meningitis, malaria and severe head injury. Hypovolemia can lower the CPP and lead to worse ICP due to autoregulatory vasodilatation.
  - Fluids may be restricted especially if SIADH suspected or the serum sodium fails to rise despite the patient receiving hypertonic saline; however, euvolemia must be maintained at all times.
  - The fluid infusion rates can be tailored based on perfusion indices, CVP, serum Na, osmolality, urine output.

- Free water must be strictly restricted: avoid hypotonic fluids such as 1/5th normal saline in 5% dextrose (Isolyte P) or ½ NS in 5% dextrose. The dextrose will be metabolized with a resultant hypotonic fluid that can aggravate cerebral edema and ICP. Concentrate all IV meds (antibiotics, sedatives).
- Isotonic fluids such as normal saline with added potassium is recommended as maintenance fluid.
- Maintain euglycemia. Add glucose to the maintenance fluid at sufficient concentrations to maintain serum glucose between 100-150 mg%.
- Enteral feeds should be started at the earliest (isocaloric formula).

- **Anti-seizure medications**

  Convulsions can cause massive increases in CBF; consequent increase in ICP can lead to secondary brain damage and may precipitate or be precipitated by cerebral herniation.

  Apart from generalized tonic-clonic seizures (GTCS), some comatose children may have non-convulsive seizures (NCS) manifesting with subtle signs such as eyelid twitching, eye deviation or nystagmus.

  - A bedside EEG may be informative. If in doubt, empiric treatment of seizures may be justified and can result in improvement of consciousness.
  - Monitor drug levels of anticonvulsants.

Initial stabilization and basic level ICP Rx

- Stabilize vitals, early controlled intubation and ventilation, pCO_2 35-40 mmHg
- Elevate head end by 30°, avoid jugular compression
- Mannitol bolus 0.5-1 gm/kg, maintain high serum osmolarity with hypertonic saline, Na^+ 145-160
- Full sedation and analgesia, MAP high normal
- Maintain euglycemia, euvoloemia, euthermia

↓

Escalated ICP Rx

- pCO_2 30-35 mmHg, continue osmotherapy
- Thiopentone infusion, maintain MAP with pressors
- Hypothermia (32-34°C) × 24 hours
- Repeated imaging
- Consider surgical options

↓

Treatment of acute neurological deterioration or spikes in ICP > 20 mmHg for > 10 mins

- Rule out systemic causes (hypoxemia, hypercarbia, DOPE, hypotension), check Na^+, glucose
- *Briefly* hyperventilate for 5-10 mins, aim for pCO_2 25-30 mmHg *(most immediate and effective therapy)*
- Drain 5-10 ml CSF via EVD drain if present
- Bolus dose of sedative (midazolam ± fentanyl)
- Mannitol 0.5-1 gm/kg bolus
- Treat seizures (convulsive or non-convulsive)
- Repeat imaging for correctable lesions

Fig. 37.1 Sequential treatment approach to a patient with raised ICP

Evaluation and treatment of underlying disorder

A systematic approach is required to determine the causes of raised ICP (See ICP Part 1 for Neuroimaging).

- **Lumbar puncture (LP) in a comatose child with suspected ICP**

  The potential benefits of early LP include making an early diagnosis of CNS infection and identification of the pathogen and drug sensitivities.

  Contraindications for LP include signs of cerebral herniation, low GCS, focal neurological signs, or cardio-respiratory compromise.

  In an unconscious child, the decision is controversial with some authors stating that the risk of herniation far outweighs the benefit of knowing the pathogen from an early LP. Therefore, if the decision for LP is taken, it must be performed with great care.

  As alluded to earlier, the absence of papilledema or a normal CT scan in the acute phase does not rule out raised ICP.

- **Choice of empiric antimicrobials**

  If a CNS infection is suspected in a febrile child presenting in acute coma and seizures, empiric antimicrobials should include acyclovir in addition to a third-generation cephalosporin until further confirmatory tests are available.

  The need for *empiric antimalarials* and anti-mycoplasma therapy (IV macrolide) should be carefully assessed.

Conclusion

- Patients presenting with altered mental status and potential raised ICP have many challenging issues.
- A systematic approach to stabilization and diagnosis may be rewarding in a large percentage of these children.
- The family needs to be counseled with honesty and sensitivity, explaining that survival and long-term prognosis may be difficult to state with certainty, especially in the initial stages of illness.

Table 37.2 **Summary of ICP treatment**
Modalities of intracranial hypertension therapy may be classified according to the mechanism and predominant brain compartment that is targeted

A. Therapeutic measures to decrease cerebral blood volume	
1. Head elevation 30° (unless hypotensive) and in midline, avoid jugular compression	Promotes cerebral venous drainage
2. Moderate hyperventilation (pCO_2 in mid 30s)	Decreases cerebral blood flow, has potential for cerebral ischemia if pCO_2 < 30 mmHg
3. Minimize intrathoracic pressure (PEEP) unless hypoxemia present	Promotes cerebral venous drainage
4. Sedation and analgesia, particularly for noxious stimuli like tracheal suctioning: facilitated by sedative-narcotic infusions	Prevents spikes in cerebral metabolic rate and consequent reflex rise in CBF
5. Prevention of seizures, don't overlook non-convulsive seizures (NCS)	Prevents rise in cerebral metabolic rate and consequent reflex rise in CBF

contd

6. Maintain normothermia (35.5-37°C)	Prevents rise in cerebral metabolic rate and consequent reflex rise in CBF.
Hypothermia (32-34°C) if ICP refractory or severe	Hypothermia ↓ $CMRO_2$ and thereby ↓ CBF without causing ischemia
7. High dose barbiturates	Lowers cerebral metabolic rate and decreases CBF without causing ischemia
B. Therapeutic measures to decrease CSF volume	
1. CSF withdrawal via an external ventricular drain (EVD)	One of the most effective methods of rapid reductions in ICP, can be drained until improvement in ICP or clinical signs noted
2. Decrease CSF production with acetazolamide	More effective in chronic communicating hydrocephalus, less useful in acute setting
C. Therapeutic measures to decrease brain volume	
1. Osmotherapy ▪ Mannitol ▪ Hypertonic saline (3%)	Mannitol acts immediately by reducing blood viscosity and improving CBF. Later and more sustained effect is decreased brain edema by establishing an osmotic gradient
2. Steroids	Useful only in localized vasogenic edema such as that around tumors, granulomas and abscesses

REFERENCES

1. Himmelseher S, Durieux ME. Revising a Dogma: Ketamine for Patients with Neurological Injury. Anesth Analg 2005; 101:524-34.
2. Tasker RC. Head and spinal cord trauma. In: Nichols DG, ed: Rogers' Textbook of Pediatric Intensive Care, 4th ed. Lippincot Williams and Wilkins, Baltimore, 2008.
3. Mayer SA, Chong JY: Critical care management of increased intracranial pressure. J Intensive Care Med 2002; 17: 55-67.

38

Approach to a Comatose Child

A child presenting with coma is one of the most difficult diagnostic and management problems that may be encountered by a pediatrician. The gravity of the situation, the need to avoid further neurological damage, the wide range of possible causes call for a calm orderly approach to the situation at hand. Regardless of the etiology, initial management includes immediate attention to the ABCs in order to sustain life and prevent loss of brain function.

DEFINITION

Coma or altered mental status implies a disorder of consciousness: it may be applied to a state or continuum of worsening consciousness from being fully alert and responsive to deep unresponsive coma.

PATHOPHYSIOLOGY

Comatose states are indicative of diffuse impairment of cerebral functions, failure of brainstem activating functions or both.

This may be caused by supratentorial lesions affecting deep diencephalic structures or subtentorial or metabolic lesions diffusely affecting brainstem function. Although it common practice to divide the etiology of coma as metabolic and structural causes, strict compartmentalization is not always possible as structural causes of coma may be associated with metabolic dysfunction, e.g., the Syndrome of Inappropriate Anti-Diuretic Hormone (SIADH) complicating head injury.

See Table 38.1 for etiology of coma in children.

EVALUATION OF A CHILD IN COMA

A. Immediate considerations

- Assess and optimize airway, breathing and circulation in order to ensure that the brain is being adequately perfused.
- Obtain an immediate bedside capillary blood glucose level and correct if low.
- Brief relevant history of chronic and recent illnesses, trauma, medications in the home.
- Consider naloxone 0.1 mg/kg in suspected narcotic ingestions.

B. Secondary considerations

A complete neurological examination is necessary with particular attention to 5 physiological variables. These may give valuable information about the level of the lesion in the brain, nature of involvement and direction of progression of the disease process.

These are:

- The level of consciousness
- Pattern of respiration
- Size and reactivity of the pupils
- Spontaneous and induced eye movements
- Motor responses

Table 38.1 **Etiology of coma in children** (The mnemonic "TIPS from the Vowels" is a useful method to remember the most common of the wide range of possible causes)

	Conditions	Comments
T	Trauma, head injury	Shaken baby syndrome: May present with non-specific history, retinal hemorrhages
I	Intussusception	Mental status changes may precede abdominal finding
	Insulin hypoglycemia	Hypoglycemia secondary to accidental ingestion of oral hypoglycemic agents Ketotic hypoglycemia following prolonged fasting in thin built children
	Inborn errors of metabolism	Coma may be associated with vomiting and seizures
P	Psychogenic	Common in adolescents
S	Seizures	Post-ictal states, non-convulsive status may masquerade as undifferentiated coma
	Shock, stroke	Coma secondary to poor brain perfusion, arterial and venous infarcts
	Shunt	Blocked or infected ventriculoperitoneal shunts
A	Alcohol ingestion, Abuse (Battered baby)	
E	Electrolytes	Disturbances of sodium, calcium, magnesium
	Encephalopathy	Hypertensive, Reye syndrome, hepatic failure, urea cycle defects, lead, porphyria
I	Infections	Encephalitis, meningitis, malaria
O	Overdose, ingestion	Consider with unexplained loss of consciousness
U	Uremic encephalopathy	

a) **Level of Consciousness**

Numerous scoring systems have been developed to assess the level of consciousness. By far the most useful is the **Glasgow Coma Score** (GCS), which was originally used to predict the outcome after head injury in adults. The **modified GCS** is applicable to younger patients and is the most frequently used general means of neurological assessment (see Table 38.3).

An alternative method for assessing the level of consciousness is the **AVPU** score. This score, like the GCS, is also useful for the serial observation of the trends in the level of coma.

A: alert

V: responds to voice

P: responds to pain
U: unresponsive

b) **Respiratory Pattern**

The control of respiration is governed by centers located in the brainstem (lower pons and medulla) and modulated by forebrain cortical centers. Respiratory pattern abnormalities signify either metabolic derangements or neurologic insult.

Several characteristic respiratory patterns exist:

- *Cheyne Stokes Respiration (CSR)*
  This is a pattern of periodic breathing where hyperpnea alternates with apnea. The depth of breathing alters from breath to breath with a smooth rise to a peak and a smooth fall (decrescendo).
  CSR results from deep hemispheric or diencephalic dysfunction and may also be seen in children with metabolic abnormalities.
- *Central neurogenic hyperventilation*
  Sustained regular, rapid and deep respiration. May be seen in children with brainstem dysfunction.
- *Apneustic breathing*
  This pattern of breathing is characterized by inspiratory pauses lasting 2-3 seconds often alternating with end-expiratory pauses. Apneustic breathing is characteristic of pontine infarction and anoxic encephalopathy.

c) **Pupillary Size and Reactivity**

Pupillary reactions are controlled by a balance between the sympathetic and parasympathetic nervous system. As brainstem centers controlling consciousness are anatomically adjacent to those controlling pupils, pupillary changes are a valuable guide to the presence and location of brain lesions.

Additionally, *metabolic disturbances affect pupillary pathways late*. Consequently, the presence or absence of the pupillary reaction to light

Table 38.2 Laboratory evaluation of a patient in coma

Routine investigations	**Specific investigations** (where clinically indicated)
White blood count, coagulation screen	EEG, ECG
CXR	CSF analysis
Neuroimaging Head US, CT or MRI	Serum ammonia, lactate, pyruvate in suspected metabolic disorders
Arterial blood gas, blood glucose, serum electrolytes, calcium, magnesium	Thyroid function tests
Liver, renal function tests	Toxin screen, lead levels
Serum and urine osmolality	Skeletal survey
Urine for sugar, ketones, pH	GI contrast studies
Infection screen, virology	

is one of the single most important differentiating features to distinguish between structural and metabolic disorders.

d) **Induced Eye Movements**

Two specific eye movements are helpful in evaluating comatose children. One is the oculocephalic or the doll's eye response. This is performed by holding the eyelids open and rotating the head from side to side. The normal or positive response is conjugate deviation of the eyes in the opposite direction to which the head is turned.

The *oculovestibular or the calorie test* is performed by elevating the patient's head to 30° and slowly injecting 50 ml of ice water with a syringe. (Rule out perforated eardrums, wax in canal, and fracture base of skull.)

There may be three types of response:

i. Normal awake patients with intact brainstem: Nystagmus with the slow component towards the irrigated ear and fast component towards midline.

ii. Unconscious patient with intact brainstem: fast component abolished, eyes move towards stimulus and remain tonically deviated for > 1 minute.

iii. Unconscious patient with brainstem dysfunction/brain dead patient: No response to stimuli, i.e., eyes remain in the midline.

e) **Motor Examination**

Assessment of muscle strength, tone and tendon reflexes should be done for normality and symmetry. The ability of the patient to localize stimuli as well as the presence or absence of abnormal posturing helps in the assessment of severity of the neurological derangement.

Decorticate posturing with flexion of the upper extremities and extension of the lower extremities suggests involvement of the cerebral cortex and preservation of brainstem function.

Decerebrate posturing with rigid extension of the arms and legs is indicative of cortical and brainstem damage.

The *flaccid patient* with no response to painful stimuli has the gravest prognosis with injury sustained to deep brainstem lesions.

MANAGEMENT OF A COMATOSE PATIENT

(See also chapter on treatment of ICP, part 2)

The main goals of care include optimizing cerebral blood flow (CBF)/cerebral perfusion pressure (CPP) and minimizing factors that can aggravate neuronal injury or trigger intracranial pressure (ICP) elevation.

1. **Assess the Airway, Breathing and Circulation (ABCs)**

   The airway should be stabilized and an assessment made for the need for intubation. Even if spontaneously breathing with normal gas exchange, many comatose children will benefit from intubation, especially if they have intracranial hypertension, evidence of herniation and irregularities in respiration (Table 38.4). The blood pressure should be kept at the higher range of normal (for age). This requires ensuring appropriate fluid and inotrope management.

2. **Assess and treat for immediately correctable cause of coma**

   Perform bedside capillary glucose test and correct if low; send samples to lab for routine haematological and biochemical testing.

3. **Assessment of the depth of coma**

   The standard assessment tool is the Glasgow Coma Score (GCS) in older children and modified GCS in children < 5 years old or the AVPU (Table 38.3).

4. **Assessment and treatment of raised ICP (see chapter on ICP therapy)**
The focus of contemporary ICP management has changed in recent years in two important aspects: firstly, increasing emphasis on CPP (cerebral perfusion pressure) management in addition to ICP control and secondly, the increasing recognition of the potential for overzealous hyperventilation to aggravate cerebral ischemia by reducing CBF.

5. **Anti-seizure medications in coma**
Convulsions can cause massive increases in CBF; consequent increase in ICP can lead to secondary brain damage and may precipitate or be precipitated by cerebral herniation. Apart from generalized tonic-clonic seizures (GTCS), some comatose children may have non-convulsive seizures (NCS) manifesting with subtle signs such as eyelid twitching, eye deviation or nystagmus. A bedside EEG may be informative. If in doubt, empiric treatment of seizures may be justified and can result in improvement of consciousness.

6. **Neuroimaging**
Urgent imaging is indicated in afebrile coma and the presence of focal signs or papilldema, as

Table 38.3 The Glasgow Coma Score

Eye opening response (< 5 years)	> 5 years	
Spontaneous	Spontaneous	4
To speech	To speech	3
To pain	To pain	2
None	None	1
Verbal response		
Alert, coos, words - normal	Oriented	4
Irritable cry	Confused	3
Cries to pain	Inappropriate words	2
Moans to pain	Incomprehensible sounds	1
No response to pain	None	
Motor response		
Normal spontaneous movements	Obeys commands	6
Localizes (>9 months)	Localizes to supraorbital stimulus	5
Withdraws	Withdraws	4
Abnormal flexion (decorticate posturing)	Abnormal flexion (decorticate posturing)	3
Abnormal extension (decerebrate response)	Abnormal extension (decerebrate response)	2
None	None	1

Table 38.4 Signs of cerebral herniation

1. Glasgow coma score < 8
2. Abnormal pupil size and reaction (unilateral or bilateral)
3. Absent doll's eye movements
4. Abnormal tone (decerebrate/decorticate posturing, flaccidity)
5. Hypertension* with bradycardia*
6. Respiratory abnormalities (hyperventilation, Cheyne-Stokes breathing, apnea*, respiratory arrest)
7. Papilledema (rare, especially in infants)

* Cushing's triad occurs late as a premorbid event.

the diagnosis includes stroke, intracranial bleed. tumor or hydrocephalus. A CT scan may provide information about the cause of altered mental status and the presence of intracranial hypertension; however, a normal CT scan does not rule out raised ICP.

An MRI may be more specific for early changes of herpes simplex encephalitis (where CT may be normal), posterior fossa and white matter pathology. A cranial ultrasound may miss subdural collections or even extensive infarcts and a CT or MRI is an essential investigation in a deeply comatose infant even when the anterior fontanelle is open.

7. **Lumbar Puncture (LP) in a comatose child**

The potential benefits of early LP include making an early diagnosis of CNS infection and identification of the pathogen and drug sensitivities. Contraindications for LP include signs of cerebral herniation, low GCS, focal neurological signs, or cardiorespiratory compromise. In an unconscious child with potential raised ICP. the decision is controversial with some authors stating that the risk of herniation far outweighs the benefit of knowing the pathogen from an early LP.

8. **Choice of empiric antimicrobials**

If a CNS infection is suspected in a febrile child presenting in acute coma and seizures, empiric anti-microbial should include acyclovir in addition to a third generation cephalosporin until further confirmatory tests are available. The need for empiric anti-malarials and anti-mycoplasma therapy (IV macrolide) should be carefully assessed.

9. **Fluid therapy**

There is accumulating data that hypovolemia worsens outcome in children with meningitis, malaria and severe head injury. Hypovolemia (fluid restriction, diuretics) can lower the CPP and lead to worse ICP due to autoregulatory vasodilation. What must be restricted are hypotonic fluids such as $1/5^{th}$ normal saline in 5% dextrose (Isolyte P). The dextrose will be metabolized with a resultant hypotonic fluid that can exacerbate cerebral edema and ICP. Enteral feeds should be started at the earliest.

10. **Prognosis**

The prognosis of a child in coma depends on the cause of altered mental status. In general, children have a better prognosis than adults. Prolonged coma after hypoxic-ischemic insult carries a poor prognosis, but children surviving infectious encephalopathies have a good outcome. Cortical blindness often recovers. Neuroimaging may be useful in predicting prognosis: poor outcome is to be expected if there are largespread areas of low densities, suggesting global ischemia.

REFERENCES

1. Kirkham FJ. Non-traumatic coma in children. Arch Dis Child 2001;85:303-312
2. Ranjit S. Emergency and Intensive Care Management of a Comatose Patient with Intracranial Hypertension: Current Concepts. Indian Pediatrics 2006;43:409-415

39

Protocol for Management of Status Epilepticus

Status epilepticus (SE) is an emergency that requires prompt recognition and treatment. Children with prolonged seizures are at risk for neuronal injury and respiratory and/or hemodynamic compromise due to both prolonged seizures and high-dose anticonvulsants; some patients may even develop multiorgan dysfunction and die.

STATUS EPILEPTICUS (SE): DEFINITION

- Continuous seizures lasting at least 5 minutes OR two or more discrete seizures between which there is incomplete recovery of consciousness.
- The time for SE has been shortened to 5 minutes from 30 minutes as:
  - Seizures that do not cease spontaneously in 5-10 minutes are unlikely to terminate without intervention.
  - Neuronal injury risk increases with increasing duration of seizures.
  - The longer seizures persist, the greater the risk of drug refractoriness.
- SE lasting > 60 minutes, despite optimal therapy with the first and second line drugs (benzodiazepines and phenytoin) may be defined as refractory SE (RSE).

☞ **REMEMBER** Do not mistake extensor posturing for seizures! Posturing can occur due to many causes including the post-ictal state, HIE, cerebral hypoperfusion due to shock, etc. Evaluate the patient and treat cause where possible.

RISK FACTORS FOR REFRACTORY STATUS EPILEPTICUS

- Lack of pre-existing epilepsy.
- Acute encephalitis causing status.
- Focal motor seizures at onset.

MANAGEMENT OF SE

A. Goals of treatment

1. Stabilize patient: Ensure adequate cardio- respiratory function.
2. Correct the correctable: temperature, hypoglycemia, abnormal electrolytes.
3. Prompt control of seizures.
4. Prevent recurrences: Evaluate and treat specific cause.
5. Prevent complications

B. Pitfalls in management

- Inadequate oxygenation and ventilation during stabilization.
- Difficult venous access and delay in drug administration.
- Inadequate doses of anticonvulsants.
- Failure of vigorous intravenous therapy early in seizure, thereby allowing progression to refractory status.

☞ **REMEMBER** With regard to toxicity, the rate of administration of drug is more important than the total dose administered, i.e., small amounts of drug administered rapidly may be more toxic than a larger amount administered slowly.

C. Stabilization (0-5 minutes)

Airway and breathing

- Position: Left lateral to prevent aspiration unless bag-mask ventilation required.
- Maintain airway patency by chin lift. If chin lift unsuccessful in maintaining airway patency, oral airway may be placed.
- Gentle oral suction with large bore Yankauer sucker.
- Pass nasogastric tube to prevent emesis and secondary aspiration, keep NG tube open.
- Supplemental oxygen by appropriate sized face mask.
- Check for inadequate oxygenation and ventilation
  - Evidence for obstructed airway, gurgling, stridor.
  - Inadequate chest rise.
  - Poor air entry.
  - Central cyanosis.
  - O_2 saturation < 90%.
  - Irregular respiration/apnea.
- Correct inadequate oxygenation and ventilation.
  - Optimize airway positioning and patency.
  - Commence bag-mask ventilation.
  - Ensure tight seal by holding a well fitting face mask with both hands and avoiding pressure on soft tissues of jaw.
- If bag-mask ventilation not producing adequate chest rise, proceed to intubation.
- *Indications for intubation in SE*
  - Inability to maintain airway despite above interventions.
  - Inadequate oxygenation and ventilation despite mask ventilation.
  - Raised ICT requiring controlled hyperventilation.
  - Refractory SE requiring general anesthesia.
  - Lower threshold for intubation if transport required.

Drugs for intubation

- Intubating a seizing child may be difficult and should preferably be carried out by using sedatives and muscle relaxants, provided the caregiver is experienced in intubation.
- The most effective agent in this scenario is thiopental, although dose-associated hypotension should be anticipated and avoided.
- Benzodiazepines and narcotic combination (midazolam + fentanyl) are alternative choices.
- For muscle relaxation, a short-acting, nondepolarizing agent such as rocuronium is preferred. Succinylcholine should be avoided due to the risk of hyperkalemia associated with ongoing seizure activity. Repeated doses of muscle relaxants should not be given, as it may mask seizure activity.

Circulation

- Assess perfusion and blood pressure.

> ☞ **REMEMBER** Re-assess perfusion after seizures controlled as active seizures may mask signs of shock and drugs used to control seizures may cause hypoperfusion.

- In early SE, perfusion usually adequate with tachycardia and raised BP due to stress induced catecholamine release.
- Prolonged status can result in poor perfusion and shock due to catecholamine depletion.
- Vascular access
  - May be difficult in the fitting child.
  - If no IV access, give midazolam intramuscularly.
  - Consider intraosseous route early (same dose and side effects as with IV route).

D. Initial investigations

- Glucose (bedside capillary dextrostix and lab sugar), electrolytes, ionised calcium, magnesium.
- Blood and urine specimens should be obtained for culture, especially in febrile children.
- After stabilization of the vitals, a head CT scan may be considered in the appropriate clinical scenario.

- Once a mass lesion or cerebral edema has been excluded, lumbar puncture may be performed in patients with suspected intracranial infections.
- Serum antiepileptic drug (AED) levels should be measured in children on chronic therapy.
- Other investigation as per suspected etiology.

E. Treat specific etiology and inciting factors, where possible

- Correct hypoglycemia, hyponatremia and hypocalcemia, if present.
- Broad spectrum high dose antibiotics and acyclovir should be administered empirically to patients who present with new-onset SE and fever. Empiric antimalarials may be considered if cerebral malaria considered possible.
- Fever may precipitate and/or aggravate seizures; fever may also occur because of seizures. Correct hyperthermia aggressively.
- Pyridoxine (50-100 mg IV) may be considered in all children < 18 months.

F. Principles of pharmacological therapy

- Several principles guide the choice of medications in SE.
- Firstly, the aim is to use agents that can be administered rapidly IV and penetrate the blood brain barrier quickly with minimal side effects.
- Second, employing medications with different mechanisms of action or acting at different receptors may be more effective than employing many drugs that act at the same receptors.
- Thirdly, in an ICU setting, where intubation and ventilator management are available, respiratory depression may need to be tolerated, but hypotension should be avoided, because the autoregulation of cerebral blood flow may be abnormal despite the maintenance of systemic blood pressure with vasopressors.

G. Sequence of drug therapy in SE

1. 1st line drugs: Immediate control of seizures with agents with rapid onset such as the benzodiazepines.
2. 2nd line drugs: Prevent recurrences with phenytoin and/or other 2nd line drugs (e.g., levetiracetam, phenobarbitone).
3. 3rd line drugs/RSE drugs: Treatment of refractory seizures with agents that have cerebral protective properties such as:
   - Midazolam infusion
   - High dose phenobarbitone
   - Thiopentone infusion

1. Drugs for immediate control of seizures: The benzodiazepines

- All benzodiazepines have the potential to cause adverse respiratory and hemodynamic consequences and the caregiver must be prepared to anticipate these risks and support the ABCs as required in order to enable early and safe control of seizures.
- Respiratory consequences of prolonged seizures and anticonvulsant drugs include depression of the central respiratory drive, decrease in airway patency (risk of airway obstruction) and protective reflexes (risk of aspiration).
- Drug induced hypotension occurs due to 3 reasons: Peripheral vasodilatation, negative inotropy and sedation induced blunting of the stress related catecholamine release.
- The risk of hypotension is higher in the hypovolemic patient, with multiple doses of benzodiazepines and following co-administration of barbiturates.

a) **Lorazepam**

- Lorazepam is the benzodiazepine of choice in SE as it is the most effective agent in its class for rapid seizure control and the least risk of respiratory depression.
- The drug has a long duration of action in view of the following properties:
  - Less lipophilic

- Less protein bound
- Less volume of distribution

- Lorazepam has a short elimination half-life.
- Large doses as bolus or infusion can cause metabolic acidosis due to solvent in the IV preparation.
- Dose: 0.05 to 0.1 mg/kg (max 4 mg)
- May be repeated Q10-15 minutely for 3 doses.
- For continuous infusion, the reconstitution should not exceed 2 mg/10 ml

b) **Midazolam**

- Midazolam is an alternative to lorazepam for immediate control of seizures.
- It has a short onset of action, rapidly penetrates the blood brain barrier and has a short duration of action.
- It may be used intramuscularly if IV access unavailable.
- It is also commonly used as an infusion in refractory SE.
  - 4 times as potent as diazepam.
  - Stable in aqueous solution, no active metabolites.
  - Dose: 0.05-0.1 mg/kg Q10 minutely for 3 doses (max single dose 5 mg).
  - Onset of action: 1.5-5 minutes, duration 1-5 hours.
  - IM dose 0.2 mg/kg.

c) **Diazepam**: With advent of newer agents, this drug is used less frequently.

Consider pyridoxine 100 mg IV for patients < 18 months

2. Second line drugs to prevent recurrence

- Options are:
  IV phenytoin/fosphenytoin, IV levetiracetam, IV valproate and IV phenobarbitone.
- An effective sequence of second line drugs to attain rapid control of seizures while minimizing cardiorespiratory complications is to commence with
  Phenytoin (20+10 mg/kg) →IV levetiracetam/IV Valproate →standard dose phenobarbitone (20 mg/kg).
  See algorithm for treatment of SE.
- The distinction between standard dose vs high dose phenobarbitone must be recognized.
- High dose phenobarbitone is used for management of refractory status epilepticus (RSE) while standard phenobarbitone (20 mg/kg) is used as a 2nd line agent.

Table 39.1 Summary of drugs for status epilepticus

1st line drugs	2nd line drugs	3rd line drugs/RSE drugs	Add-on drugs for difficult seizures
Lorazepam*	Phenytoin or Fosphenytoin*	Midazolam infusion*	Topiramate
Midazolam	IV Levetiracetam	High dose phenobarbitone	
Diazepam	IV Valproate	Thiopentone infusion	
	Phenobarbitone (standard dose)	Propofol infusion	

Pyridoxine 100 mg/IV for children < 2 yrs.
* Drug of choice, RSE: Refractory Status Epilepticus

a) **Phenytoin**

- Widely used as a second line agent for controlling seizures along with benzodiazepines in SE and to maintain a prolonged anti-seizure effect.
- Inhibits spread of electrical discharges from the epileptiform focus.
- Best for GTCS, focal, post-traumatic seizures: Less effective for absence and febrile seizures.
- Dose: IV loading dose 18-20 mg/kg, effective in 70-90% of patients with SE (max dose 1000 mg)
  Repeat dose of 10 mg/kg bolus up to a total load of 30 mg/kg can be tried if unresponsive to initial loading dose.
- Peak effect 10-30 minutes after completion of infusion.
- Proper administration of phenytoin is critical.
  - Dissolve only in saline.
  - Rate of administration 1 mg/kg/minute.
  - 20 mg/kg to be diluted in 20 ml saline and infused over 20-30 min by infusion pump.
  - Only intravenous route may be used for loading dose, absorption after intramuscular dose is erratic.
- Side effects
  - Highly caustic to veins in view of alkaline pH, can cause tissue necrosis if extravasation occurs.
  - Hypotension, bradycardia, heart block can occur if given rapidly (mainly due to the solvent propylene glycol in IV preparation).
  - Ataxia, blurred vision, dizziness at toxic levels.
- Monitor phenytoin levels (therapeutic level 15-25 mcg/ml in the presence of normal protein levels).
- Valproate, a highly protein-bound drug, can displace phenytoin and increase its free level.
- Hypoalbuminemia will also increase free drug.
- Phenytoin correction for hypoalbuminemia = measured phenytoin/[(0.2 x measured albumin) + 0.1]
- In liver disease, administer a smaller load of 10-15 mg/kg, maintenance of 5 mg/kg, correct drug levels for serum albumin.

b) **Phosphenytoin/Fosphenytoin**

- Water soluble pro-drug of phenytoin
- Administered as phenytoin equivalents (PE) where 1 mg PE of fosphenytoin = 1.5 mg phenytoin.
- The infusion may be given at faster rates of 3 mg/kg/minute up to 150 mg/min phosphenytoin as it is not formulated with propylene glycol.
- Infusion related phlebitis and soft tissue damage less common with fosphenytoin.
- Can be given intramuscularly.
- In a patient who is already on phenytoin, fosphenytoin may displace phenytoin from albumin-binding sites and increase the free drug.

c) **Levetiracetam**

- Newer drug acting via non-GABAergic mechanism.
- Rapidly emerging as an effective second line agent in SE refractory to phenytoin in view of its safe cardio-respiratory profile, rapid attainment of a steady state level and minimal drug-drug interactions with other AEDs.
- Levetiracetam may be more effective than phenobarbital, given the different mechanisms of action, and may be more attractive as it has less side effects.
- Available as an intravenous and oral preparation.

- Can be used in liver dysfunction as it is not metabolized in the liver.
- The drug is excreted by the kidney; reduce dose in renal failure.
- IV dosing: 20-30 mg/kg load followed by 10 mg/kg/dose Q6-12H, increase to 10-20 mg/kg Q6H to a maximum of 80 mg/kg/day, not exceeding 3 gm/day.
- Side effects: Neuropsychiatric symptoms, leucopenia and albuminuria.

d) **Sodium valproate**

- Intravenous valproate is an alternative 2nd line agent in SE.
- Several studies suggest that intravenous valproate acid exhibits high efficacy in promptly treating RSE, with few adverse reactions.
- The initial bolus may be 20-30 mg/kg bolus administered at a rate of 4 mg/kg/minute.
- If seizures are terminated, continue intermittent maintenance doses twice daily.
- If seizures persist or recur, a continuous infusion of 5 mg/kg/hr may be efficacious.
- A few reports state that higher infusion rates of 3-4 mg/kg/minute may be successful.
- Serum level decreases if patient is on drugs such as meropenem or amikacin.
- Monitor liver function test 2-3 times a week. Stop the drug if the ALT increases by more than 3 times baseline value.
- Side effects of valproate
  - Liver dysfunction
  - Bleeding risk: Coagulopathy, thrombocytopenia, hypofibrinogenemia
  - Valproic acid may induce encephalopathy, with or without elevated ammonia levels: This must be considered in patients with persisting encephalopathy.
  - Pancreatitis (rare).

e) **Standard dose phenobarbitone**

- Effective agent for neonatal seizures and in seizures unresponsive to phenytoin in infants and older children.
- May be given both intravenously and intramuscularly.
- Compatible with all fluids.
  Loading dose 15-20 mg to be diluted in 20 ml NS and infused over 5-10 minutes.
- Rate not to exceed 100 mg/minute.
- Maximum loading dose 1000 mg.
- Peak effect 10-20 minutes after IV loading dose.
- Maintain serum levels 20-40 mcg/ml.
- Side effects
  - CNS depression, respiratory depression
  - Hypotension, particularly with prior benzodiazepine use and in hypovolemic patients.

TREATMENT OF REFRACTORY STATUS EPILEPTICUS (RSE)

- Patients with RSE are at high risk of neurological sequelae, complications of drugs, multiorgan failure and death.
- The goals of therapy are to terminate clinical and electrographic seizure activity along with meticulous supportive care.
- The limitations of high dose RSE regimens (e.g., barbiturate or benzodiazepine) are usually related to cardiovascular toxicity rather than to any predefined upper dose.
- Commonly used agents include:
  - Midazolam infusion.
  - High dose phenobarbitone.
  - Thiopentone infusion.

Midazolam infusion

- Preferred benzodiazepine in RSE as its metabolites are cleared quickly.
- The advantages of midazolam include a rapid onset of action, a short half-life, stability in aqueous solution and a lower incidence of cardiovascular depression and need for vasopressors than with thiopentone.

- The major disadvantage of midazolam is the need for escalating doses due to tachyphylaxis that can occur after 4-5 days. Withdrawal effect (tremors) may also occur after 5 days.
- Loading dose: 0.15 mg/kg followed by infusion of 1-10 mcg/kg/minute.
- Preparation of infusion: 3 mg/kg midazolam in 50 cc normal saline. 1 cc/hour = 1 mcg/kg/min.
- Start at 2 mcg/kg/minute after bolus of 0.15 mg/kg. If seizures recur, re-bolus with 0.15 mg/kg and increase infusion rate by 1 mcg/kg/minute every 15 minutes until control achieved.
- Generally, if seizures not controlled at 10 mcg/kg/minute, higher doses are unlikely to be successful and furthermore, complication rates usually increase incrementally above this rate. However, some reports suggest higher maximum rates of up to 24 mcg/kg/min.
- Once control achieved, maintain same dose for 24 hours.
- Taper the infusion over 12-24 hours.
- Ensure adequate therapeutic levels of other AED so as to minimize the chances for seizure recurrence when midazolam weaned.
- Wean by 20% per day if infused for more than 5 days and by 10% per day if infused for more than 10 days in order to prevent withdrawal.

Barbiturates

Drugs such as thiopental and phenobarbital are widely used medications for RSE that may also have neuroprotective effects.

The main drawback of all of the barbiturates in high doses is the high risk of respiratory and cardiovascular depression and hypotension.

High dose phenobarbitone

- Among the barbiturates, multiple dose phenobarbitone has the lowest risk of hypotension and respiratory depression even when levels are supra-therapeutic.
- Phenobarbitone may be given in repeated boluses of 10 mg/kg until seizure control is achieved.
- There appears to be no maximum dose beyond which further doses are ineffective, thus dosing is toxicity limited.
- Bedside EEG monitoring is extremely useful to enable therapy of both motor and electrical seizures.
- Serum levels are irrelevant when multiple doses of phenobarbitone are employed. Levels >1000 mol/L have been reported.

Thiopentone infusion

- This is general anesthesia which is reserved only for RSE refractory to midazolam and high dose phenobarbitone.
- The drug accumulates in fatty tissue leading to prolonged recovery times. The hepatic metabolism of thiopentone exhibits saturable kinetics, resulting in increasing accumulation during high dose infusions. Thiopentone is metabolized to pentobarbital, which accounts for 10-15% of active barbiturate levels during thiopental therapy.
- Patients receiving thiopentone usually require intubation and ventilation.
- Side effects of thiopentone sodium
  - Hypotension due to peripheral vasodilatation and negative inotropy.
  - Loss of airway patency, risk of aspiration and hypoventilation/apnea.
  - Controlled ventilation, central venous and invasive arterial access are essential to monitor and support the hemodynamics. Volume resuscitation and inotropes/pressors may be required.
  - High dose thiopentone may be immunosuppressive. Can also cause ileus and feed intolerance.

- Special precautions
  - Ensure that a dedicated venous access for thiopentone is used and no other drugs/fluids are co-infused via thiopentone line.
  - Central access preferred as the drug has an extremely alkaline pH and can cause skin necrosis if it extravasates.
  - Inadvertent arterial injection can lead to distal necrosis and gangrene.
  - Thiopentone is stable in solution when mixed with distilled water and saline. Precipitates with glucose containing fluids.
  - Bedside EEG continuous or at least twice daily.
- Dose
  - Loading dose 3-5 mg/kg slowly.
  - Infusion 1-5 mg/kg/hr.
  - Start with 1 mg/kg/hr, if fits persist or recur, gradually increase to 5 mg/kg/hr.
- Preparation of thiopentone
  - Each vial has 500 mg dry powder.
  - Add 50 ml distilled water, so 1 ml = 20 mg (2% solution).
- How to titrate thiopentone
  - The infusion should be titrated so as to achieve burst suppression on background EEG in order to attain sustained cessation of seizures.
  - Due to the long elimination half-life, gradual tapering of thiopentone is usually not necessary and the infusion may be ceased 12-24 hours after EEG targets reached.
- Thiopentone is sometimes given as bolus of 5 mg/kg in patients with refractory seizures, this may be especially useful prior to transport. Dose associated hypotension should be anticipated and prevented.

Other agents used for RSE: Propofol infusion

- Major advantage of this agent is rapid recovery with lesser duration of hypoventilation when compared to thiopentone on account of its short elimination half-life.
- Side effects
  - Hypotension due to peripheral vasodilatation and negative inotropy.
  - Bradycardia can occur despite hypotension: this leads to further compromise of cardiac output.
  - Propofol infusion syndrome: This is usually seen when high dose infusion is used for > 48 hr. The syndrome is characterized by hypotension, bradycardia, metabolic acidosois, rhabdomyolysis and renal failure.
- Propofol dose
  - Loading dose of 1-4 mg/kg slowly as titrated boluses till seizures controlled.
  - Infusion 2-5 mg/kg/hr.

Newer antiepileptic drugs: Topiramate

- Topiramate is an attractive drug acting via non-GABAergic mechanism.
- It is particularly attractive as it possesses neuroprotective properties and attenuates seizure induced neuronal injury.
- Metabolized by liver p450 pathway and excreted by kidneys, hence decrease dosage in liver and/or renal failure.
- Effective in partial onset and generalized tonic-clonic seizures.
- Side effects
  - Metabolic acidosis because it is carbonic anhydrase inhibitor.
  - Hyponatremia, particularly if used with carbamazepine.
  - Topiramate may enhance the hepatotoxic effects of valproic acid.
  - Renal calculi
- Dose: 1–3 mg/kg/day, maximum up to 9 mg/kg/day.

H. Non-pharmacological approaches

- In RSE non responsive to above agents and IV

STATUS EPILEPTICUS ALGORITHM

1st line drugs

On presentation to hospital, support ABCs

Unabated seizures at 5 min; **Lorazepam** 0.1 mg/kg IV or IO, max 4 mg, can repeat 10 minutely x 3 doses OR midazolam 0.2 mg/kg IM

↓

2nd line drugs

Fosphenytoin 30 mg/kg IV, max 1 gm, dilute in NS over 10 minutes, along with 2nd dose lorazepam (1.5 mg fosphenytoin= 1 mg phenytoin equivalents) *May repeat 15 mg/kg fosphenytoin load if seizures persist*

↓

Unabated seizures 20 min after phenytoin load-**Levetericetam** 20 mg/kg at 5 mg/kg/min **OR IV Valproate** 20 mg/kg (5 mg/kg/min) followed by infusion

↓

Phenobarbitone 20 mg/kg (2 mg/kg/min) repeat 10 mg/kg if seizures persist

↓

RSE drugs

Midazolam 0.15 mg/kg bolus then 2 mcg/kg/min. If seizures persist, repeat 0.15 mg/kg bolus & increase infusion rate by 2 mcg/kg/min as needed, max 24 mcg/kg/min or 20 mg/hr

↓

Consider multiple dose phenobarbitone 10 mg/kg *irrespective of serum levels*

↓

If RSE not controlled, Consider **Thiopentone** infusion 4 mg/kg, then 1–6 mg/kg/hr with EEG monitoring

---

- **A** : Support airway. Rapid Sequence. Intubation if compromised airway or breathing at any point
- **B** : 100% oxygen, assess ventilation, SpO_2 monitor
- **C** : cardio-respiratory monitor, check pulses, establish IV access *(Seizures can mask signs of shock)*

Investigations

- In all patients: Glucose, electrolytes, calcium, magnesium.
- Depending on clinical setting: CT scan, drug levels, toxin screen, metabolic screen, blood cultures and antibiotics as appropriate

- History - AMPLE
- Treat raised ICP if suspected (early intubation important)
- Keep normothermic, rectal paracetamol if febrile
- Consider **pyridoxine** 100 mg IV push if < 18 months

Early referral to PICU if any of the following:

- Airway / ventilation / cardiovascular compromise
- Seizure>30 min
- Seizure refractory to 2nd line medications.
- Need for Midazolam or Thiopentone infusions

Midazolam infusion

- Monitor ABC, may need intubation, ventilation and pressor support. Consider arterial BP monitoring
- Consider EEG at least BD
- If no seizures (clinical or EEG) for 24 hrs, wean by 1 mcg/ kg/min Q 2 hrly
- If seizures recur, consider previous midazolam infusion rate that achieved burst suppression pattern
- Stop midazolam infusion once thiopentone is started

RSE therapy:

Continue pharmacological coma for 24 hr after last seizure with EEG goal of burst suppression pattern anesthetics, resective surgery has been tried. Most effective in focal seizures.

- Hypothermia (moderate) has an impressive anticonvulsant activity in patients with refractory NCSE and RSE.

I. Non-convulsive status epilepticus (NCSE)

- NCSE consists of continuous electrographic seizures with no motor movements.
- NCSE is fairly common in critically ill children with neurological illness and usually follows prolonged convulsive SE.
- NCSE may present as vacant stares, unresponsiveness, nystagmoid eye movements, tachycardia, apnea, automatic behavior, unilateral clonus or chewing movements of mouth. Pupillary responses may be abnormal (dilatation, asymmetrical size and/or reaction).
- Suspect NCSE if a patient fails to regain consciousness 30-60 minutes after cessation of convulsive status seizures.
- 50% of NCSE are detected in the first one hour and 20% of NCSE may occur 24 hours after convulsive SE. Hence prolonged continuous EEG recording is required for the diagnosis of NCSE.
- Functional outcome of NCSE in patients with pre-existing seizure disorder is good.
- Treatment of non-convulsive status is same as convulsive status. IV phenobarbitone or valproate are preferred and anesthetic drugs are usually avoided.

REFERENCES

1. Elizabeth J, Donner EJ et al. Status Epilepticus. In: Pediatric Critical Care, 3rd ed. Fuhrman & Zimmerman (Eds). Mosby Elsevier Philadelphia 2005.
2. Abend NS, Dlugos DJ. Treatment of Refractory Status Epilepticus: Literature Review and a Proposed Protocol. Pediatr Neurol 2008; 38:377-390.
3. The anesthetic and intensive care of status epilepticus. Holtkamp M. Current Opinion in Neurology 2007; 20:188-193.
4. Karine J, Lawrence J. Advances in the management of seizures and status epilepticus in critically ill patients. Crit Care Clinics 2007; 22:637-659.
5. Hirsch LJ. The Status of Intravenous Valproate for Status epilepticus, Epilepsy Curr. 2007 July; 7(4): 96-98.

40

Head Injury

Head injury is a common clinical problem in the pediatric population.

- Most head injured children have minor head injuries and will have good clinical outcomes.
- However, it is important to identify promptly the small number that are at risk of developing intracranial complications following head trauma and subsequently deteriorate, resulting in severe neurological deficits, even death.
- *Although children have better survival rates than adults with TBI, the long term sequelae are more devastating in children due to their age and developmental potential.*

Why do children suffer greater damage following TBI?

- Greater head to torso ratio →higher angular biomechanical forces
- Higher brain water content
- Incomplete axonal myelination
- Immature brain has increased susceptibility to delayed cell death.

Significant cervical spine injury may be associated with brain injury, although less commonly in children compared to adults

- Care to stabilize and support the cervical spine during all maneuvers involving the neck (such as intubation and shifting from bed to stretcher, etc) is essential in order to avoid potential spinal injury that can lead to catastrophic consequences such as paraplegia and respiratory muscles paralysis.
- These precautions must be continued until the *"Cervical spine is cleared"* (see below).

RISK FACTORS FOR SIGNIFICANT BRAIN INJURY

- Significant mechanism of injury (high velocity injuries, e.g., motor vehicle accidents, fall from height)
- Altered LOC: Irritable, GCS < 13
- Skull fracture, particularly if depressed
- Penetrating injuries
- Evidence of base of skull fracture (raccoon eye, Battle sign, CSF rhinorrhea, hemotympanum)
- Focal neurological signs
- Severe worsening headache, persistent vomiting
- Post-traumatic seizure
- Patients with blood dyscrasias or on anticoagulant therapy.

90-95% of all head injuries are mild and may be discharged after parents are educated regarding danger signs and prevention.

Children with moderate and severe head injury will require rapid evaluation and resuscitation at the Emergency Department in conjunction with the neurosurgeon.

TBI PATHOPHYSIOLOGY

- The pathophysiology of head injury is divided into two events: *Primary Injury and Secondary Injury.*
- *Primary injury* occurs within seconds of the traumatic event and no specific therapy is available apart from prevention.
- *Secondary injury* includes the endogenous evolution of brain damage or intracranial hypertension and secondary extracerebral insults such as hypotension, hypoxia, hypercarbia.
- Secondary insults can be modified or prevented by appropriate interventions.
- *The goals of ER and PICU care are to optimize neurological outcome by preventing secondary injury/insults.*

SEVERITY OF TBI

Mild TBI

- No loss of consciousness (LOC)
- One or less episodes of vomiting
- Stable, alert conscious state
- May have scalp bruising or laceration
- Normal examination otherwise

Moderate TBI

- LOC < 5 minutes
- Alert or responds to voice. May be drowsy
- Two or more episodes of vomiting
- Persistent headache
- Up to one single brief (< 2 min) convulsion occurring immediately after the impact
- May have a large scalp bruise, hematoma or laceration
- Normal examination otherwise

Severe TBI

- LOC > 5 minutes
- Decreased conscious state – responsive only to pain or unresponsive
- CSF leak from nose or ears
- Localizing neurological signs (unequal pupils, lateralising motor weakness)
- Signs of increased intracranial pressure:
  - Uncal herniation: Ipsilateral dilated non-reactive pupil due to compression of the oculomotor nerve
  - Central herniation: Brainstem compression causing bradycardia and hypertension
- Penetrating head injury
- Seizures (other than single brief [< 2 min] convulsion occurring immediately after the impact)

CAUSES OF RAISED INTRACRANIAL PRESSURE (ICP) AFTER TBI

Intracranial

- Focal impact damage
- Focal or diffuse cerebral edema
- Hematoma
- Diffuse axonal injury
- Seizures

Systemic

- Hypotension/ischemia
- Hypoxia/hypercarbia
- Hyperthermia
- Agitation

CEREBRAL EDEMA

Cerebral edema is a consistent reaction of the brain to a variety of insults.

- While it may not be apparent at the outset, cerebral edema usually develops over 24-72 hours and results in increased intracranial pressure (ICP).
- There are 3 types of cerebral edema:
  - *Vasogenic:* Protein rich edema fluid due to blood brain barrier defect, inflammatory or traumatic in origin.
  - *Cytotoxic:* Neuronal swelling due to disruption of intracellular machinery and/or cellular membrane function. Cause may be traumatic, inflammatory or hypoxic ischemic.
  - *Interstitial:* Increased intraventricular pressure due to obstruction of normal CSF pathways.

Patients with head injuries usually have a mixed type of edema: cytotoxic and vasogenic.

TYPES OF HEAD INJURIES

A blow to the skull results in compression injury to the adjacent brain (coup) and stretching on the opposite side (contre-coup). This may result in contusion, shearing injuries and rupture of intra-axial or extra-axial vessels, leading to hemorrhage.

1. **Vault fractures**
   These are indicative of the severity of the injury. Uncomplicated fractures are not of great significance, except that temporal bone fractures may predispose to extradural hematoma.
   - *Depressed skull fractures*
     These may require surgery to elevate the bone fragment. These are well demonstrated on CT.
   - *Base of skull (BOS) fractures*
     - These are not always visible on CT, but blood in the sinus cavities (e.g., sphenoid sinus) suggests their presence.
     - If the patient has clinical evidence of BOS fracture (e.g., CSF rhinorrhea or bleeding from the external auditory meatus), a normal CT does not exclude such a fracture.
     - Recognition of BOS fracture is important as such patients are prone to developing meningitis and require antibiotic prophylaxis.
2. **Intracranial air**
   This indicates an open head injury, such as due to a basal fracture communicating with sinuses or a penetrating injury to the vault (e.g., a bullet wound). Again it indicates the need for antibiotics.
3. **Intracranial hematoma (Fig. 40.1)**
   a. *Extradural hematoma (EDH)*
   - These arise between the inner table of the skull and the dura.
   - They usually develop from injury to the middle meningeal artery or one of its branches, and therefore are usually temporo-parietal in location.
   - The expanding hematoma strips the dura from the skull; this attachment is quite strong such that the hematoma is confined, giving rise to its characteristic biconvex shape, with a well defined margin.
   - It may present as primary depressed consciousness or LOC following a lucid interval.
   - The bleeding is usually acute and so of high attenuation on CT.
   - There is often significant mass effect with compression of the ipsilateral lateral ventricle and dilatation of the opposite lateral ventricle due to obstruction of the foramen of Munro.

   b. *Acute subdural hematoma (SDH)*
   - Clinical presentation depends on the size and location and the presence of associated injury.
   - SDH can have severe consequences due to mass effect, requiring urgent surgery.
   - Differentiating SDH vs EDH is therefore not so important in the acute situation.
   - The blood is again of high attenuation, but may spread more widely in the subdural space, with a crescentic appearance and a more irregular inner margin.
   - Associated brain parenchymal injury is common.

   c. *Traumatic subarachnoid hemorrhage (t-SAH)*
   - This may occur alone or in association with other intracerebral or extracerebral hematomas.
   - The presence of a t-SAH signifies a significant mechanism of injury and prognosis for recovery may be guarded.
   - Increased attenuation is seen in the CSF spaces, over the cerebral hemispheres

(look closely at the Sylvian fissure), in the basal cisterns or in the ventricular system.

- SAH may be complicated by hydrocephalus.
- Confusion can sometimes arise between SAH due to trauma and due to a ruptured aneurysm or arteriovenous malformation (AVM); the patient may collapse and hit his head as a result of a bleed and the history (from the patient or a witness) is important.

d. *Intracerebral hemorrhage: Hemorrhagic contusion*

- These occur due to stretching and shearing injury, often due to impaction of the brain against the skull on the side opposite to the injury.
- Thus they may be seen directly opposite the impact site, ranging from a subcutaneous hematoma, fracture, or extradural hematoma (contre-coup injury).
- The inferior frontal lobes and anterior temporal lobes are common sites after a blow to the back of the head.

4. **Diffuse Axonal Injury (DAI)**

- DAI can result in multiple contusions and petechial hemorrhages throughout the cerebral hemispheres.
- These occur due to shearing injury with rupture of small intracerebral vessels, and in a comatose patient with no other obvious cause, they imply a severe diffuse brain injury with a poor prognosis.
- DAI may be present in up to 50% of severe TBI.
- Petechial hemorrhages are often very small and visible at the grey/white matter interface.
- Larger hemorrhages may occur in severe trauma, and they may not be apparent on a scan performed immediately after the injury, only becoming prominent after a day or two.
- MRI is more sensitive to diffuse brain injury, particularly in the absence of hemorrhage.
- Typical presentation of DAI is a significant mechanism of injury, a deeply comatose patient and a CT that shows cerebral edema, poor grey-white differentiation ± petechial hemorrhages but no discrete hematoma/contusions.

INITIAL ASSESSMENT & MANAGEMENT OF A PEDIATRIC HEAD TRAUMA PATIENT

- A brief history of the event must be obtained *after the initial assessment* (see below). Useful information includes the following:
  - Type and mechanism of injury, e.g., height of fall or speed of the vehicle, etc.
  - Time of injury

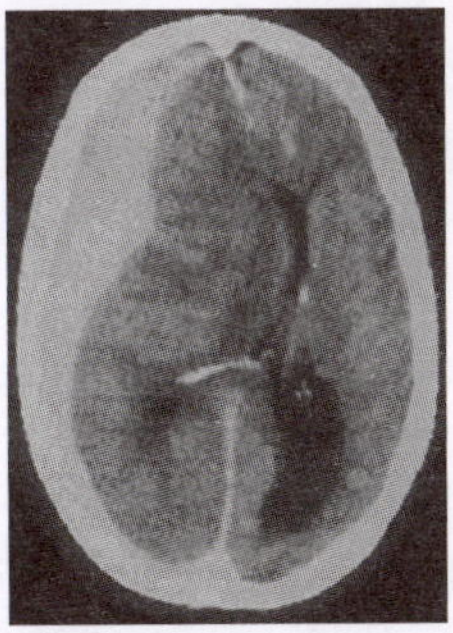

Subdural hematoma

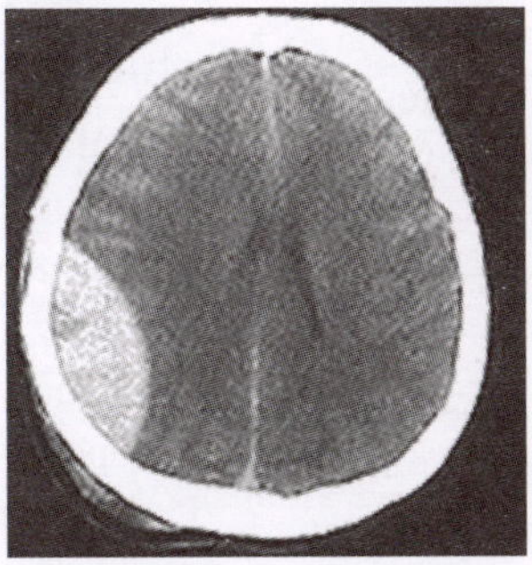

Epidural hematoma

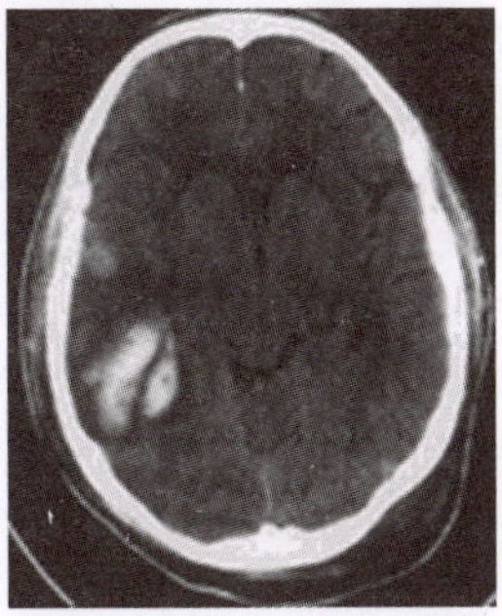

Temporal contusion

Fig. 40.1 Types of intracranial hematomas

- GCS at scene
- Need for resuscitation at scene
- Past medical history and possible medical reason for accident (seizure, arrhythmia, blood dyscrasias)
- Symptoms that have occurred since the injury has occurred, including any loss of consciousness, ENT bleed, focal deficits, etc.
- Treatment received before arrival

- The progression of symptoms provides invaluable information to assist the physician in clinical decision making.
- Consider the possibility of *non-accidental injury* during secondary survey especially in infants with head injury.

The primary survey (see also chapter on Major Trauma)

- *This is an important first step in all patients with trauma and constitutes a rapid, focused initial physical examination aimed at identifying and stabilizing any life-threatening injuries.*
- Relief of airway obstruction, correcting inadequate oxygenation and ventilation and restoring normal circulation takes priority over detailed neurological evaluation.
- The order of assessment is:
  - **A**irway with cervical spine precaution: Assess whether airway is patent/unprotected/obstructed. *See indications for intubation*
    - Assess/stabilize cervical spine: Look for pain, deformity, tenderness, bruising.
    - As stressed previously, overzealous attempts at intubation with the neck extended, unsupported and without strict cervical precautions can exacerbate potential spinal injury and result in devastating consequences such as paraplegia and respiratory muscles paralysis. *See below: Clearing of the cervical spine*
  - **B**reathing: Assess respiratory rate, chest movements, air entry, evidence of external injury like chest contusions or rib fracture, crepitus.
  - **C**irculation with hemorrhage control: Assess heart rate, BP, peripheral pulse volume, CRT, temperature
  - **D**isability: Neurological examination (level of consciousness, GCS, pupillary size and reaction); respiratory pattern, motor tone, focal neurological deficits, abnormal posturing
  - **E**xposure: Undress the patient completely to determine the extent of other organ systems injury, prevent hypothermia.

> Prevent secondary brain insults by maintaining a patent airway, adequate ventilation and oxygenation and avoiding hypotension

Indications for intubation in TBI

1. Airway compromise
   - Soft tissues of mouth and pharynx obstructing airway (usually due to low GCS, seizures)
   - Inability to clear secretions, blood, vomitus
2. Breathing
   - Inability to maintain normal O_2 saturations despite high flow oxygen
   - Lung contusion, flail chest etc
   - Hypoventilation, hypercarbia.
3. Neurological
   - GCS < 8-9 or fall in GCS by > 3 points
   - Features of herniation
4. Need for transport
   - Lower threshold for intubation prior to transport or CT, specially if the patient is agitated.

Technique of intubation

- Spinal immobilisation (removal of the anterior flap of spinal collar, manual in-line axial support of neck by assistant)
- Assume full stomach and use rapid sequence intubation technique (RSI)
- Thiopentone is the induction agent of choice. Use the minimum dose required to induce anaesthesia (3-5 mg/kg). *Beware of large doses of induction agent in under-resuscitated children, as they may become profoundly hypotensive.*

- Recent literature supports use of ketamine in head injury patients: This agent has the added advantage of maintaining hemodynamic stability.
- Premedication with lignocaine 1 mg/kg, analgesia with fentanyl 2-3 mcg/kg and paralysis with vecuronium 0.2 mg/kg.
- Intubation by experienced personnel mandatory. *Avoid muscle relaxants if airway deemed difficult or expertise unavailable.*
- *Use only oral route for both endotracheal tube and gastric tubes* (nasal tubes may migrate intracranially if ethmoid fracture present).
- Once intubated, all patients must be kept sedated.
- A hard collar, blocks and tape are essential to ensure the cervical spine is immobilised.
- All patients should be log rolled to protect the thoracic and lumbar spine.

Hypotension/Shock in TBI

Implications

- Hypotension after TBI can lead to a much higher mortality and worse neurological outcome in survivors. *(Prevent as far as possible, treat aggressively if hypotension occurs.)*
- Raised ICP (hypertension/bradycardia) can mask signs of shock.
- Serious blood loss and hypotension from head injury alone are uncommon, except in infants with large scalp hematomas.
- Drugs used for sedation can precipitate shock.

Causes of Shock

- Other organ injury with overt or concealed blood loss
- Spinal shock (combination of bradycardia with hypotension)
- Cardiac contusion, tamponade

Indications for CT scan

- *A CT scan without contrast is the imaging modality of choice in head trauma.* The CT should include the cranio-cervical junction to look for atlanto occipital dislocation.
- Indications for CT are:
  - Significant mechanism of head injury
  - GCS < 13 at any time after injury
  - GCS 13-14 two hours after injury
  - Focal neurological signs
  - Persistent vomiting/headache
  - ENT bleed/CSF discharge
  - Post traumatic seizures
  - Polytrauma
  - Suspicion of child abuse (iTBI: inflicted traumatic brain injury)

Clearing of the cervical spine

- The cervical spine may be cleared clinically and the collar removed if the following preconditions are met:
  - Fully alert and orientated
  - No drugs or alcohol
  - No neck pain/local swelling/tenderness
  - No abnormality on neuro exam
  - No significant other 'distracting' injury (another injury which may 'distract' the patient from complaining about a possible spinal injury).
- If the above criteria are not fulfilled, then C-spine protection is mandatory until cervical imaging performed.

Imaging of the cervical spine

- As stated previously, "spine" precautions must be continued in severe TBI in order to prevent worsening of potential cervical cord injury until the cervical spine is deemed to be clear.
- Indications for imaging:
  - Altered level of consciousness, intoxication
  - Neck/back pain or tenderness
  - Sensory/motor deficits
  - Painful distracting injuries outside spinal region

- The *three standard spine X-rays* are: AP, lateral, odontoid (open mouth view)
  - This should include C1 to C7 / T1 intervertebral space.
  - Look for changes in vertebral body alignment, intervertebral spaces and soft tissue
  - A *CT cervical spine* is indicated when the spine cannot be adequately visualized on standard films (e.g., in an intubated patient) or an abnormality is suspected. A CT is sensitive for bony injuries.
- Spine MRI is sensitive for soft tissue injuries: (spinal cord, ligamentous injury, hematoma)

Goals for management of severe TBI in the PICU (See chapter on Intracranial Hypertension, Part 2)
- Optimize cerebral perfusion pressure and cerebral oxygen delivery
- Lower elevated ICP
- Prevent secondary injuries

Monitoring in the PICU

(See chapter on Intracranial Hypertension, Part 2)

- Heart rate, invasive arterial blood pressure and CVP monitoring
- ABG Q4H, capnography
- Precise hourly fluid balance monitoring. An indwelling urinary catheter is usually necessary.
- Hemogram, infection screen, coagulation screen, blood crossmatch and type.
- Blood glucose Q2-4H, electrolytes every 6-12 hours
- Serum osmolality Q12H, BUN daily
- Cranial imaging as necessary.
- ICP monitoring: This aids in titrating and targeting therapy in a rational manner and can facilitate earlier ICP reducing treatment before florid signs of herniation.
  - Likewise, overtreatment and attendant complications may be avoided
  - Indication: Severe head injury (GCS < 9), mass effect on CT scan.
  - An external ventricular drain (EVD) may be inserted by the neurosurgeon provided the ventricles are visible on CT.
  - Advantages of an EVD include its reliability, accuracy, ability to calibrate as needed and low cost. Its outstanding advantage over other methods of ICP measurement is the ability to drain CSF as required, thus affording a key therapeutic option as well.
  - Other ICP monitoring methods: Parenchymal monitor (Camino), subdural bolt.
- See Fig. 40.2 for estimation of high ICP based on admission CT, systolic BP and pupillary changes.

TBI related complications

- Coagulopathy due to release of brain tissue thromboplastin
- Neurogenic pulmonary edema
  - This is infrequent and occurs due to surges in catecholamine mediated rise in systemic vascular resistance (SVR) and consequent increased blood volume in the pulmonary vasculature.
  - Increased vascular permeability of pulmonary vascular bed.
  - Treatment: Increase PEEP as needed to prevent hypoxemia.

Miscellaneous treatment issues of a child with severe traumatic brain injury

- Indications for antibiotics:
  - Fracture base of skull, evidence of CSF leak from ear/nose
  - Intracranial air
- Prophylactic anticonvulsants: load with 20 mg/kg of phenytoin.
- Consider gastric acid reduction.
- All patients with suspected polytrauma should have a secondary survey performed.
- If an abdominal injury is suspected, either an ultrasound or CT scan of the abdomen should be performed.

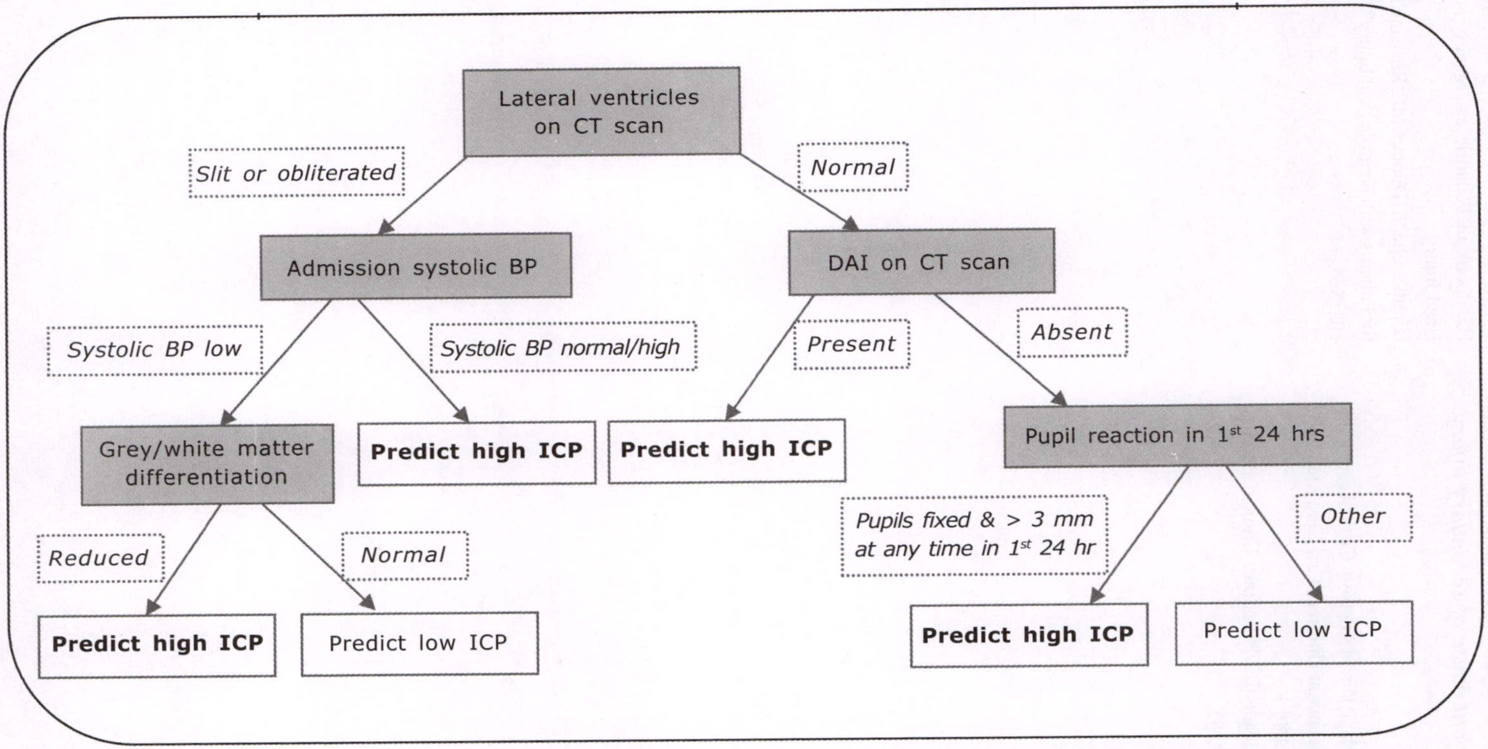

Fig. 40.2 Prediction of high ICP based on CT changes, SBP and pupils changes. DAI: Diffuse axonal injury. *Modified from*: Kochanek et al, PCCM 2009, 10 (4): 517-523

- Treat hypotension aggressively. *Hypotension is the most important cause of secondary injury.*

REFERENCES

1. Catherine A Mazzola, P David Adelson: Critical care management of head trauma in children; Crit Care Med 2002 Vol. 30, No. 11 (Suppl.)
2. Royal Childrens Hospital, Melbourne. Clinical Practice Guidelines. Head injury
3. Lalani A, Schneeweiss S. The Hospital for sick children, Handbook of Pedaitric emergency medicine. Chapter 7: Head Injury
4. Himmelseher S, Durieux ME. Revising a Dogma: Ketamine for Patients with Neurological Injury? Anesth Analg 2005; 101:524-34.

PEDIATRIC EMERGENCIES & CRITICAL CARE

Index

A

B

F

PEDIATRIC EMERGENCIES & CRITICAL CARE

M

Q

R

U

V

PEDIATRIC EMERGENCIES & CRITICAL CARE

Contributors to the 2nd Edition of *Manual of Pediatric Emergencies & Critical Care*

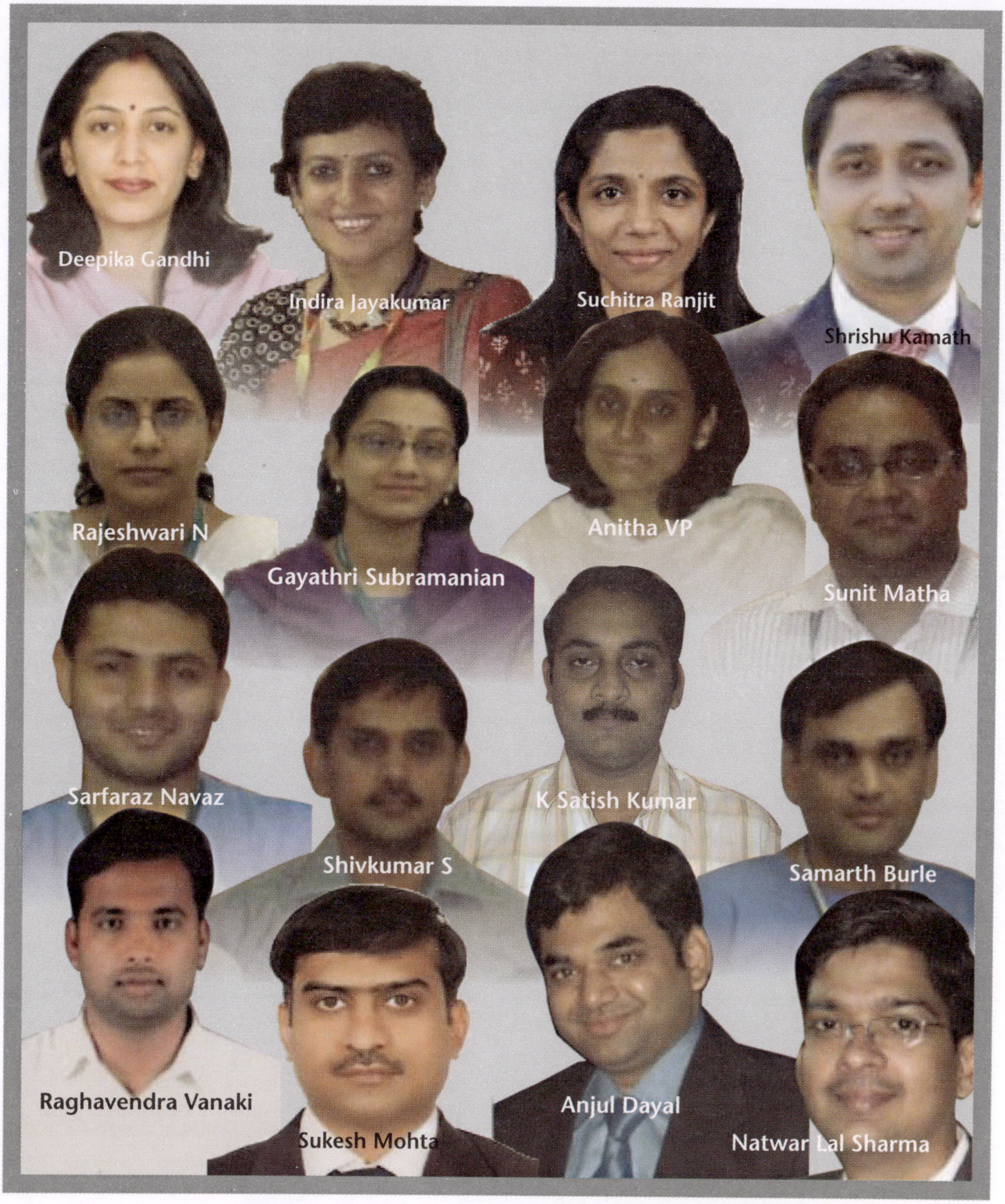

Former and current team members of the Pediatric Critical Care Group, Chennai